A Practical Approach to

# VASCULAR AND ENDOVASCULAR SURGERY

# A Practical Approach to
# VASCULAR AND ENDOVASCULAR SURGERY

*Editors*

**Jaisom Chopra** MS FRCS
Senior Consultant Vascular Surgeon
Apollo Hospitals, New Delhi, India
*E-mail: jaisomchopra@hotmail.com*

**VS Bedi** MBBS MS FVSI
Chairman and Senior Consultant
Department of Vascular and Endovascular Surgery
Sir Ganga Ram Hospital, New Delhi, India
*E-mail: bedivs@gmail.com*

*Foreword*

**John HN Wolfe**

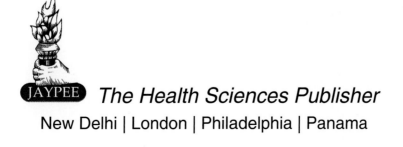

*The Health Sciences Publisher*
New Delhi | London | Philadelphia | Panama

**Jaypee Brothers Medical Publishers (P) Ltd.**

**Headquarters**
Jaypee Brothers Medical Publishers (P) Ltd.
4838/24, Ansari Road, Daryaganj
New Delhi 110 002, India
Phone: +91-11-43574357
Fax: +91-11-43574314
E-mail: jaypee@jaypeebrothers.com

**Overseas Offices**

J.P. Medical Ltd.
83, Victoria Street, London
SW1H 0HW (UK)
Phone: +44-20 3170 8910
Fax: +44 (0)20 3008 6180
E-mail: info@jpmedpub.com

Jaypee-Highlights Medical Publishers Inc.
City of Knowledge, Bld. 237, Clayton
Panama City, Panama
Phone: +1 507-301-0496
Fax: +1 507-301-0499
E-mail: cservice@jphmedical.com

Jaypee Medical Inc.
325, Chestnut Street
Suite 412, Philadelphia,
PA 19106, USA
Phone: +1 267-519-9789
E-mail: jpmed.us@gmail.com

Jaypee Brothers Medical Publishers (P) Ltd.
17/1-B, Babar Road, Block-B
Shaymali, Mohammadpur
Dhaka-1207, Bangladesh
Mobile: +08801912003485
E-mail: jaypeedhaka@gmail.com

Jaypee Brothers Medical Publishers (P) Ltd.
Bhotahity, Kathmandu, Nepal
Phone: +977-9741283608
E-mail: kathmandu@jaypeebrothers.com

Website: www.jaypeebrothers.com
Website: www.jaypeedigital.com

© 2016, Jaypee Brothers Medical Publishers

**Inquiries for bulk sales may be solicited at:** jaypee@jaypeebrothers.com

*A Practical Approach to Vascular and Endovascular Surgery*

*First Edition:* **2016**

ISBN: 978-93-5152-995-8

*Printed at* Ajanta Offset & Packagings Ltd., New Delhi

## Dedicated to

*My wife Mira*

–Jaisom Chopra

*My Late Father and My Family including
My Mother, Wife Kavita Bedi and My Children*

–VS Bedi

# Contributors

**Ajay Yadav**
MBBS MS FNB (Vascular Surgery) MRCS (Glasgow)
Senior Consultant and Director of
Vascular Cathlab
In Charge Diabetic Foot Care Center
Department of Vascular and
Endovascular Surgery
Sir Ganga Ram Hospital
New Delhi, India
E-mail: ajay.vascular @gmail.com

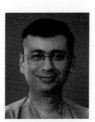

**Ambarish Satwik**
MBBS MS DNB (Vascular) FIAGES FAMS
Senior Consultant
Department of Vascular and
Endovascular Surgery
Sir Ganga Ram Hospital
New Delhi, India
E-mail: asatwik @gmail.com

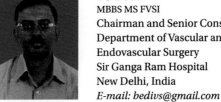

**Anand Chandrasekar**
MBBS MS DNB (Vascular Surgery)
Consultant Vascular Surgeon
Kauvery Hospitals
Trichy, Tamil Nadu, India
E-mail: drcams@rediffmail.com

**Jaisom Chopra**
MS FRCS
Senior Consultant Vascular Surgeon
Apollo Hospitals
New Delhi, India
E-mail: jaisomchopra@hotmail.com

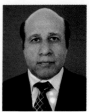

**Kamran Ali Khan**
MBBS MS MRCS (Edinburgh) DNB MNAMS
DNB Trainee (Vascular Surgery)
Department of Vascular and
Endovascular Surgery
Sir Ganga Ram Hospital
New Delhi, India
E-mail: khan22k@yahoo.co.in

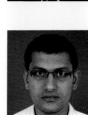

**VS Bedi**
MBBS MS FVSI
Chairman and Senior Consultant
Department of Vascular and
Endovascular Surgery
Sir Ganga Ram Hospital
New Delhi, India
E-mail: bedivs@gmail.com

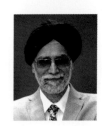

# Foreword

Vascular surgery has been arguably the most rapidly developing specialty over the last 40 years. Consider at that time, Duplex Ultrasound was almost unavailable and even the measurement of foot Doppler Pressures was in its infancy. No digital subtraction angiography, no MRI, no CAT scan angiography; these are now the basis of accurate diagnosis following a careful clinical assessment of the patient. No investigation can replace the bedside judgment of an experienced clinician.

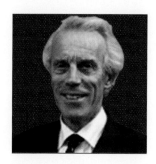

The safety of complex arterial operations has improved dramatically allowing more demanding treatment to become available. Carotid end-arterectomy is now a routine procedure in the right hands that has not been surpassed by endovascular techniques. Major amputations have been significantly reduced by distal bypass operations and endovascular intervention.

General surgeons using silk sutures but referral to specialist units repaired aneurysms and slicker techniques have resulted in tumbling mortality rates. The introduction of endovascular stent grafts has transformed the results of complex thoracoabdominal aneurysms.

These explosive advances can also be attributed to a complex array of innovations in those specialties that are so important to the surgeon: interventional radiologists, anesthetists, intensivists, cardiologists, renal physicians, diabetic physicians, and neurologists among others.

All these advances need to be corralled and explained succinctly for a general readership and Dr Jaisom Chopra and Dr VS Bedi are to be congratulated on doing just that. As members of The Vascular Society of India (formed in 1994), they have been seminal in spreading expertise from rudimentary beginnings by enthusiasm and inspirational leadership. This book provides an excellent guide from an Indian perspective and will be helpful in disseminating knowledge to all those who are confronted with vascular disease in all its manifestations.

**John HN Wolfe** MS FRCS FEBVS
Emeritus Consultant
St Mary's Hospital and King Edward VII Hospital
London, UK
Honorary Member
Vascular Society of India

# Preface

Diagnosis, treatment and patient safety are closely linked. The progressively better diagnostic facilities available to the physician lead to more accurate and quick diagnosis, which, in turn, is responsible for better care and less suffering to the patient.

Though there is an increasing interest in vascular surgery, a comparatively new, separate specialty in India; there are some diseases, which are treated unsatisfactorily despite all the recent advances. Vascular disease may present as a separate entity, but may also be a part of a generalized illness.

There are a few textbooks in vascular surgery and they present a detailed view of the disease process, making it difficult for the general physician to scan through the text to manage his patient.

The purpose of this textbook is to provide the medical students, the non-vascular doctors and the postgraduate medical students with a practical running knowledge of vascular diseases. It is user friendly to the general physician who needs a quick-practical way to manage a vascular surgery patient. The text includes the latest techniques, recent endovascular practices and their indications and results. It is a practical book for any physician (cardiologist, general physician), surgeon and radiologist for quick reading.

The book is concise and still exhaustive. Since common diseases occur more commonly, more stress is placed on their diagnosis and management. There are plenty of tables, illustrations and point-wise text to make it easy to understand and manage the patient.

We hope this book inspires the medical students, postgraduate students to be passionate practitioners of vascular surgery.

**Jaisom Chopra**
**VS Bedi**

# Acknowledgments

We gratefully acknowledge the contributions of Dr VS Bedi, Chairman, Vascular Surgery, Sir Ganga Ram Hospital, New Delhi, for his contribution towards this book without which it would not have been possible to write and publish it.

We are also indebted to Shri Jitendar P Vij (Group Chairman), Mr Ankit Vij (Group President) and Mr Tarun Duneja (Director-Publishing) of M/s Jaypee Brothers Medical Publishers (P) Ltd, New Delhi, India, for their patience during the writing of this book and making this book a reality that will help the vascular-oriented among us.

—**Jaisom Chopra**

The most gratifying moment in the process of writing a book is probably when the work is compiled and one can look back into 'thanks giving.' I first thank the God for giving me the required will and strength to accomplish this project. With great pleasure, I take this opportunity to thank all those whose efforts made this book possible.

I wish to express my deep and heartfelt gratitude for my colleagues and juniors in the Department of Vascular and Endovascular Surgery at Sir Ganga Ram Hospital, New Delhi, for their constant motivation. Working with such multi-talented personalities and an excellent team has indeed been an honor and it is hard to pen down words for the enormous care, empathy and affection they bestowed upon me!!

I am greatly indebted to Dr Sandeep Agarwal, Dr Ajay Yadav, Dr Ambarish Satwik, Dr Dhruv Agarwal and my residents for their valuable suggestions, unmatched enthusiasm, constructive criticism and constant efforts.

I would like to thank all the staff from my department, for their unfailing support. Mrs Asha Rawat and Mr Paramjeet Arneja need a special mention for their readiness to offer a helping hand at every step.

Thanks to Ms Shivangi Pramanik from M/s Jaypee Brothers Medical Publishers (P) Ltd, New Delhi, India, for her constant backing and last-minute help in compiling this work.

I express my highest regards to my parents, for their prayers and blessings. I spare a 'bouquet of thanks' for my wife and family, for their everlasting patience.

Last but not least, my sincere thanks to all my patients without whose participation this book would not have been possible.

I dedicate this work to my fraternity of Vascular and Endovascular Surgery!

—**VS Bedi**

# Contents

# 1

# History and Examination of the Arterial System

*Jaisom Chopra*

History and examination in medical practice help us not only to reach at a provisional diagnosis but also to outline the appropriate investigations so that we can arrive at a final diagnosis. It is mandatory to first perform a general and systemic-orientated examination by combining history of present illness, past history, and personal history along with a thorough physical examination. In the arterial system, it is vital to reach at an early diagnosis and to start appropriate treatment so as to salvage the extremity or save a life. A casual approach wherein detail and accuracy are lacking may delay therapeutic decisions.

## ■ VASCULAR HISTORY

Those suffering from the arterial disease have characteristic clinical features helping us to arrive at a diagnosis even before conducting a physical examination.

## Demographics

The patient's age gives us a strong indication on what could be the cause of peripheral arterial disease.
- 20–40 years – Buerger's disease and large vessel vasculitis such as Takayasu's disease
- After 40 years – atherosclerosis
- After 65 years – Temporal arteritis and arterial aneurysmal disease.

Strong female predilection is seen in Raynaud's syndrome, lupus vasculitis, and Takayasu's arteritis.

## ■ PRESENTING COMPLAINTS

The nature of symptoms offers a clue to the diagnosis. There are three important questions we have to consider:
1. Are we dealing with an acute arterial disease or a chronic arterial problem?

2. Is it involving a larger artery or a small artery?
3. Is it occlusive or aneurismal disease?

## Acute Arterial Disease

This generally presents as an emergency where there is danger of not only loss of limb but also even loss of life (Fig. 1).

It is typically of sudden onset with the patient experiencing the classical 5 "Ps":
1. **P**ain is severe and of sudden onset
2. **P**allor—the limb goes pale and later with time cyanosed
3. **P**ulseless—the pulses are absent distal to the site of blocked artery
4. **P**aresis—the limb goes numb with loss of sensation
5. **P**aralysis—there is reduced movement, which is a late sign.

Another finding is not a part of the classical 5 "Ps" but could be included as the sixth—Perishing with cold.

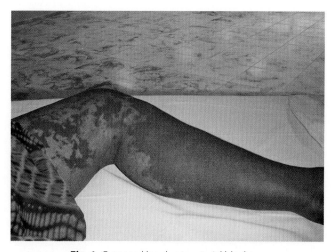

**Fig. 1** Cyanosed leg due to arterial blockage

This condition is an emergency because we have only six golden hours to correct the outcome before irreversible changes occur. The patient and the doctor must act immediately and decisively.

## Chronic Arterial Disease

There is decreased blood supply due to gradual narrowing progressing to blockage of the artery. The patients present with reproducible ischemic muscle pain known as claudication that occurs during exercise and is relieved by rest.

The most common cause is atherosclerosis. These patients are mostly smokers and present to the doctor years after the origin of the problem. If ignored and left untreated, they develop constant pain even at night while resting (rest pain), which is a precursor to ulcers and gangrene.

At this stage, there is a high risk of amputation. Abrupt deterioration of symptoms is generally due to superadded thrombosis or embolus.

## Large Artery Occlusive Disease

It again can be acute or chronic. In the acute form, the extremity distal to the site of blockage becomes very painful, pale, and cold compared with the other side, numb with reduced power.

In the chronic form, there is pain on walking (claudication) distal to the site of blockage with absent pulses. If aorta is involved, then both extremities are affected, but beyond the aortic bifurcation, only one limb is involved.

## Small Artery Occlusive Disease

Raynaud's syndrome is a vasospastic disease with sensitivity to cold and presents as a classic triphasic response—pale digits followed by cyanosis on exposure to cold, turning red on heating the part. Generally, wrist pulses are palpable. Raynaud's phenomenon is also seen in embolic occlusions from more proximal arteries such as subclavian and axillary. When tissue necrosis along with Raynaud's phenomenon occurs in the upper extremity, there generally is a proximal fixed obstructive lesion.

It is important to know whether the disease is intermittent or fixed. A good history tells us whether the disease is intermittent due to vasospasm or fixed due to a proximal occlusion.

Large artery (subclavian) involvement in the upper extremity is mostly asymptomatic. Chronic stenosis of the brachial artery presents as muscle fatigue or arm claudication.

In thoracic outlet syndrome, there are recurrent bouts of pain or numbness with activity involving a dermatological pattern.

## Claudication

Claudication means limping in Latin and is classically cramping pain or weakness on exercise and relieved by

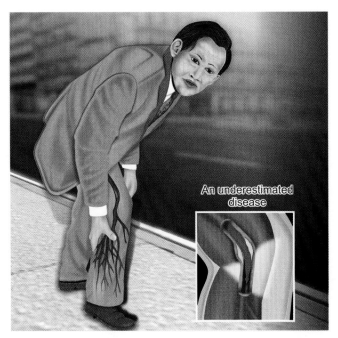

**Fig. 2** Calf claudication due to reduced blood supply to the leg muscles

rest. It is restricted to the muscles groups such as buttock, thigh, or calf and is due to reduced blood supply. It is more prominent in the calf muscles because these muscles are metabolically more active. The amount of exercise needed to bring on the pain is inversely proportional to the degree of arterial narrowing brought about by the atherosclerotic disease. The pain presents one segment below the site of occlusion or stenosis. Thus, aortic disease presents with pain in both buttocks and legs. Iliac disease presents as pain in the same side thigh muscles and leg, while superficial femoral arterial occlusion presents as calf pain. As the disease is multifocal, symptoms are more prominent distal to the most significant arterial narrowing or area with poorest collateral support (Fig. 2).

### Upper Extremity Claudication

This is seen in subclavian artery stenosis. If stenosis is proximal to the vertebral artery origin, the subclavian steal may be seen.

### Differential Diagnosis of Claudication

The conditions listed in Table 1 present as pseudoclaudication (false claudication) and may be mistaken for true claudication.

Night cramps are the most common nonvascular cause of leg pain due to exaggerated neuromuscular response to stretch.

The non-atherosclerotic causes of true claudication are listed in Table 2.

**Table 1** Differential diagnosis of pseudoclaudication at different sites in the leg

| Condition | Description | Effects of exercise and stopping activity | Other specific features |
|---|---|---|---|
| **Calf pseudoclaudication** | | | |
| Nocturnal cramps | Cramping calf pain at night relieved in few minutes | Occurs at rest | Relieved by postural change |
| Chronic compartment syndrome | Bursting pain in athletes or cyclists | Caused by strenuous exercise and subsides gradually | Elevation speeds recovery |
| Venous claudication | Bursting calf pain in extensive proximal deep venous thrombosis (DVT) (iliofemoral) | Walking increases and then pain gradually subsides on elevation | Elevation speeds recovery and signs of chronic venous insufficiency |
| Radiculopathy (herniated disc) | Sharp pain radiating down back of leg in a patient with back problems | Increased by postural change and not relieved by rest | May be relieved by postural change |
| Symptomatic Baker's cyst | Tenderness and swelling behind knee | Worse on activity and not relieved by rest | Signs of inflammation at back of knee |
| **Hip/buttock pseudoclaudication** | | | |
| Hip arthritis | Ache related to the level of activity | Worse with activity and not relieved by rest | More relief by non-weight bearing. weather-sensitive symptoms |
| Neurogenic claudication (spinal cord compression) | Weakness more than pain | Symptoms on standing and relieved by rest | May have back problems |
| **Foot pseudoclaudication** | | | |
| Arthritic/ inflammatory processes | Continuous ache related to activity | Increased by weight bearing but may continue at rest | |

**Table 2** Causes of true intermittent claudication other than arterial narrowing

Collagen vascular disease

Giant cell arteritis (Takayasu's and temporal)

Buerger's disease

Embolism (proximal sources)

- Heart (Left ventricular [LV] thrombus, paradoxic embolus)

- Aneurysms

Dissection

- Traumatic

- Inherited disorder of collagen metabolism

Adventitial cystic disease

Popliteal artery entrapment

Retroperitoneal fibrosis

Drugs

- Ergot derivatives

- 5HT1A/D agonists

## Rest Pain

As arterial insufficiency progresses, the blood supply becomes insufficient to supply the basal needs of the sensory nerves. There is severe continuous pain at night that begins over the metatarsal heads. It is relieved by dependency and worsened by elevation above the level of the heart. It is a sign of threat to the limb if no intervention is undertaken.

Metatarsalgia mimics rest pain, the difference being it is worsened by dependency and relieved on standing.

## Neuropathic Pain and Causalgia

This is a burning sensation in the extremity. Neuropathic pain is seen in diabetics whose nerves are involved in a glove and stocking distribution. In causalgia mostly upper extremities are involved and is triggered by some event which may be trivial or a major occurrence like myocardial infarction (MI), DVT of hip fracture.

## Erythermalgia

Erythermalgia presents with redness and burning sensation in the extremity typically worsened by heat. It may be a primary condition or secondary to myeloproliferative disorders, diabetes, lymphoma, hypertension, and drugs such as calcium channel blockers and bromocriptine.

## ■ MODE OF ONSET OF ILLNESS

- Acute arterial insufficiency typically presents as the 5 Ps—pain, pallor, poikilothermia, paresthesias, and paralysis.
- Chronic arterial insufficiency shows progressive limitation of symptoms, which is very gradual.
- Abrupt onset of pain with pallor is suggestive of embolic occlusion, though with arterial thrombosis, it is less dramatic. It is important to differentiate embolic from thrombotic arterial occlusion as responsible for limb ischemia (Table 3). The symptoms becoming worse or better depend on collateral pathway. Thrombus superimposed on the previous arterial plaque leading to acute ischemia often occurs and is more common in the superficial femoral artery.

**Table 3** Differentiating between embolism and thrombosis

|  | Embolism | Thrombosis in situ |
|---|---|---|
| History | Abrupt onset of pain<br>Previous cardiac event | Onset may or may not be abrupt. Symptoms acute but not abrupt |
| Physical examination | Cold mottled and paralyzed with clear demarcation<br>Normal contralateral limb | Cool bluish limb (slow progression) without clear demarcation<br>Abnormal contralateral pulse |
| Etiology | Cardiac thrombus (75–85%)<br>Aortic atheroma<br>Proximal aneurysm | Native artery plaque rupture<br>Graft occlusion |
| Prior vascular intervention | Usually none | Often yes |

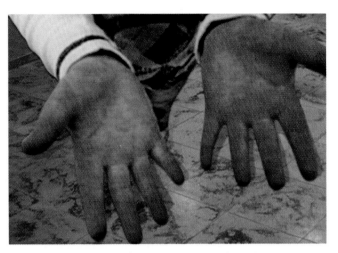

**Fig. 3** Cyanotic fingers due to Raynaud's syndrome

This thrombosis may be due to reduced blood flow as in reduced cardiac output seen in congestive heart failure (CHF) or MI.

The site of involvement often gives a clue to the diagnosis:

- Bilateral claudication in lower limbs—atherosclerosis and Buerger's disease.
- Foot claudication—small vessel disease—Buerger's or thromboembolism.
- Bilateral upper limb involvement—vasculitic disorder.
- Ulcer or gangrene in unilateral hand of acute onset—embolism from heart, proximal vessel, or aneurysm.

## Past Medical History

Always ask the patient whether he has any other illness apart from pertaining to vascular disease. Make a note of the risk factors such as smoking, hypertension, diabetes, tobacco abuse, dyslipidemia, strokes, blood clot, or amputation.

Has the patient had any other vascular intervention in the past (percutaneous or surgical) that may have occluded?

## Personal History

- Occupation—usage of vibratory tools should raise the suspicion of Raynaud's syndrome, although work involving repeated trauma to the hand may cause hypothenar-hammer syndrome (Fig. 3).
- Smoking has a strong association with Buerger's disease so much so that if one does not smoke, we may have to reconsider the diagnosis.
- Sexual dysfunction is common in patient with PAD.

## Drug History

This is very important. Migraine medication and ergot derivatives cause vasospasm.

### β-blockers Worsen Raynaud's

Toxic vasculitis is associated with sulfonamide, allopurinol, phenytoin, carbamazepine, chlorthalidone, methylthiouracil, spironolactone, and tetracycline.

## Family History

A family history of premature arterial disease suggests some inherent disorder in the mechanism of thrombosis, lipoprotein metabolism, and hyperhomocysteinemia.

A family history of sudden death from aneurysmal rupture or of joint or skin laxity would suggest collagen disorder. This could occur in Marfan's syndrome or Ehlers–Danlos syndrome.

## ■ PHYSICAL EXAMINATION OF THE ARTERIAL SYSTEM

Examine the patient region-wise from head to toe (Fig. 4).

## General Examination

This can lead to the diagnosis.

- Arm span greater than height as seen in patients with longer pubis to head distance than pubis to foot. These are present in arachnodactyly and chest deformities—Marfan's syndrome.
- Yellowish orange papules over neck and flexure areas with angioid streaks in the retina—pseudoxanthoma elasticum.
- Coarctation of the pararenal aorta with proximal stenosis of the renal arteries—neurofibromatosis and cafe-au-lait spots.

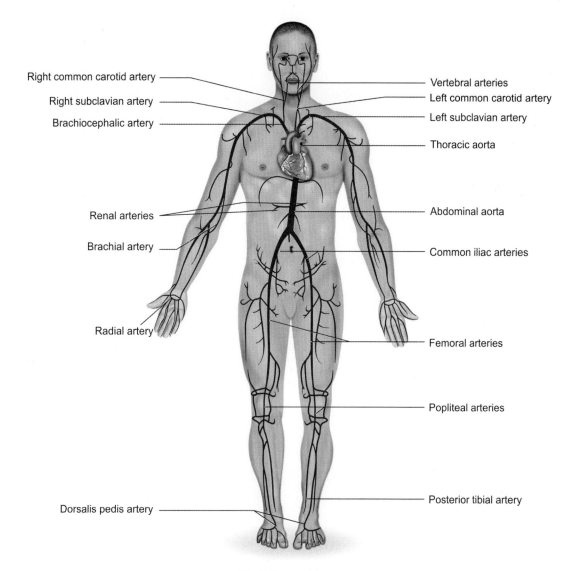

Right common carotid artery

Right subclavian artery

Brachiocephalic artery

Vertebral arteries

Left common carotid artery

Left subclavian artery

Thoracic aorta

Renal arteries

Abdominal aorta

Brachial artery

Common iliac arteries

Radial artery

Femoral arteries

Popliteal arteries

Posterior tibial artery

Dorsalis pedis artery

**Fig. 4** The arterial tree

- Tendinous xanthomas—seen subcutaneously or over the extensor tendons in patients with type II hyperlipoproteinemia.
- Tuberoeruptive xanthomas—on extremities and palms and associated with systemic atherosclerosis.
- Cutaneous telangiectasias are often associated with arteriovenous (AV) malformations.
- Nevus vinosus (port-wine stain) that does not regress is associated with three syndromes:
  - *Sturge–Weber syndrome:* Port-wine stain in trigeminal distribution and associated with seizures and vascular malformation of the retina and leptomeninges.
  - *Klippel–Trenaunay syndrome:* Port-wine stain involving an extremity with associated venous varicosities and absent deep venous system.
  - *Parke–Weber syndrome:* A subset of Klippel-Trenaunay syndrome with arteriovenous malformation and a tendency for congestive heart failure.

## Examination of the Head, Neck and Chest

### Inspection

The oral mucous membrane and conjunctiva of the eyes are examined for clues of systemic vascular disease.
- Subconjunctival hemorrhage and petechiae suggest infective endocarditis.
- Blue sclerae are seen in osteogenesis imperfecta and aneurysmal disease.
- Hollenhorst's plaques are seen in the retina of those with monocular symptoms and transient ischemic attacks (TIAs).

### Neck and Chest

- Pulsatile neck masses suggest aneurysms or kinking of arteries at the root of the neck. This is more common on the right side and is seen in elderly hypertensive or with carotid body tumor.
- Carotid artery aneurysm is the most common in the common carotid artery and seen below the angle of the mandible.
- Aneurysms of the internal carotid artery are not visible, as they lie below the fascia.
- Supraclavicular pulsations are from subclavian artery or its thyrocervical branch.

### Palpation

Palpating the pulses is the most important part of any arterial examination and the following points are to be stressed:

- Pulse volume—if expansile indicates aneurysmal dilatation, although if diminished it may show proximal occlusion or stenosis.
- Condition of the arterial wall—if hard is atheromatous.
- Record the pulse volume on a scale: 0 – absent; 1 – trace; 2 – moderately reduced; 3 – mildly reduced; 4 – bounding.

*The common carotid artery* is felt in the carotid triangle lying anterior to the sternomastoid muscle against the carotid tubercle of the sixth cervical vertebra. The carotid pulses are felt strongly in occlusion of the internal carotid artery.

*The superficial temporal artery* is felt in front of the tragus of the ear, and if prominent, it excludes significant stenosis of the common or external carotid artery of that side.

An expansile lesion in the neck is certainly aneurysmal and must be distinguished from kinking of the carotid. Here, the pulsations are along the axis of the artery, although they are at right angle to the artery in an aneurysm.

*Carotid body tumor* is at the angle of the mandible and is mobile laterally but fixed along the vertical axis of the artery as it is fixed by the carotid sheath. It is a painless mass.

*Vertebral artery* cannot be palpated.

### Auscultation

Auscultation should be performed over all superficial arteries and swellings. Carotid bruits in the neck may originate in the chest along the aorta. Noninvasive vascular studies are a must to assess the lesion. Bruits over the subclavian suggest stenosis.

## Examination of the Lower Extremity

### Inspection

Always place the contralateral limb alongside to assess changes by comparison. These changes are seen distal to the site of occlusion.

In the initial stages of acute ischemia, there is paresthesia with reduced sensation to light touch and position that progress to complete anesthesia. With further ischemia, paralysis and cyanosis followed by gangrene occur (Fig. 5).

In chronic ischemia, there is reduced subcutaneous fat, shininess, hair loss, and nail changes, which are brittle with transverse ridges and ulcerations (Fig. 6 and Table 4).

The dependent foot may turn purple—dependent rubor is due to filling of dilated capillaries with deoxygenated blood.

In microembolization, there are palpable pulses with cyanotic toes known as the blue toe syndrome.

Capillary filling time—the limb is pale on elevation and takes time to become pink on dependency (20–30 s). It may progress to dependent rubor.

Vascular (Buerger's) angle—it is the angle at which the limb turns pale on elevation, usually 30° in critical ischemia.

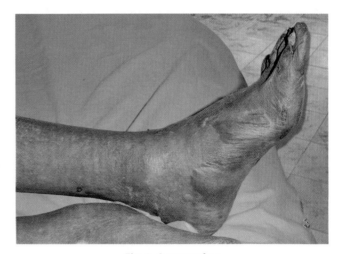

**Fig. 5** Gangrene foot

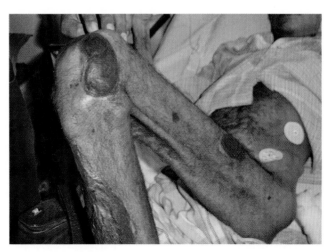

**Fig. 6** Chronically ischemic lower limb

**Table 4** Urgency of treatment in various grades of limb ischemia

| Category | Description | Motor/sensory findings | Arterial Doppler signals |
|---|---|---|---|
| I – Viable | Not immediately threatened | None | Audible |
| IIa – Marginally threatened | Salvageable if promptly treated | Minimal sensory deficit or none | Often audible |
| IIb – Immediately threatened | Salvageable with immediate revascularization | Mild to moderate weakness Sensory deficit extends beyond toes and is associated with rest pain | Usually inaudible |
| III | Major tissue loss or permanent nerve damage inevitable | Profound motor paralysis with extensive sensory deficit | Inaudible and venous sounds also absent |

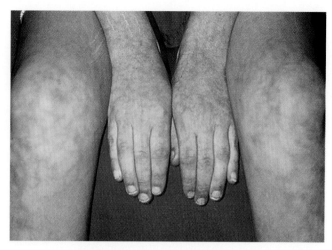

**Fig. 7** Livedo reticularis hands and knees

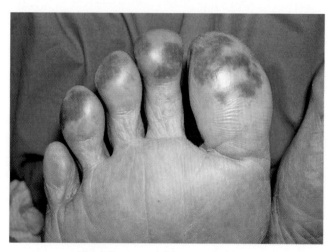

**Fig. 8** Pernio or chilblains involving toes

Venous filling time—the limb is elevated for a while and laid flat. The veins should fill within 5 s, but in ischemic limb, they take considerably longer.

Examination of gangrenous area—the extent is according to the level of occlusion and it may be wet (diabetics) or dry. The line of demarcation must be noted.

Livedo reticularis – mottled discoloration (fishnet) of the skin as seen in atheroembolism. It may be seen in young females (20–40 years) with Raynaud's and hypertension. It is also noticed in vascular collagen disease—systemic lupus erythematosus (SLE), polyarteritis nodosum (PAN), hyperviscosity syndrome, and drugs such as amentidine.

Pernio—seen in females with bluish red lesions on the toes and shin. There is burning and severe itching. The lesions last less than 10 days. Chronic pernio is called chilblains and seen on toes on exposure to cold (Figs 7 and 8).

## Palpation

Skin temperature—Use the back of the hand to assess the degree of warmth and coolness that will help us to differentiate between healthy tissue and ischemic one.

Capillary filling time—press finger pulp firmly on hard surface and note the time for pallor to disappear. Elevate the leg to empty the capillaries. Now make it dependent. Normally, capillaries fill in less than 5 s, but in ischemia, they would take less than 20 s.

Pulses—those below the occlusion will be absent unless there are excellent collaterals in which case it may be diminished but does not disappear. The dorsalis pedis is felt lateral to the tendon of extensor hallucis longus but is absent in 10%. The posterior tibial artery lies behind the medial malleolus midway between the malleolus and the tendon Achilles. The anterior tibial artery lies midway between the two malleoli against the lower end of the tibia, above the ankle joint, and lateral to the extensor hallucis tendon. The popliteal artery is palpated behind the knee by making the patient prone and flexing the knee. It may also be felt with the patient lying supine with the knee flexed to 40° and the artery felt against the upper end of the tibia by rolling the fingers from side to side. The femoral artery is felt just below the inguinal ligament midway between the pubis and the anterior superior iliac spine.

## Neurological Evaluation

In advanced limb ischemia, light touch, two-point discrimination, vibratory perception, and proprioception are lost well before deep pain and pressure. Motor involvement is a sign of advanced limb threatening ischemia. Diabetic individuals have pre-existing sensory deficits that add to the confusion (Table 4).

## Evaluation of the Upper Extremity

### Inspection

Severe pallor is seen in severe ischemia or during attack of Raynaud's syndrome. Note nail bed changes such as hemorrhages, cyanosis, ulceration, and gangrene. Abnormally dilated capillaries, as seen by the capillary microscope, are seen in progressive systemic sclerosis (PSS)/calcinosis, Raynaud, esophagus, sclerosis telangiectasiae (CREST), while abnormal capillary rarefaction may suggest collagen vascular disease such as SLE or rheumatoid arthritis in patients presenting with secondary Raynaud's syndrome.

### Palpation

Temperature—use the back of the hand to determine the warmth or coolness that points to the viability and ischemia.

Capillary filling time—press the finger pulp against a hard surface and note the time for pallor to disappear. Subclavian aneurysms are palpated in the supraclavicular fossa.

Pulses—subclavian artery is felt above the middle of the clavicle. Brachial artery is felt in the medial upper arm between the bellies of the biceps and the triceps and at the elbow medial to the biceps tendon. Radial and ulnar arteries are felt at the lateral and medial volar aspects. Ulnar artery may be absent in 3% from birth. Absent radial and ulnar pulses in young adults suggest Takayasu's arteritis.

### Auscultation

Blood pressure is recorded in both upper extremities, and if a difference of over 10 mm Hg is noted, it is considered abnormal. Low blood pressure in both upper extremities is an indication to see blood pressure in lower extremities.

Thoracic outlet syndrome maneuvers—the radial artery pulse is felt digitally or with Doppler at rest and after the provocative maneuver. A positive test is diminution of the pulse after the maneuver. Adson's test—patient sitting upright is asked to take a deep breath and look upwards while turning the head to the affected side. Hyperabduction maneuver—the symptomatic extremity is hyperabducted to 180°. The pulse disappears to reappear when normal position is restored. Costoclavicular maneuver—patient thrusts both shoulders backwards and downwards maximally. EAST maneuver (external rotation-abduction stress test) may be the most reliable test. The patient is in a "stick up posture", with arms extended, externally rotated, and behind the head. He then makes fists repeatedly for 3 minutes after which the pulse is felt. Branham's sign—done for AV fistula. Pressure of the artery proximal to the fistula will reduce the swelling, disappearance of bruit, and reduction in pulse rate.

## Examination of the Abdomen

This is a must in any vascular examination.

### Inspection

Pulsations are normally not seen, but in aortic dilatation, they may visible in a thin subject.

### Palpation

Normal aorta is the size of the width of the patient's thumb. In aneurysm, the pulse is expansile and larger than a full centimeter. If one cannot feel the upper end of the aneurysm due to the costal margin or xiphoid, then we are dealing with a suprarenal aneurysm or a thoracoabdominal aneurysm. Tenderness over the aneurysm is a bad sign and implies impending rupture.

### Auscultation

Bruits present should raise the doubts of atherosclerotic aneurysmal disease or a stenosis in the aorta or renals. Renal arteries bruits are normally systolic-diastolic in nature. A diastolic bruit indicates severe stenosis, as there is continued flow during diastole. These bruits are in the lower abdomen and femoral areas.

## ■ ASSESSING THE OUTCOMES AND IMPROVEMENTS IN ARTERIAL DISEASE

The clinical categories of limb ischemia are summarized in Table 5.

Patients with irreversible ischemia are treated with urgent amputation rather than with attempted revascularization, as large quantities of muscle metabolites released into the circulation cause sepsis, multiple organ failure, and ultimate death. Patients presenting with severe limb ischemia (class IIb) progress to class III in 6 hours when irreversible changes are seen leading to amputation. The time frame may not allow diagnostic investigations and angiography. The clinical categories of chronic limb ischemia are outlined in Table 6.

**Table 5** The clinical categories of acute limb ischemia

| Categories | Description | Neuromuscular findings | Doppler study |
|---|---|---|---|
| I | Viable | No sensory or muscle weakness | Audible arterial and venous signals |
| IIa | Threatened marginally | Minimal | Often inaudible arterial and audible venous signals |
| IIb | Threatened immediately | Mild to moderate associated with pain | Usually inaudible arterial and audible venous signals |
| III | Irreversible | Profound deficit | No arterial or venous signals |

**Table 6** The clinical categories of chronic limb ischemia

| Grade | Category | Clinical description | Objective criteria |
|---|---|---|---|
| 0 | 0 | Asymptomatic; no significant disease | Normal treadmill or stress tests |
| I | 1 | Mild claudication | Completes treadmill exercise Airway pressure (AP) >50 mm Hg but 25 mm Hg <BP |
| I | 2 | Moderate claudication | Between category 1 and 3 |
| I | 3 | Severe claudication | Cannot complete treadmill exercise AP after exercise <50 mm Hg |
| II | 4 | Ischemic rest pain | Resting AP <40 mm Hg. Flat or barely pulsatile ankle wave form. Toe pressure (TP) <30 mm Hg |
| III | 5 | Minor tissue loss. Focal gangrene or non-healing ulcer | Resting AP <60 mm Hg ankle wave forms flat. TP <40 mm Hg |
| III | 6 | Major tissue loss extending to the ankle. Foot no longer salvageable | Same as category 5 |

Table 7 gives the follow-up parameters to assess the improvement in peripheral artery disease (PAD) patients.

# ■ CONCLUSION

- A detailed history and thorough examination of arterial system is needed for accurate diagnosis, diagnostic planning, and therapy.
- Differential diagnosis of upper extremity lesions is more in number than lower extremity lesions.
- Atherosclerosis is the most common form of disease in lower extremity and presents as intermittent claudication.

**Table 7** Follow-up parameters to assess the improvement of peripheral vascular disease

**Clinical parameters**

*Patient-based parameters*
- Mortality
- Limb salvage
- Ankle brachial indices
- Absolute and initial claudication distance.

*Procedure-based parameters*
- Technical success
- Primary and secondary patency rates (percutaneous and graft)
- Procedural morbidity and mortality

*Surrogate markers*
- Perfusion-related end points
  - Doppler blood flow
  - $TcPO_2$
  - Skin perfusion by laser Doppler perfusion
  - Reactive hyperemia perfusion by various modalities
- Vessel-related end points
  - Contrast angiography
  - Intravascular ultrasound

*Biomarkers*
- C-reactive protein (CRP)
- CD40 ligand
- Asymmetric dimethylarginine (ADMA)

**Quality of life instruments**

*General health (SF-36v2)*

*PAD-specific questionnaire*
- Walking impairment questionnaire
- PAD-physical activity recall (PAD-PAR)

# PRACTICAL POINTS

- Symptoms due to vasospasm are intermittent and the extremity is normal between the attacks.
- Tissue necrosis in the upper extremity is always due to arterial occlusion even if there are symptoms of Raynaud's syndrome.
- Acrocyanosis and pernio mimic critical limb ischemia and need to be differentiated from more serious disorders.
- Aortoiliac disease has aching discomfort in the hips and thighs along with weakness of the lower extremity.
- Renal artery bruits are hemodynamically significant and are systolic-diastolic.
- Thoracic-outlet syndrome maneuvers such as Adson's test are positive in normal people.
- The most common expansile lesion of the neck could be aneurysm or kinking or carotid artery.

# 2

# Noninvasive Vascular Imaging for Vascular Disease

*Jaisom Chopra*

## ■ INTRODUCTION

- A complete history and examination followed by an accurate noninvasive testing is required for a successful patient work-up in vascular surgery.
- These diagnostic methods must be safe, accurate, painless, and reproducible.
- Methodical testing improves the outcome through proper patient selection.

## ■ BASIS OF VASCULAR ULTRASOUND

This is the first line of investigation in vascular imaging. There is a "frequency shift" of the emitted sound wave beam. This shift is the difference between the frequencies of transmission and reflection. The frequency is measured in megahertz (MHz) and cannot be heard by the human ear. The emitted ultrasound beam is reflected by the flowing blood back to the transducer, which converts it into a gray scale image on the screen. This Doppler waveform being converted to the gray scale image is known as duplex ultrasonography. Modern ultrasound machines add color to the gray scale image. The peak flow velocity needs the ultrasound beam to be parallel to the blood flow in the vessel. As ultrasound images are captured in real time, they show the structure of the body's organs and their movement as well as the blood flowing through the blood vessels. This is a noninvasive test helping doctors to diagnose and treat the medical condition. This provides pictures of the body's arteries and the veins (Fig. 1).

## ■ COMMON USES OF THE PROCEDURE

It is useful to evaluate body's circulatory system. We do vascular ultrasound to:
- Monitor blood flow throughout the body to the organs and the tissue.

- Locate blockages and stenosis and abnormalities such as plaque and emboli to plan proper treatment.
- Detect blood clots in the veins (deep vein thrombosis—DVT) of the legs and the arms.
- Determine if the site of puncture for angiography is atherosclerotic or not.
- To evaluate the success of bypass by seeing the outflow.
- Determine an enlarged artery (aneurysm).
- Determine site of incompetent valves and severity of varicose veins.

*Doppler ultrasound helps physician to see and evaluate:*
- Blocks to the blood flow (clots)
- Narrowing of the blood vessels due to plaque
- Tumor and congenital malformation.

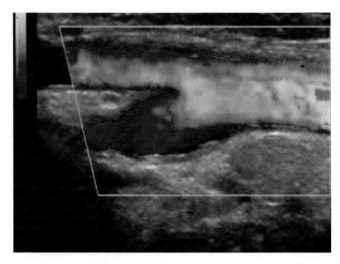

**Fig. 1** Color Doppler showing blood flow through common femoral artery and bifurcating into superficial femoral and profunda femoris artery

## How should One Prepare?

Wear comfortable clothes. In abdominal ultrasound, overnight fasting is needed. These are very sensitive to movement.

## What does the Equipment Look Like?

It has a console containing a computer and electronics, a video display screen, and transducer to scan the body and the blood vessels. This sends high-frequency sound waves into the body and then records the returning echoes from the tissues in the body. The ultrasound image is visible on the screen. The image is created on the basis of the amplitude (strength) frequency, the time it takes to return from the patient to the transducer, and the type of the body structure the sound waves travel through (Fig. 2).

## How does the Procedure Work?

The inaudible high frequency sound wave bounces back or echoes. By measuring these echo waves, it is possible to determine:

- How far the object is from the skin surface
- The exact size of the object
- The shape of the object and
- The consistency of the object (solid, filled with fluid or both)
- It detects changes in organs, tissues, vessels, and abnormal masses such as tumors
- It detects the velocity of blood flow measuring the speed and direction of the blood flow through the vessel. The movement of the cells causes a change in pitch of reflected sound waves (Doppler effect). The computer collects and processes the sounds, creating color pictures representing the flow of blood through the vessel (Figs 3 and 4).

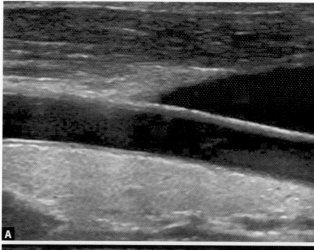

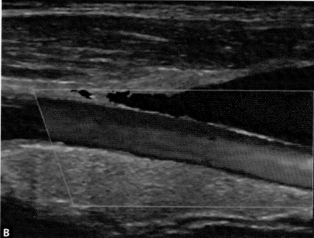

**Figs 3A and B**  (A) Ultrasound; (B) Color Doppler study

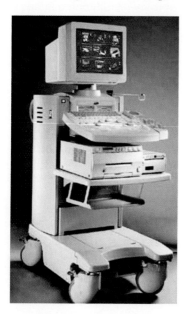

**Fig. 2** Ultrasound machine

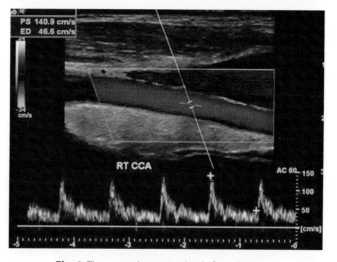

**Fig. 4** The artery showing pulsatile flow shown on graphic recording

## How is the Procedure Performed?

With patient lying, a water-based gel is applied generously to the area of the body to be studied. This helps make contact with the skin without air pockets. The transducer is pressed firmly against the skin of the patient (Figs 5A and B).

*Caution:* In visualization of very superficial veins in thin people, the probe is held just in contact with the jelly, but no pressure is applied that would immediately obliterate the vein.
    The examination takes 30–45 minutes.

## What are the Benefits?

- It is noninvasive and painless
- Widely available, easy to use, and cheap compared with other modalities
- Does not use ionizing radiations
- Gives very clear images that do not show up on the X-rays.

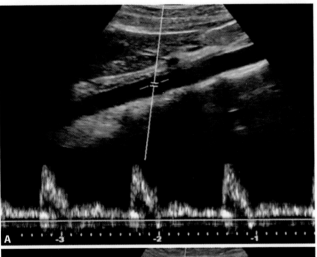

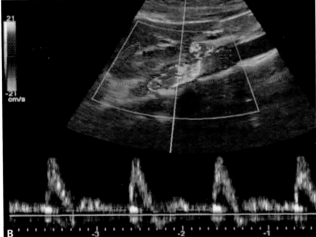

**Figs 5A and B** (A) Arterial ultrasound; (B) Color Doppler study

## What are the Risks?

No harmful effects on humans.

## What are the Limitations of Vascular Ultrasound?

- Vessels deep in the body are harder to see than the superficial ones. For deep vessels not clearly visualized on ultrasound, computed tomography (CT) or magnetic resonance imaging (MRI) may be needed to see them.
- Small vessels are more difficult to see and evaluate than larger ones.
- Calcification seen in atherosclerosis and diabetic individuals may obstruct the ultrasound beam.
- It may be difficult to differentiate between an occluded vessel and one over 90% closed. The weak blood flow in the latter may not be detected by ultrasound.
- The test is operator dependent and best performed by a person experienced in vascular ultrasound.

## ■ DIAGNOSTIC EVALUATION OF LOWER EXTREMITY ARTERIAL DISEASE

### Lower Extremity Arterial Vascular Testing

The evaluation of patients suffering from peripheral artery disease (PAD) includes taking proper history, including risk factors, physical examination, and use of noninvasive tests. These tests need minimal training and thus are routinely performed in the clinics and outpatient departments (OPDs).

### The Overall Approach to Lower Extremity Diagnostic Testing—The Steps

- First of all prove that the patient is suffering from PAD by performing ankle-brachial index (ABI) in every patient suspected of having PAD.
- Once PAD is proven, further location of PAD is needed. This is carried out by noninvasive physiological testing using segmental limb pressures and pulse volume recording (PVR).
- If there is doubt about claudication, then exercise treadmill test followed by ABI may be very helpful and may prove PAD that was not seen at rest (Table 1).
- If specific information regarding the exact site of the arterial stenosis or occlusion is needed, then complete duplex ultrasonography may be needed from the infrarenal aorta to the tibials.

**Table 1** Noninvasive testing for peripheral artery disease

| Vascular laboratory examination | Information obtained | Clinical indication | Limitations |
|---|---|---|---|
| Segmental limb pressures (SLP) | Localizes disease to specific segments in limbs. Could predict wound healing | Moderate to severe claudication with limb ischemia needing revascularization | Inaccurate in diabetic individuals with noncompressible arteries. Requires special cuffs |
| Pulse volume recording (PVR) | Localizes disease to specific segments in limb. Could predict wound healing | Moderate to severe claudication with limb ischemia needing revascularization Useful in calcified arteries | Needs an experienced technologist. Mainly qualitative information |
| Segmental Doppler wave-form | Localizes disease to specific segments in limbs. Easy to perform and interpret | Moderate to severe claudication with limb ischemia needing revascularization | Not accurate in calcified arteries. Less accurate than pulse volume recording |
| Exercise ABI | Confirms diagnosis of peripheral arterial disease when ABI <90 mm Hg | Atypical symptoms of exertional limb discomfort. Performed postoperative to see effects of treatment | Needs treadmill and close observation |
| Arterial duplex ultrasonography | Identifies site of atherosclerosis—stenosis or occlusion. Helps plan open surgery or endovascular intervention | Advanced claudication or critical limb ischemia needing revascularization Postcatheterization access site complications such as pseudoaneurysm, hematoma, and arteriovenous fistula | Needs skilled operator and expensive equipment. Prolonged examination time. Calcified arteries cause shadowing preventing Doppler velocities. Provides anatomy and not functional limitation |

# ■ ANKLE-BRACHIAL INDEX

## Definition

It is the ratio of the blood pressure in the lower legs to the blood pressure in the arms. If the pressure in the legs is lower than that of the arms, it indicates arterial occlusive disease (Fig. 6).

## Method

The blood pressure cuff is inflated in the arm and the calf above the systolic pressure level and deflated. A hand-held Doppler probe placed over the dorsalis pedis or the posterior tibial arteries at the ankle and the brachial artery in the arm records the first sound of the arterial signal, just as we record the usual blood pressure. This is the systolic pressure at the ankle and the arm. Then, we divide the ankle pressure by the arm pressure to get ABI.

$$ABPI_{Leg} = \frac{P_{Leg}}{P_{Arm}}$$

This test has a sensitivity of 90% and a specificity of 98% if the arterial stenosis is more than 50% as proven on an angiogram.

## Problems with Ankle-Brachial Pressure Index (ABPI)

• It is unreliable in calcified arteries (hardened and therefore not compressible). This produces falsely high pressures and therefore gives false negative results. This is found in diabetic individuals (41% patients with diabetes have PAD), renal failure patients, and heavy smokers.

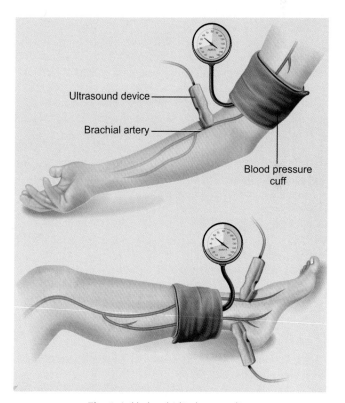

**Fig. 6** Ankle-brachial index recording

ABPI less than 0.9 and more than 1.3 must be investigated further.
• In mild PAD, resting ABPI may be unreliable. Exercise ABPI is more reliable. This is a treadmill (6-min test) that increases the sensitivity of ABPI but unsuitable for obese

**Table 2** Correlating ABI with the severity of the disease

| ABPI value | Interpretation | Action | Nature of ulcer if present |
|---|---|---|---|
| Above 1.2 | Hardened arteries—PAD | Refer routinely | Venous ulcer—compression bandaging |
| 1.0–1.2 | Normal range | None | Venous ulcer |
| 0.9–1.0 | Acceptable | None | Venous ulcer |
| 0.8–0.9 | Minimal arterial disease | Manage risk factors | Venous ulcer |
| 0.5–0.8 | Moderate arterial disease | Routine vascular referral | Mixed ulcers use reduce compression bandage |
| Below 0.5 | Severe arterial disease | Urgent vascular referral | Arterial ulcers—no compression bandage used |

or with comorbidities such as obesity, cardiac disease, and abdominal aortic aneurysm (AAA).

- Lack of protocol standardization.
- Skilled operators to increase reliability.

The ankle pressure is always higher at the ankle because it reflects the foot arteries, while the brachial artery has some distance to go before the hand.

Table 2 gives the severity of PAD and the best management of various types of leg ulcers.

ABPI is an independent predictor of mortality, as it reflects the burden of atherosclerosis.

Whenever PAD is suspected, three tests must be done:
1. ABI testing
2. Carotid Doppler ultrasound
3. Echocardiogram.

In the following conditions, PAD should be suspected and ABPI must be done:
- Being a current or former smoker
- Diabetes
- Overweight
- High blood pressure
- High cholesterol.

If one is already having PAD, then the test is done to know whether the treatment is working or the condition has worsened.

## Risks

There are no risks involved. One may find some discomfort on blood pressure cuff being inflated, but the inconvenience is temporary. With severe pain in the legs or arms, one may avoid doing ABI and go for other tests.

## What Preparation is Needed?

No preparation is needed. Only loose clothes are worn around the arms and the ankles to allow the blood pressure cuff to be put.

## ■ EXERCISE ANKLE-BRACHIAL INDEX

This noninvasive test is extremely helpful in unclear cases wherein ABI at rest is borderline or mildly reduced and wherein patient has mild discomfort not typical of claudication (pseudoclaudication). The exercise is at 2 miles/h at an incline of 12% for 5 minutes. A decline in mercury by 15 mm Hg is a positive test. In normal people with no PAD after exercise, the ankle systolic pressure rises or remains the same (Fig. 7).

## ■ SEGMENTAL LEG PRESSURES

Here six cuffs are tied on each leg—upper thigh, lower thigh above knee, calf, above ankle, transmetatarsal level of the foot, and big toe. After calculating the ABI, each segment is inflated in turn and the systolic pressure noted using a probe at the ankle artery (Fig. 8).

## Results

- A reduction in pressure of over 30 mm Hg between two consecutive cuff levels in one leg means a stenosis in the artery proximal to the cuff is present.
- If there is a reduction in the pressure by 20–30 mm Hg between the two legs at the same level cuffs, then there is a significant stenosis or occlusion above the cuff on the affected side.

## ■ PULSE VOLUME RECORDING

These are plethysmographic changes that detect the changes of the volume of the blood as it flows through the extremity.

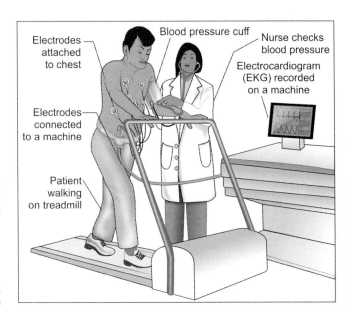

**Fig. 7** Exercise ABI

the severity and the site of the disease. Normal waveform is triphasic with a forward and reverse diastolic component. In severe disease, the reverse component is lost and waveform becomes biphasic. When forward flow becomes continuous, the waveform becomes monophasic. In severe disease, the waveform is attenuated. Patterns of arterial flow are recorded using a continuous Doppler over the femoral, popliteal, posterior tibial, and dorsalis pedis arteries (Fig. 10).

## ■ DUPLEX ARTERIAL ULTRASOUND

It is very often performed and is accepted as a reliable method to record arterial stenosis or occlusion. The sensitivity of the method to record occlusion and stenosis is 95% and 92%, while the specificity is 99% and 97%, respectively.

A 5–7.5 MHz transducer is used to image the vessels above and below the inguinal ligament. The vessels are studied in the sagittal plane and the Doppler velocities are studied using a 60° Doppler angle.

### Advantages of Duplex Arterial Ultrasound

- Classification of arterial disease—Vessels are classified into five categories—(i) normal, (ii) up to 19% stenosis, (iii) 20–49% stenosis, (iv) 50–99% stenosis, and (v) total occlusion. These categories are determined by changes in the Doppler waveform as well as increasing the peak systolic velocity. If the artery has to be classified as 50–99% stenosis, then the peak systolic velocity must be increased by 100% in comparison to the normal segment of the artery proximal to the stenosis (Fig. 11).
- Color Doppler may be used as a guide to gain arterial access by the interventionist.
- It is very helpful in finding the areas of vascular trauma, specifically iatrogenic.
- Pseudoaneurysms occur in 7.5% of the femoral interventions and could lead to distal embolization, compression of the adjacent structures such as the nerve and the vein, rupture, and hemorrhage. Duplex ultrasound can reliably and accurately determine these lesions and help in the direct compression of insertion of ultrasound-guided thrombin injection to repair it without surgical intervention (Fig. 12).
- **Graft surveillance**
  - Those who have had bypass surgery using a vein graft may develop stenosis at a number of sites. Once the graft thromboses, secondary patency rates are very poor. It is important to detect the stenosis and correct it prior to thrombosis as the salvage rate is 80%. Thus, a well-organized graft surveillance program is essential to preserve the graft patency.
  - In vein bypass grafts, the following protocol is recommended—7 days after surgery followed by 1 month and then 3 monthly intervals for first year.

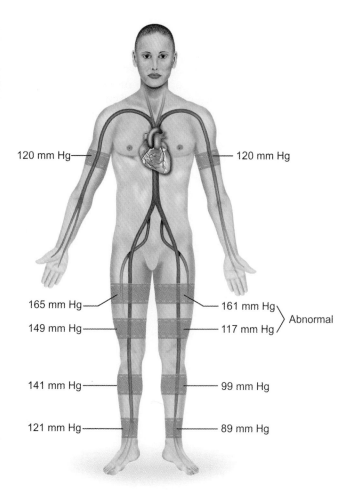

120 mm Hg

120 mm Hg

165 mm Hg

161 mm Hg

149 mm Hg

117 mm Hg

⟩ Abnormal

141 mm Hg

99 mm Hg

121 mm Hg

89 mm Hg

**Fig. 8** Segmental limb pressures

With the blood pressure cuffs at the six locations on each leg as described in the segmental pressure section, the tracing is recorded at each level. The recording in a normal patient is similar to the intra-arterial recording with a rapid systolic upstroke and a rapid down stroke with a prominent dicrotic notch. The BP cuff is inflated to 65 mm Hg (Fig. 9).

In arterial disease, the waveform is dampened and widened. As disease progresses, the waveform becomes flatter or nonpulsatile.

The limitations of the procedure are high cost, prolonged examination time, and difficulty in interpreting a very severe lesion.

## ■ DOPPLER VELOCITY WAVEFORM ANALYSIS

It can be used instead of pulse volume recording (PVR), though it is more operator dependent. Used with segmental length pressure (SLP), it provides more information about

**Lower extremity arterial-PVR**

**Right**

Above knee                    Not interpreted

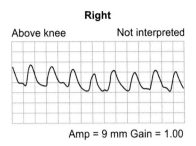

Amp = 9 mm Gain = 1.00

Calf                              Not interpreted

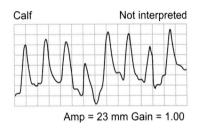

Amp = 23 mm Gain = 1.00

Ankle                            Not interpreted

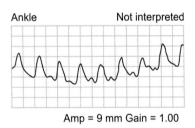

Amp = 9 mm Gain = 1.00

Toe                              Not interpreted

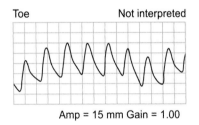

Amp = 15 mm Gain = 1.00

**Left**

Above knee                    Not interpreted

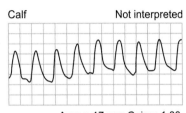

Amp = 11 mm Gain = 1.00

Calf                              Not interpreted

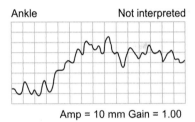

Amp = 17 mm Gain = 1.00

Ankle                            Not interpreted

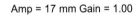

Amp = 10 mm Gain = 1.00

Toe                              Not interpreted

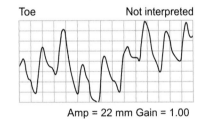

Amp = 22 mm Gain = 1.00

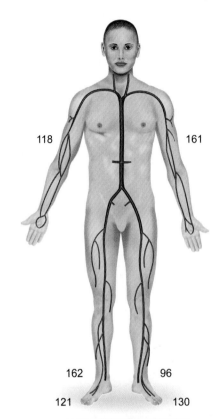

118                161

162                96
121                130

| Right |      | Left |
|-------|------|------|
| 1.01  | ABI  | 1.01 |
| 0.75  | TBI  | 0.75 |

**Fig. 9** Segmental limb recordings

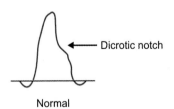

←— Dicrotic notch

Normal

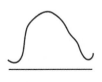

Moderate disease

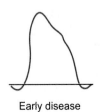

Early disease

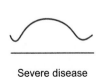

Severe disease

**Fig. 10** Segmental volume plethysmography in peripheral vascular disease

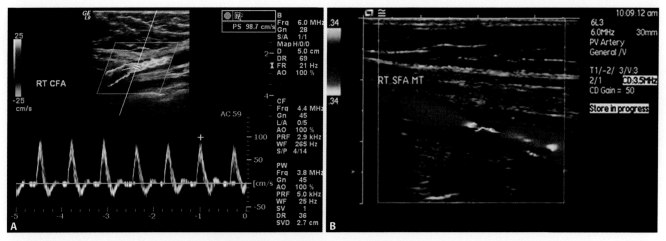

**Figs 11A and B** (A) Normal artery; (B) Tight stenosis in artery

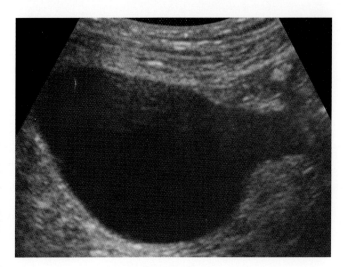

**Fig. 12** False aneurysm

If well functional, then the surveillance is done at 6-month interval.

- Ankle pressures and waveform studies should be performed every time. If stenosis is considered, then prompt angiogram or magnetic resonance angiography (MRA) should be conducted.
- The two graft anastomosis, proximal, mid and distal ends of the graft are studied using a 5–7.5 MHz transducer held at 60°. The peak systolic and end diastolic velocities are obtained at each of these five segments and compared with the segment of the graft proximal to the area under review. If the ratio of the peak systolic velocity in the area studied is two times that of the proximal normal segment, then it suggests a 50–75% reduction is diameter. If in addition the end diastolic velocities are over 100 cm/s, it suggests a reduction in diameter of over 75%.

## COMPUTED TOMOGRAPHIC ANGIOGRAPHY

It is a minimally invasive medical test that helps physicians to diagnose and treat medical conditions (Fig. 13).

Computed tomographic angiography (CTA) uses the following:
- X-rays with catheters
- CT
- MRI
- Contrast material.

Iodine-rich contrast is injected into the vein, and as it flows throughout the blood vessels in various organs of the body, it is scanned. The images produced by the machine are processed through a special computer and software to view it in different planes and projections.

## Uses of CTA

Computed tomographic angiography is used to study the blood vessels and organs of the body such as:
- Brain
- Neck
- Lungs
- Heart
- Abdomen
- Legs (Fig. 14).

It helps diagnose and evaluate blood vessel diseases such as:
- Injury
- Aneurysms (Fig. 15)
- Blockages (including those from clots or plaques)
- Blood supply to tumors and abnormal blood vessels
- Congenital anomalies of the heart and blood vessels

Computed tomographic angiography is ordered in the following conditions:
- Identify aneurysms in aorta and other arteries
- Detect atherosclerotic disease in carotid that can cause transient ischemic attacks (TIAs) and cerebrovascular accidents (CVA)

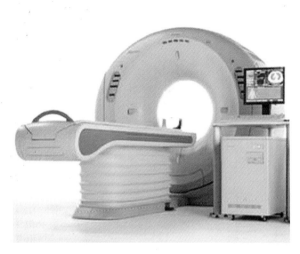

**Fig. 13** Computed tomography scan machine

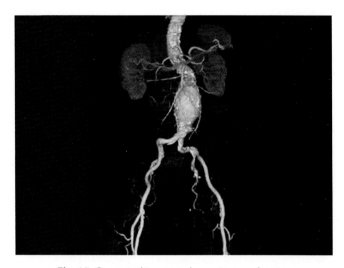

**Fig. 15** Computed tomography angiogram showing abdominal aortic aneurysm

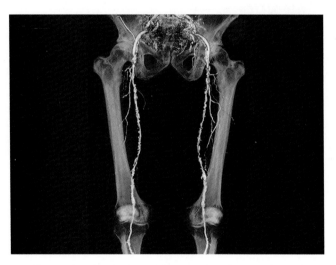

**Fig. 14** Computed tomography angiogram showing diseased superficial femoral artery bilaterally

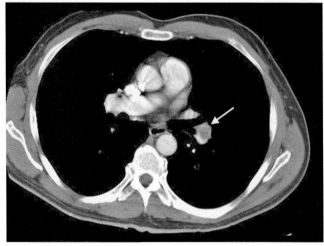

**Fig. 16** Computed tomography angiogram showing clot in pulmonary artery

- Identify aneurysms or arteriovenous (AV) malformations in the brain
- Detect stenoses or occlusions in leg arteries and plan endovascular or surgical intervention
- Detect renal artery disease and prepare for kidney transplant
- Detect injury to arteries in trauma patients
- Evaluate arteries feeding tumors prior to surgery of chemo-embolization or selection internal radiation therapy
- Identify dissection in aorta or other vessels
- Show extent of atherosclerosis in coronary arteries and plan bypass or stenting
- Sample blood from specific veins to detect endocrine disease

- Detect clots in pulmonary artery in pulmonary embolism (PE) (Fig. 16).
- *Look for congenital abnormalities in blood vessels:* In preparation for the test:
  - The patient must be nil orally for 6 hours prior to the test if contrast is to be used.
  - The history of any allergies must be known.
  - If breastfeeding, pump out the milk prior to the test and keep it for use after the contrast is cleared from the body that takes 24 hours.

Breath-hold spiral CT angiography is being increasingly used to diagnose PAD. This has a sensitivity of 93% and a specificity of 96% and an overall accuracy of 96% compared with digital subtraction angiography (DSA).

## Limitations of CTA

- Allergic to iodine
- Advanced kidney disease of severe diabetes—contrast may be harmful
- Very obese people.

## Risks

- Slight chance of cancer due to exposure to radiation. The benefit of an accurate diagnosis outweighs the risk.
- If there is a history of allergic reaction, then steroids may be given few hours prior to test or a day before. Another option is doing MRA instead of CTA.
- Leakage of contrast below the skin may lead to damage of the skin, blood vessel, and nerve.

## Benefits versus Risks

- CTA may eliminate the need for surgery or it may be performed more accurately.
- Stenosis or occlusion of blood vessels is visualized and corrective therapy performed.
- CTA may give accurate details about small vessels than MRA.
- CTA is less cumbersome, faster, and less invasive than conventional angiography.
- By CTA, arterial and venous phases can be seen, which is not possible on conventional angiography.
- CTA has a lower cost than conventional angiography.

## ■ MAGNETIC RESONANCE ANGIOGRAPHY

Magnetic resonance angiography (MRA) is a medical test helping physicians to diagnose and treat medical conditions related to blood vessels (Fig. 17). In MRA, a powerful magnetic field, radiowaves, and a computer produces detailed images. MRA does not use ionizing radiations (X-rays) (Fig. 18).

## Common Uses

It examines blood vessels in various parts of the body such as:
- Brain
- Neck
- Heart
- Lungs
- Abdomen
- Pelvis
- Legs.

Physicians use the procedure to:
- Identify aneurysms in chest and abdomen
- Detect carotid artery disease that may cause TIA or stroke
- Identify small aneurysms and AV malformations in brain
- Detect peripheral disease causing narrowing or occlusion and help prepare for endovascular or surgical intervention

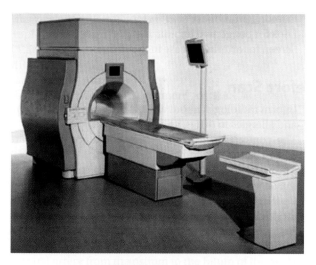

**Fig. 17** MRI machine

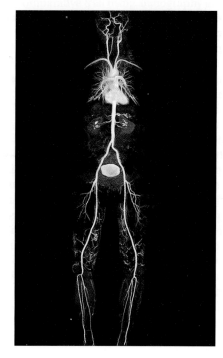

**Fig. 18** Magnetic resonance angiography showing the arterial tree in the human body

- Detect renal artery disease and visualize blood flow to prepare for kidney transplant
- Detect arterial injury in various parts of the body
- Evaluate arteries feeding tumor prior to surgery or embolization or selective internal radiation therapy
- Identify aortic dissection in chest or abdomen
- Show extent of coronary artery disease and plan stenting or coronary artery bypass graft (CABG)
- Sample blood from specific veins to detect endocrine disease

## PRACTICAL POINTS

- ABI is the first step to perform in suspected PAD.
- Segmental limb pressures and PVR provide information about the location of the disease.
- Exercise tests helps exclude disease in patients with lower limb discomfort and pseudoclaudication.
- RAS is detected by duplex ultrasound. An RAR more than 3.5 corresponds to 60–99% stenosis.
- Duplex ultrasound is useful to screen and follow-up AAA.
- CT is superior to ultrasound in visualizing aortic wall integrity—dissection, calcification, venous abnormalities, retroperitoneal blood, anatomic extent of aneurysmal disease, and in the diagnosis and follow-up of endoleaks.

## Limitations of CTA

- Allergic to iodine
- Advanced kidney disease of severe diabetes—contrast may be harmful
- Very obese people.

## Risks

- Slight chance of cancer due to exposure to radiation. The benefit of an accurate diagnosis outweighs the risk.
- If there is a history of allergic reaction, then steroids may be given few hours prior to test or a day before. Another option is doing MRA instead of CTA.
- Leakage of contrast below the skin may lead to damage of the skin, blood vessel, and nerve.

## Benefits versus Risks

- CTA may eliminate the need for surgery or it may be performed more accurately.
- Stenosis or occlusion of blood vessels is visualized and corrective therapy performed.
- CTA may give accurate details about small vessels than MRA.
- CTA is less cumbersome, faster, and less invasive than conventional angiography.
- By CTA, arterial and venous phases can be seen, which is not possible on conventional angiography.
- CTA has a lower cost than conventional angiography.

## ■ MAGNETIC RESONANCE ANGIOGRAPHY

Magnetic resonance angiography (MRA) is a medical test helping physicians to diagnose and treat medical conditions related to blood vessels (Fig. 17). In MRA, a powerful magnetic field, radiowaves, and a computer produces detailed images. MRA does not use ionizing radiations (X-rays) (Fig. 18).

## Common Uses

It examines blood vessels in various parts of the body such as:
- Brain
- Neck
- Heart
- Lungs
- Abdomen
- Pelvis
- Legs.

Physicians use the procedure to:
- Identify aneurysms in chest and abdomen
- Detect carotid artery disease that may cause TIA or stroke
- Identify small aneurysms and AV malformations in brain
- Detect peripheral disease causing narrowing or occlusion and help prepare for endovascular or surgical intervention

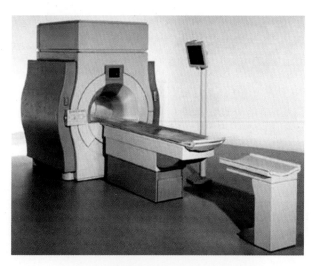

**Fig. 17** MRI machine

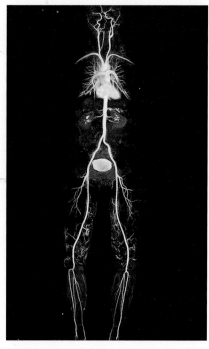

**Fig. 18** Magnetic resonance angiography showing the arterial tree in the human body

- Detect renal artery disease and visualize blood flow to prepare for kidney transplant
- Detect arterial injury in various parts of the body
- Evaluate arteries feeding tumor prior to surgery or embolization or selective internal radiation therapy
- Identify aortic dissection in chest or abdomen
- Show extent of coronary artery disease and plan stenting or coronary artery bypass graft (CABG)
- Sample blood from specific veins to detect endocrine disease

- Examine pulmonary arteries for PE
- Look for congenital anomalies
- Screen for arterial disease in families.

## Before Scan

- Inform radiologist about allergic diseases such as asthma and allergies to drugs, iodine, food, and so on.
- The contrast used in MRA is gadolinium, which rarely causes allergic reaction.
- Must inform about previous surgeries, as metal staples may have been used.
- Radiologist must be informed about pregnancy, as the fetus will be in a powerful magnetic field.
- Breastfeeding mothers must pump out the milk and keep it to be given to the baby. It takes 24 hours for the dye to clear.
- It is safe to perform MRA in patients with metal implants except:
  - Internal implanted defibrillator or pacemaker
  - Cochlear (ear) implant
  - Clips on brain aneurysms
  - Metal coils placed in blood vessels.

Although not a contraindication to MRA, the radiologist must be informed about:

- Artificial heart valves
- Implanted drug infusion ports
- Metallic joint prosthesis
- Implanted nerve stimulators
- Metal pins, screws, plates, stents, or surgical staples.

Metal objects implanted in orthopedic surgery pose no problems in MRA unless recently implanted. A plane X-ray is indicated prior to MRA if a metal object is implanted. Trauma with bullets or shrapnel injury must be informed. Tooth fillings and braces rarely are a problem, but the radiologist must be aware, as they could interfere with images.

The magnetic field is created by passing electric current through wire coils.

The differentiation between normal and diseased tissue is better with MRI than with CT, X-ray, or ultrasound.

The blood vessels with contrast appear as white.

## Benefits versus Risks

- Catheter-based DSA is the gold standard for evaluating vascular disease. MRA is fast becoming the noninvasive investigation of choice to replace DSA. MRA is especially adapted to visualization of the lumen and the wall of the artery in question.
- Clinical use—it is used to study arteries in the head, neck, thorax, abdomen, and extremities. It has been less successful in studying coronary arteries then conventional angiography and CT angiography. Mostly, underlying disease is atherosclerosis, but aneurysms and AV malformations can also be diagnosed by MRA.

- The advantage over conventional angiography is that it is noninvasive.

Compared with both CT angiography and conventional angiography:
  - Less ionization radiations are given to the patient
  - The contrast used for MRA is less toxic because less quantity is used compared with the other two modalities.
- The disadvantages are:
  - The higher cost
  - Limited spatial resolution
  - Longer time taken
  - Patients with pacemaker, metal clips from previous surgery, or metal in the eyes.

## ■ NONINVASIVE EVALUATION OF EXTRA-CRANIAL CAROTID ARTERY DISEASE

Significant internal carotid artery stenosis increases the risk of TIAs and strokes as well of myocardial infarction (MI) and cardiovascular death. Thus, it is important to diagnose this condition noninvasively.

## Duplex Ultrasonography

It provides excellent accuracy and reproducibility and is the investigation of choice. It identifies accurately plaques, stenosis and occlusions of the internal, common, and external carotid arteries. It also identifies flow direction in the vertebral arteries. The indications for this test are:

- TIAs
- CVA
- Cervical bruit
- After surgical or endovascular revascularization
- Patients who are at a high risk for carotid stenosis.

The carotid vessels are located in two planes—longitudinal and transverse noting plaques and alterations in flow. Doppler waveform and velocity are noted in common (CCA), internal (ICA), and external (ECA) carotid arteries (Fig. 19). These velocities are noted using a constant Doppler angle of 60°. This helps to determine the degree of stenosis (Fig. 20). The sensitivity is 85% and the specificity is 90%. It is 93% accurate in locating carotid occlusion. The limitations of this test are:

- Overestimation of ICA stenosis due to severe contralateral ICA disease
- Underestimation of ICA stenosis due to tight ipsilateral CCA stenosis
- Identifying ECA as the ICA
- Mistaking severe stenosis as occlusion.

## Magnetic Resonance Angiography

The MRA along with MRI of the brain provides excellent information on:

- Extracranial carotid circulation
- Symptomatic disease unexplained by duplex ultrasound
- Patients with suspected intracranial disease.

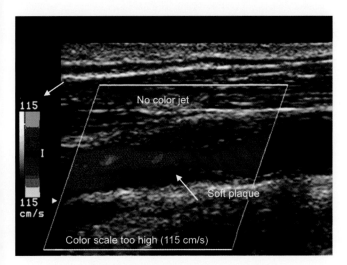

**Fig. 19** Color Doppler showing carotid artery stenosis

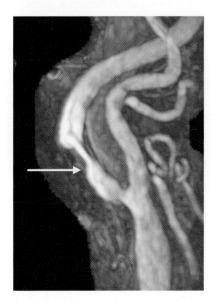

**Fig. 20** Tight stenosis of internal carotid artery on magnetic resonance angiography

## ■ NONINVASIVE EVALUATION OF RENAL ARTERY STENOSIS

Atherosclerotic renal artery stenosis (RAS) can be the cause of:
- Resistant hypertension
- Deterioration of renal function
- Recurrent "flash pulmonary edema"
- Long-term ill effects of poorly controlled hypertension
- If bilateral RAS or stenosis in a solitary kidney—develop end-stage renal disease
- Long-term survival in such patients is very poor.

The diagnosis of RAS is made on:
- Duplex ultrasound
- CT angiogram
- MRA
- Radionuclide scans.

The investigation and treatment of RAS is given in Flow chart 1.

## Renal Artery Duplex Ultrasonography

This is an excellent test but only in experienced hands. The principle it is based on is comparing the peak systolic velocities within the renal arteries and the aorta called the renal:aortic ratio (RAR). The ultrasound findings are compared with angiography or MRA. The peak systolic velocity in the aorta is measured at the level of the superior mesenteric artery. The entire renal artery from the ostium to the hilum of the kidney is visualized. RAR over 3.5 means a RAS 60–99% (Fig. 21).

In a large comparative trial using angiography and duplex ultrasound, the sensitivity was 98%, the specificity 99%, and the positive predictive value 99% while negative predictive value 97%. It is useful for:
- RAS
- Renal artery occlusion
- Patency of renal artery stents
- Early and late restenosis of renal artery stents
- Detect the degree of stenosis prior to stenting.

Patients have both renal artery and renal parenchymal disease. The addition of restrictive indices within the parenchyma may help us determine which patients will benefit from revascularization.

The limitations of this technique are:
- Bowel gas preventing proper identification of renal arteries.

## Magnetic Resonance Angiography

This is extremely useful test in the workup of secondary hypertension due to RAS. Gadolinium-enhanced MRA provides three-dimensional (3D) images with multiplane images of renal arteries (Fig. 22).

## ■ EVALUATION OF AORTIC ANEURYSMAL DISEASE

The diagnosis of aneurysmal disease depends upon:
- Palpating a pulsatile abdominal mass
- Family history of aortic aneurysms in first-degree relatives
- Incidentally found on abdominal imaging performed for other unrelated causes.

Management is based on:
- The transverse diameter of the aneurysm
- Site of the aneurysm—suprarenal or infrarenal
- General health of the patient.

**Flow chart 1** Algorithm for detection of renal artery stenosis

Clinical history and physical examination suggestive of RAS (Refer to Table 1) → No → Screening for RAS not recommended

↓ Yes

Screening test (Duplex ultrasound, spiral CT, MRA)

No significant RAS

No further tests indicated

↓

Significant RAS (>50%) detected on screening test

Well controlled BP, no renal impairment

Renal size <7 cm, no evidence of renal function in affected kidney

Indications for revascularization present (Refer to Table 2)

↓

Medical therapy, seconday atherosclerosis prevention measures

Revascularization not indicated

Perform hemodynamic assessment

Gradient across >20 mm Hg, and/or RI <80, EDV >90 mm Hg

Gradient across stenosis <20 mm Hg and/or RI >80, EDV <90 mm Hg

↓

Proceed with revcascularization

Revascularization unlikely to improve outcomes so not indicated

*Abbreviations:* RAS, renal artery stenosis; CT, computed tomography; MRA, magnetic resonance angiography; RI, renal artery resistance index; EDV, end diastolic velocity.

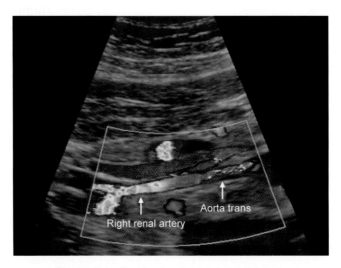

**Fig. 21** Color Doppler showing renal artery stenosis

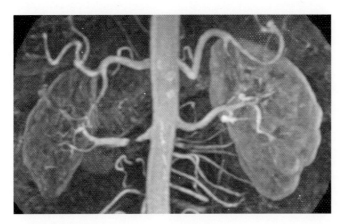

**Fig. 22** Magnetic resonance angiography showing tight right renal artery stenosis

Investigative techniques are:
- Ultrasound study
- CT angiogram
- MRA.

CT angiogram and MRA are preferred because they provide anatomical and spatial details needed for endovascular management and the postoperative follow-up of these patients.

## Computed Tomographic Angiography

It is of value in determining:
- Growth rate of the aneurysm
- Timing of the surgery
- Precise extent of the aneurysm
- Aneurysmal wall integrity
- Location and amount of calcification within the wall
- Venous anomalies
- Retroperitoneal blood
- Aortic dissection
- Infection of inflammation of the wall
- Proximal and distal extent of the aneurysm
- Shows other intra-abdominal pathology
- Diagnosing and follow-up of endovascular leaks.

Limitations of CT angiography are:
- Need for nephrotoxic iodinated contrast
- Increased radiation exposure
- Increased cost.

It is performed by:
- Rapid intravenous bolus injection
- Timed breath held spiral CT acquisition during peak arterial opacification
- 3D reformatting using maximal intensity projections (MIPs)
- Curved planar reformation
- Shaded surface displays.

## Magnetic Resonance Imaging

The advantages are:
- No iodinated contrast—risk of nephrotoxicity
- No catheter-based arteriography—risk of atheroembolism.

It provides information regarding the extent of the aneurysm and the involvement and relationship with the great vessels. It is quick taking less than 30 s for 3D contrast. It is also of value in follow-up of endovascular stents provided the stents are made of Nitinol that can be visualized.

## Duplex Ultrasonography

This is the most common test conducted primarily and provides reliable information regarding the size of the AAA and its periodic surveillance of expansion. A low-frequency (3.5 MHz) transducer is used. After an overnight fast, the test is done in supine reverse Trendelenburg position and aorta seen in the sagittal plane throughout its length and then in the coronal plane to record the transverse measurements in suprarenal, juxtarenal, and infrarenal positions. The normal infrarenal aortic diameter varies with age and sex being about 2 cm. The average growth rate is 0.21 cm per year. The chances of rupture are 0% per year if less than 4 cm diameter, 1% per year if 4–5 cm, and 11% per year if 5–6 cm. This screening has reduced the rupture rate by 49%. Recently, it is being used for detection of endoleaks (Fig. 23).

Limitations are:
- Obesity
- Bowel gas.

## ◼ CONCLUSION

- Vascular laboratory provides an accurate and noninvasive technique for arterial disorders.
- History and examination provide information to the type of test needed.
- Duplex ultrasound is the mainstay of noninvasive vascular imaging.
- MR and CT are very useful in evaluating AAA and cerebrovascular disease.

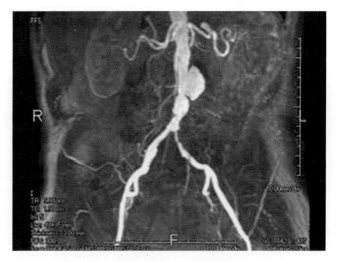

**Fig. 23** Magnetic resonance angiogram showing abdominal aortic aneurysm

## PRACTICAL POINTS

- ABI is the first step to perform in suspected PAD.
- Segmental limb pressures and PVR provide information about the location of the disease.
- Exercise tests helps exclude disease in patients with lower limb discomfort and pseudoclaudication.
- RAS is detected by duplex ultrasound. An RAR more than 3.5 corresponds to 60–99% stenosis.
- Duplex ultrasound is useful to screen and follow-up AAA.
- CT is superior to ultrasound in visualizing aortic wall integrity—dissection, calcification, venous abnormalities, retroperitoneal blood, anatomic extent of aneurysmal disease, and in the diagnosis and follow-up of endoleaks.

# 3

# Diagnostic Catheter-based Vascular Angiography

*Jaisom Chopra*

## ■ INTRODUCTION

- Direct visualization of blood vessels by placing a catheter into the artery or vein percutaneously and giving iodinated contrast.
- It is the gold standard to determine the severity and extent of peripheral artery disease (PAD) (Fig. 1).
- Digital subtraction angiography (DSA) allows high quality images using small amounts of contrast (Fig. 2).
- Angiography is invasive and indicated in patients considered for revascularization.

## ■ ANATOMIC CONSIDERATIONS

### Access for Vascular Angiography

- This site should be as close to the suspected lesion as possible (Figs 3A and B).

- Iliac and common femoral artery occlusions are approached from the contralateral femoral artery.
- In cases there are no pulses palpable in either groin, then the upper limb approach is indicated.
- For lesions above the groin, a retrograde femoral artery approach is done.

### Retrograde Common Femoral Artery Access

This is the most common site accessed. The pulse, if present, is palpated below the inguinal ligament.

The common femoral artery lies midway between the pubis and the anterior superior iliac spine. In peripheral arterial disease, the site and level of arterial puncture is located under fluoroscopy. If no pulses are palpable, then ultrasound is used to locate the artery and puncture it (Fig. 4).

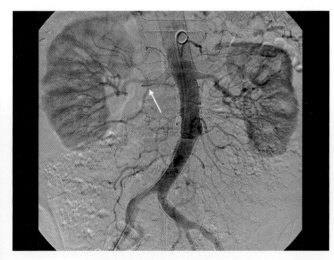

**Fig. 1** Conventional angiogram

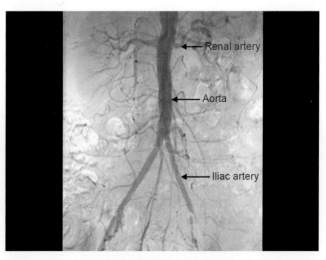

**Fig. 2** Digital subtraction angiography

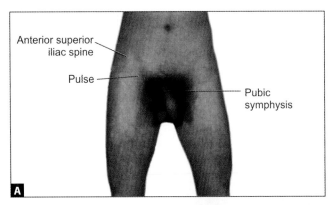

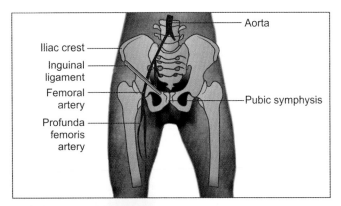

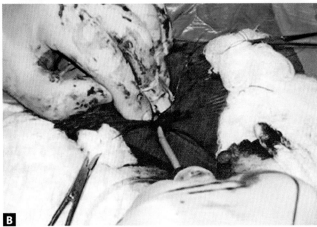

**Figs 3A and B** (A) Location of femoral vessels in groin; (B) Femoral puncture and sheath introduced

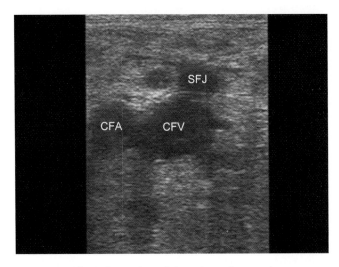

**Fig. 4** Femoral vessels in groin on ultrasound

*Abbreviations:* CFA, common femoral artery; CFV, common femoral vein; SFJ, saphenofemoral junction.

Color Doppler should be used to puncture the concerned artery. The advantages are:
• Puncture under direct vision
• Clean puncture in the middle of the artery anteriorly
• Can visualize plaque within the artery and avoid dissection
• Can detect intimal injury if it accidently occurs.

## Brachial/Radial Artery Access

### Indications
• This is considered in cases with bilateral iliac artery occlusion or aortic occlusion and no palpable pulses in the groins.
• It is also considered in superior mesenteric, renal, or celiac arteries in which the acute angle calls for brachial approach.
• The left brachial approach minimizes the risk of stroke that may be present from the right brachial side due to embolization.

### Risks Involved
• The risks of injury and thrombosis are much higher from the brachial route than from the femoral route.
• Thrombosis is reduced by injecting 5000 U heparin into the sheath.
• If radial artery is punctured, 0–100 mL of intra-arterial nitroglycerin is used to reduce spasm. This is in addition to heparin.

# Popliteal Artery Access

This is rarely done for angiography but for interventions. The patient lies prone and the superficial femoral artery (SFA) must be occluded. It is only to visualize below knee vessels (Fig. 5).

## ■ FUNDAMENTALS

- Angiography is the direct contrast containing iodine into the bloodstream.
- All contrasts in use depend on the iodine content and the osmolality (concentration).
- Iodine produces radiographic contrast by blocking X-rays.

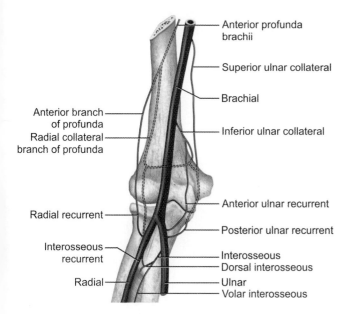

**Fig. 5** Brachial artery anatomy related to bony structures

- Thus, visualization is improved by increasing the dose of iodine, while higher the dose, the more chances of renal toxicity. So, a fine balance has to be struck.
- Also, the osmolality should be close to the body fluid. High osmolality will cause cells to shrink by drawing water out of theme whereas low osmolality will cause edema of the cells by drawing water into them.
- The goal is to use lowest dose and volume of the contrast for adequate clinical angiography.

*The low osmolality agents are better but more expensive. They should be used in:*

- Previous contrast reactions
- Bronchial asthma
- Congestive heart failure
- Active significant arrhythmias
- Aortic stenosis
- Pulmonary hypertension
- Significant renal failure (creatinine > 2 mg%).

The recommended iso-osmolal agent is iodixanol (Visipaque; Amersham, Princeton, New Jersey, USA).

In known renal dysfunction or patients with known allergic reactions, gadolinium is used with DSA.

## ■ CLINICAL ASPECTS OF ANGIOGRAPHY

For safe injection of contrast, it is important to know:

- Appropriate catheters
- Angulations
- Injection rates (Table 1).

## Lower Extremity Angiography

- This is still considered the gold standard (Fig. 6).
- An abdominal/pelvic aortogram is performed using a straight pigtail catheter placed at L1–L2 level above the aortic bifurcation, which is generally at L3 (Fig. 7).

**Table 1** Angiograms of different body sites—the recommended catheters, angulations and injections

| Artery | Catheter | Angulation | Injection |
|---|---|---|---|
| Arch aortogram | 5 FR angulated pigtail at aortic root | 30° LAO | 10 mL/s for 3 s |
| Abdominal aortogram for mesenteric ischemia | 5 FR straight pigtail between T12 and L1 | Biplane or lateral | 20 mL/s for 2 s |
| Abdominal aortogram for renal artery stenosis | 5 FR straight pigtail between T12 and L1 | AP | 20 mL/s for 0.5 s using DSA |
| Pelvic/abdominal aortogram | 5 FR straight pigtail between L1 and L2 | AP | 15 mL/s for 1 s using DSA |
| Distal aorta for bolus chase and run-off | 5 FR straight pigtail between L2 and L3 | AP | 8 mL/s for 10 s using DSA |
| Carotids and great vessels | JR4 catheter level 1 arch. Vitek catheter for level 2 arch | Ipsilateral oblique 30° and lateral | Hand injection with DSA |
| Renal arteries | JR4 catheter | AP and ipsilateral oblique at 20°–30° | Hand injection with DSA |
| Celiac trunk | JR4, SOS, Cobra catheters | AP | Injection at 10 mL/s |
| Superior mesenteric artery | JR4, SOS, Cobra catheters | AP | Injection at 8 mL/s |
| Inferior mesenteric artery | JR4, SOS, Cobra catheters | AP | Injection at 3 mL/s |
| Pulmonary artery | Groliman catheter | LAO/RAO 30° | 20 mL/s for 2 s |

*Abbreviations:* AP, anteroposterior; DSA, digital subtraction angiography; LAO, left anterior oblique; RAO, right anterior oblique.

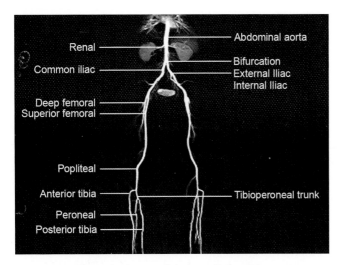

**Fig. 6** Angiogram of the lower limb arteries

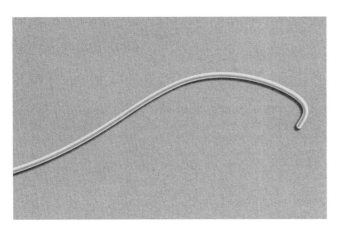

**Fig. 7** Judkins Right 4 catheter to cannulate renal, mesenteric and great vessels

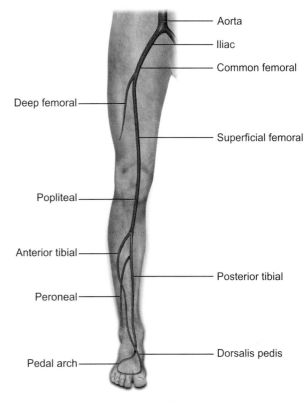

**Fig. 8** Arteries of lower limb

- This gives very good images of distal aorta, iliacs, and common femorals (Fig. 8).
- Angulated views are needed to see the iliac and femoral bifurcations without overlap.
- A pelvic DSA is performed with 10–15 mL iso-osmolal contrast at a rate of 15 cc/s.
- Now, the catheter is withdrawn to the aortic bifurcation so that the contrast fills the run-off vessels that are well visualized.
- The bolus chase is used to see the lower limb vessels.

## Upper Extremity Angiography

- It is less frequently performed because less than 5% limb ischemia affects the upper limbs (Fig. 9).
- It is performed for thoracic outlet syndrome and embolic occlusion.

- It is generally performed by retrograde femoral route using a JR4 catheter and the vasculature from the subclavian to the digital arteries is seen.
- The hand vessels are seen with the catheter in the brachial artery when DSA is performed.

It is vital to know the upper limb arterial anomalies such as incomplete palmar arch (Table 2).

## Renal Angiography

It is performed in:
- Refractory hypertension.
- Renal insufficiency.
- Renal donors.
- To assess vascularity in renal tumors.
- The catheter tip is placed between L1 and L2 vertebra.
- The renal arteries arise caudal to the superior mesenteric artery (SMA) and in a small percentage may be multiple to each kidney and may arise as low as the iliacs.
- Selective cannulation of the renal arteries is carried out by Judkins right catheter (JR4) (Fig. 10).
- Arteries with an angulated or an unusual origin may be cannulated with SOS catheters.
- These angiograms are performed with a hand-injected 3–4 mL contrast using DSA.
- The renal artery ostium is visualized with a 30° oblique view.

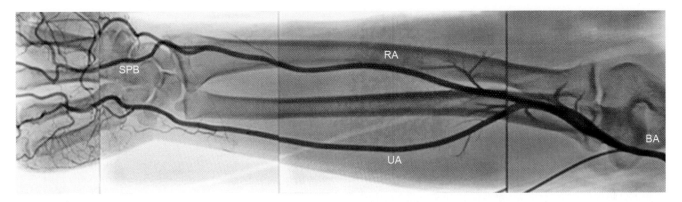

**Fig. 9** Anatomy of upper limb arteries

**Table 2** Percentages of arterial variants

| Common arterial variants | Incidence (%) |
|---|---|
| *Brachial artery* | |
| • Persistent superficial brachial artery | 1–2% |
| • Radial artery origin from proximal brachial artery | 12% |
| • Ulnar artery origin from proximal brachial artery | 1–2% |
| *Forearm arteries* | |
| • High origin of radial artery from brachial  or axillary artery | 14–17% |
| • Persistent median artery | 2–4% |
| • Persistent interosseus artery | <0.1% |
| *Palmar arch* | |
| • Incomplete deep palmar arch of hand | 3–5% |
| • Incomplete superficial palmar arch | 22% |

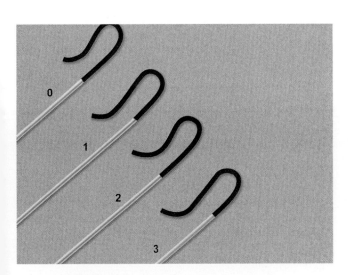

**Fig. 10** SOS catheter for renal and mesenteric

- If significant renal artery stenosis is seen, then the pressure gradient is measured prior to revascularization.
- If the gradient is more than 20 mm Hg, then it suggests significant stenosis (Fig. 11).

## Mesenteric Angiography

The indications are:
- Chronic mesenteric ischemia
- Acute mesenteric ischemia
- Uncontrolled gastrointestinal bleeding
- Origin of the mesenteric vessel—lateral view
- Selective cannulation of the celiac trunk, SMA, and inferior mesenteric artery (IMA) is done using JR4 catheter (Fig. 12).
- The typical flow rates through the celiac trunk are 10 mL/s; SMA is 8 mL/s and IMA is 3 mL/s. The rate of injecting contrast must match these flow rates for good images.
- DSA is less helpful because of the bowel gas. If performed for bleeding, then the clinically suspected vessel is first cannulated and injected (Fig. 13).
- One must be aware of the common anomalies. These are as high as 40% in the celiac trunk. Normally, the hepatic artery arises from the celiac trunk, but it may arise from the aorta, left gastric, or superior mesenteric.
- Aberrant hepatic artery is when it arises from a site other than the normal. There is no normal hepatic artery.
- Accessory hepatic artery is when a hepatic artery arises from an abnormal site apart from the normal hepatic artery.

## Cerebral Angiography

- An arch angiogram is performed prior to cannulation of the great vessels.
- There are multiple anomalies at this site and even a small plaque dislodged may have devastating consequences.
- Therefore, a low-profile performed catheter is used.
- Multiple injections with minimal contrast are used to visualize carotids and cerebral vessels.

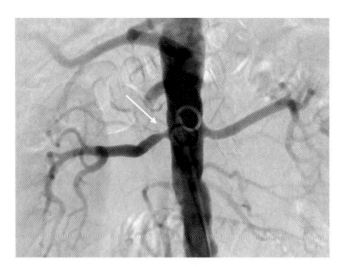

**Fig. 11** Renal angiography showing right renal artery stenosis

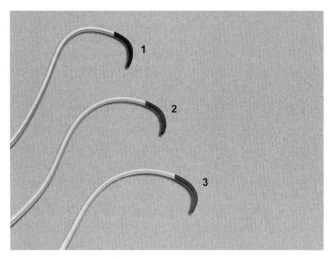

**Fig. 12** Cobra catheter for mesenteric cannulation

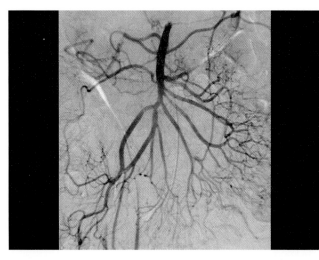

**Fig. 13** Superior mesenteric artery angiogram

- The patients must receive aspirin preoperatively and bolus of 3000–4000 U heparin is given to reduce the risk of embolization.
- The angiogram is performed at 30°–45° LAO to see the origin of the great vessels and the tortuosity of the arch (Fig. 14).
- Typical arch or level 1 arch is seen in 70%.
- Level 2—Common origin of the brachoicephalic trunk and the common carotid—15%.
- Level 3—Origin of left common carotid from the brachoicephalic—10%.

With increasing age:
- Hypertension
- Atherosclerotic changes occur in aorta
- Arch sinks deeper into the thoracic cavity and draws the origin of the great vessels along with it. Using the origin of the left subclavian artery as landmark, the arch curvature is classified into three levels. This is defined by an aortogram that helps the operator to choose the appropriate diagnostic catheter (Figs 15A and B).

This prevents scraping the arch with an inappropriate catheter and so reduces the chances of stroke and other complications. In a level 3 aortic arch, a Vitek or Headhunter catheter is used, whereas in level 2 arch, a Simmons 1 or 2 catheter is used (Figs 16 to 18).

Angiogram is performed at ipsilateral 30° oblique and a lateral view. The vertebral arteries are best visualized in an anteroposterior (AP) view, although angulated views are needed for the ostium.

- The intracranial circulation is best viewed in AP cranial and lateral projections.

## Pulmonary Angiography

Pulmonary angiography is performed in acute or chronic pulmonary embolism (PE). A radionucleide perfusion/ventilation scan is performed prior to this if possible. Venous access is via the femoral vein using 8F sheath. A Grollman catheter is used, which has a wide bore with multiple side holes, excellent torque control, and sidearm curve that helps to be directed through the tricuspid valve (Fig. 19).

The catheter tip is placed in the pulmonary trunk identified by V/Q scan and 40 mL contrast injected at 20 mL/c two views—left anterior oblique (LAO)/right anterior oblique (RAO) 30° of each lung is obtained. Biplane angiography is used. Selective angiography may be used to rule out PE (Fig. 20).

## ■ LIMITATIONS/RISKS

The complications (1%) associated with angiography are:
- Vascular injury
  - Complicatios with femoral access is 1.7% while with brachial access is 7%.
- Contrast reactions
  - The severity of anaphylactic reaction ranges from nausea, vomiting, and rash to laryngeal edema,

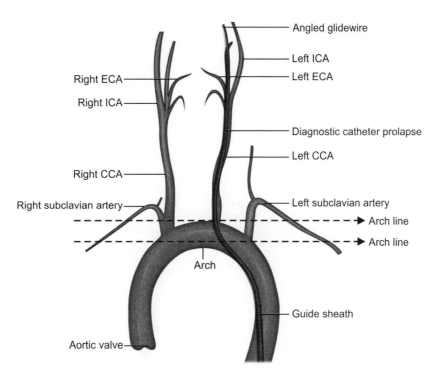

**Fig. 14** The great vessels arise above the horizontal line at the origin of the left subclavian artery

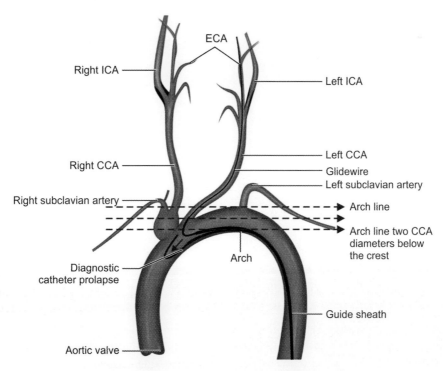

**Fig. 15A** Great vessels arise well below the arch line

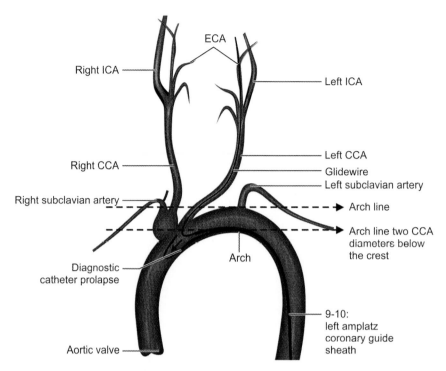

**Fig. 15B** The great vessels arise below the arch line

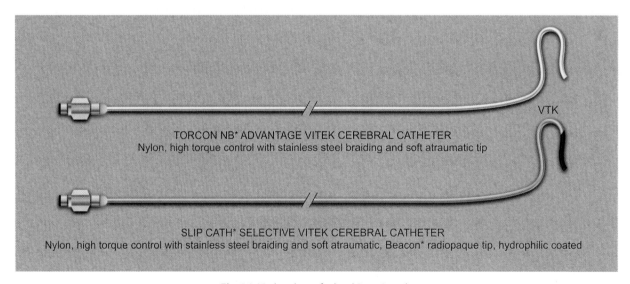

**Fig. 16** Vitek catheter for level 2 aortic arch

cardiovascular collapse, and death. The risk of death in severe anaphylactic reaction is genuine and ranges from 1 in 12,000 to 1 in 75,000.

- Renal failure
  - The incidence of renal failure ranges from 05% to 35%.
  - Thus, if there is renal compromise prior to angiography, such patients should have adequate intravenous (IV) hydration prior to angiography and may get N-acetylcysteine 600 mg orally for two doses a day prior to angiography. Then, 600 mg orally immediately before the procedure and 600 mg 6 hours after the contrast injection.
  - Alternatively, fenoldopam 0.1 µg/kg/min is started 2 hours prior to injection of contrast and continued 4 hours after the procedure.
- Stroke (< 0.07%).
- Rarely death (< 0.1%).

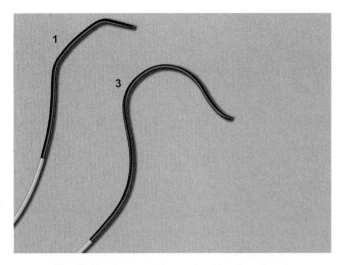

**Fig. 17** Headhunter catheter—level 1 or 2 aortic arch

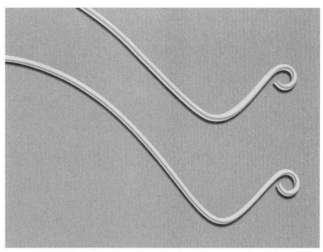

**Fig. 19** Grollman catheter for pulmonary angiography

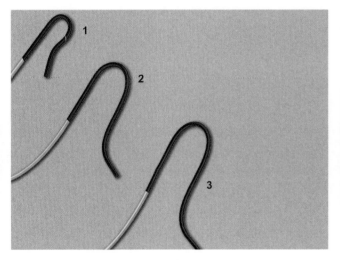

**Fig. 18** Simmons catheter—level 3 arch

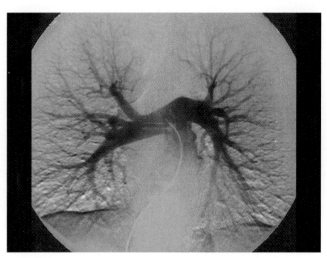

**Fig. 20** Pulmonary angiography

## ■ SPECIAL ISSUES/CONSIDERATION

The absolute contrainidication to angiography is:
- Inadequate equipment
- Untrained operator.

Relative contraindications are:
- Severe hypertension
- Uncorrectable coagulopathy
- Clinically significant iodinated contrast material sensitivity
- Severe renal insufficiency
- Congestive heart failure
- Severe anemia.

## ■ CONCLUSION

Contrast angiography is the gold standard in defining the extent and severity of vascular disease.
- It is performed in people considered for revascularization and should be preceded through history and physical examination to identify potential contraindications to surgery.
- Choosing appropriate catheters at the start of the procedure reduces the risk of complications.
- A pressure gradient o more than 20 mm Hg across a stenosis is a reliable indicator of a hemodynamically significant lesion.

## PRACTICAL POINTS

Iodixanol (Visipaque) is better tolerated than high osmolal contrast agents and has fewer contrast reactions.

- Adequate hydration to all patients with renal compromise prior to angiography.
- Lateral angiography should be performed to see the origin of mesenteric arteries prior to selective catheterization.
- Arch aortograms should be done prior to attempts at selective catheterization of great vessels.
- Selective pulmonary angiograms based on results of V/Q scans or computed tomographic (CT) scans are better than non-selective main pulmonary artery angiogram in diagnosing PE.
- Choice of appropriate arterial access site is crucial to performing safe and success angiography.

# 4

# Magnetic Resonance Angiography in the Diagnosis of Vascular Disease

*Jaisom Chopra*

## ■ INTRODUCTION

- Catheter-based digital subtraction angiography (DSA) is still the gold standard for evaluating vascular disease.
- Magnetic resonance angiography (MRA) is fast becoming the noninvasive procedure of choice for certain vascular beds. It gives us information about the anatomy of the vascular tree, the blood flow, and the vascular wall.

## ■ CLINICAL APPLICATIONS

### Cerebrovascular MRA (Fig. 1)

- It evaluates the cerebral circulation in a single sitting and gives additional parenchymal information making it the modality of choice.
- As the arteriovenous transit time is fast in the brain and because gadolinium contrast is not extracted by the brain capillaries, contrast imaging must be done very rapidly.

### Extracranial Vessels (Fig. 2)

Three-dimensional (3D) contrast MRA of carotids and thoracic aortic arch vessels is the investigation of choice to establish the presence and the absence of disease. Although DSA has a sensitivity and specificity of 95%, the reported advantages of MRA are:

- Ability to image plaque ulcerations
- No flow-related artifacts so that tortuous vessels are not degraded
- Short imaging times—coverage of aortic arch to circle of Willis takes on 30–40 s.

### *Techniques*

Three-dimensional gadolinium-enhanced MRA of the carotids is obtained in the coronal plane without breath

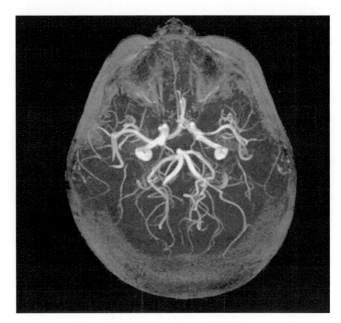

**Fig. 1** Cerebrovascular MRA

holding. This improves the sharpness of the image of the aortic great vessels and their origin. This runs the risk of moving out of the coronal plane with any movement of the neck. This also involves the digital subtraction wherein background images are deleted to improve the quality of the vessels especially in the area of stenosis.

### Intracranial Vessels (Fig. 3)

### *Techniques*

In acquired disease where there is narrowing—the sting sign—the lumen is very narrow and just short of total occlusion.

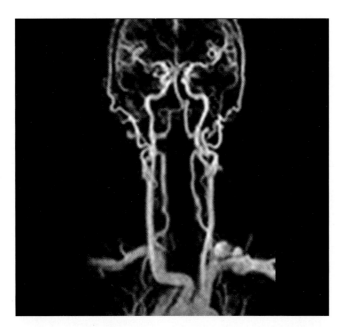

**Fig. 2** MRA extracranial vessels

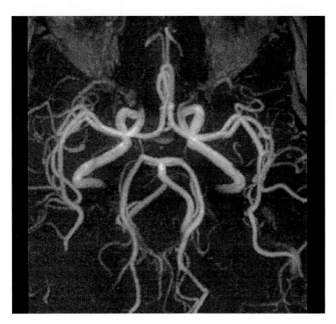

**Fig. 3** MRA intracranial vessels

The 3D sequence is sensitive to a wide range of flow velocities and shows better flow morphology. It is sensitive to any movement by the patient and so the patient has to remain still during this procedure which may pose a problem at times. That is why a fidgety head injury patient may take time because he cannot lie still.

## Indications

- MRA has sensitivity and specificity comparable to invasive angiography.
- Intracranially, it shows arterial stenosis and occlusion, aneurysms, arteriovenous malformations (AVMs), tumors, vascular compressions, and venous pathology.
- Extracranially, it shows carotid bifurcation disease, aortic arch branch vessel disease, stenosis and occlusion, atherosclerotic disease, and carotid and vertebral artery dissection.

## Thoracic MRA (Fig. 4)

Computed tomography (CT), angiography and MRA have replaced conventional angiography. The multiplanar reformations of magnetic resonance imaging (MRI) eliminate the problem of overlap seen in catheter angiography and provide a complete picture of the anatomy of the vessels and complex congenital disease in the chest. Phase-contrast MRA can measure flow and provide physiological information across stenosis and shunts.

## Indications

- Pathology of the great vessels in the chest—thoracic aorta and its branches, pulmonary artery and its branches, and large veins of the chest. Imaging of the coronary arteries and veins is possible but in experimental stages.
- Aortic disease—congenital and acquired disease of the thoracic aorta. In congenital disease—coarctation, right-sided aorta, vascular rings, and double arch. In acquired

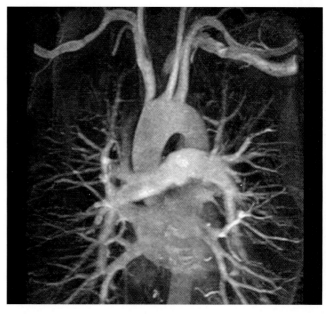

**Fig. 4** MRA thorax

disease—aneurysms, dissection, trauma, inflammatory disease (giant cell arteritis).

- Pulmonary disease—congenital and acquired disease. In congenital disease of the pulmonary artery, we see pulmonary atresia, pulmonary slings, and arteriovenous (AV) malformations. In acquired disease, we have pulmonary hypertension. There is high sensitivity and specificity to pulmonary embolism. Compression and invasion of the pulmonary vessels by tumor is seen well by MRA.
- Venous disease—magnetic resonance venography (MRV) of large veins of the chest has proved to be very useful to assess thoracic inlet syndrome, superior vena cava (SVC) syndrome, and thrombus in SVC and branches. Pulmonary vein anatomy is assessed before and after radiofrequency ablation therapy for refractory atrial fibrillation.

## Abdominal and Pelvic MRA (Fig. 5)

- Although CT angiography is still the preferred modality for abdominal aorta, but MRA has started to bypass it in various aspects of abdominal and pelvic vascular disease imaging.
- MRA images are rapid, efficient, offer high spatial and contrast resolution apart from avoiding high doses of IV contrast and ionizing radiations as seen in CTA.
- MRA also provides assessment of flow and functional stenosis severity. This is useful in renal arteries and mesenteric arteries and portal venous systems.
- Multiplanar reformations provide good images of complex anatomy.

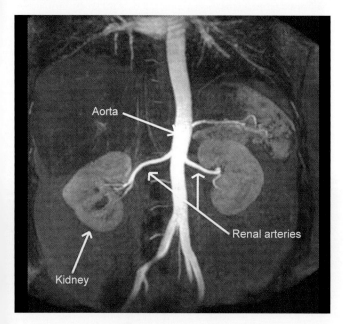

**Fig. 5** MRA abdomen

- It provides images of the lumen and wall of the vessels along with dynamic imaging of the flow through different abdominal viscera.
- Up to 50 high-quality images can be obtained in one breath that will cover the entire abdominal aorta from diaphragm to aortic bifurcation.

### Indications

- Evaluating renal artery stenosis, aneurysms, dissection, and fibromuscular disease. Not only the renal anatomy but also the function can be evaluated by MRA, which is not possible with catheter angiograms.
- Renal failure patients cannot tolerate high bolus of IV contrast, and so, MRA has a distinct advantage over catheter angiogram or CT angiogram.
- MRA is excellent for evaluating renal donor kidneys for vasculature and structure.
- MRA is excellent for evaluating renal allograft after transplantation to assess patency of anastomosis and function of allograft.
- Mesenteric MRA is used to define mesenteric ischemia, aneurysms, dissection, anatomic variations, collateral circulation, and encasement by tumor.
- MRA can evaluate the venous circulation—systemic and portal.
- Inferior vena cava (IVC) and branches are evaluated for occlusion by thrombus and tumor encasement.
- MRI evaluates liver parenchymal disease, as well as vascular supply in portal hypertension, portosystemic shunts, portal vein thrombosis, cavernous transformation, and tumor encasement.
- MRI helps assess hepatic veins in Budd-Chiari syndrome and liver tumor encasement.
- MRI is helpful in evaluating arterial and dual venous connections to the liver after liver transplant.
- MRV helps assess renal veins and extent of renal cell carcinoma.
- MRV is helpful in mesenteric vein thrombosis and acute thrombosis of ovarian veins.

## Peripheral Vascular MRA (Fig. 6)

- It helps screen at-risk persons and provides a roadmap for planning further therapy. It helps evaluate in-flow disease.
- A 3-D MRA can evaluate the pathology to the foot by a single-dose bolus-chase method. The foot vessels remain a challenge and are not well visualized.

### Indications

- MRA evaluates arteries of upper and lower limbs involved in atherosclerosis, aneurysms, inflammatory vasculitis, and embolic disease.

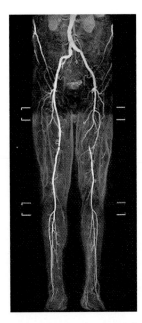

**Fig. 6** MRA peripheral vascular

- MRA helps investigate AV malformations and assess dialysis fistulas.
- MRV assesses deep vein thrombosis, vascular malformations, and post-thrombotic venous disease.

## ■ LIMITATIONS

### Susceptibility Artifacts

These are the T2 effects—dephasing due to the magnetic properties of the local environment. These include:
- Surgical clips, shrapnel, and stents
- High concentration of IV contrast
- Air-tissue interfaces such as lung vessels and bowel vessels.

They produce focal signal fall-outs—dark areas in images obscuring surrounding vessels and make them look like stenosis or occlusion. These artifacts can be minimized but not eliminated. Plane X-rays can detect location of metals.

### Motion Artifacts

In uncooperative patients or during breathing. This makes images blurred and reduces sensitivity to detect subtle findings. These are minimized by breath holding and shorter duration of examination. The involuntary motion like peristalsis and arterial pulsations cause ghosting and reduced by echocardiography (ECG) gating. Intraluminal turbulence causes spin dephasing leading to overestimation of stenosis.

## Coverage Artifacts

If parts of the vessels are not included, they appear as occluded vessels. This may happen in markedly tortuous aorta and other vessels. Vessels toward the edges of the field show drop off signals and blurring.

## Timing Artifacts

This is of prime importance. If performed too early, then the signal is weak and vessel may look diseased especially distal to a stenosis or occlusion. Delayed phase shows collateral and reformation distal to the occlusion. The delayed timing is based on the part of the body slowest to fill.

## Resolution Artifacts

This limits sensitivity to detect subtle lesions. It may give the appearance of stenosis or fail to detect intraluminal lesions partially obstructing flow.

## Non-contrast-Enhanced Artifacts

The blood flow within the plane of the image causes false occlusions and stenosis due to in-plane saturation effects. Blood turbulence in stenosis, aneurysms, and bifurcations gives a similar effect. This is also seen in tortuous vessels or with temporary retrograde flow seen during cardiac diastole. This effect is minimized by increasing the distance between the tracking saturation and the imaging plane.

## Mural and Extramural Pathology

Many extramural tissues such as fat, hemorrahage, and bowel content can mimic normal flow or masses. Lung atelectasis can mimic a mass or even inflammatory aneurysm due to abnormal periaortic enhancement. A high signal from perivascular fat due to incomplete fat suppression can mimic intraluminal flow. A high signal from a thrombus within an aneurysm can mimic normal blood flow. Vascular stenosis and perfusion defects are seen in extramural pathologies such as lung disease.

## ■ SPECIAL ISSUES

Contraindication to MRI include:
- Pacemaker
- Epicardial pacer wires
- Aneurysm clips
- Metal fragments in the eye
- Some metallic implants:
  - Many metallic implants are compatible with MRI.
  - Endovascular stents (Nitinol) are MRI compatible.
  - Pregnant patients can be scanned but without contrast.

## ■ CONCLUSION

- MRA is becoming the technique of choice for many vascular beds.
- MRA is popular because it is associated with minimal risks and gives high resolution anatomical and functional details.

- Three-dimensional contrast-enhanced MRA can be done with a single breath hold.
- By MRA, the hemodynamic significance of a stenosis can be assessed.

## PRACTICAL POINTS

- If possible, MRI should be performed holding the breath.
- Consider the possibility of an artifact to explain an unusual finding and always correlate the finding with other imaging modalities.
- Consider the possibility of slow flow if no images are seen.

# 5

# Approach to Management of Intermittent Claudication

*Jaisom Chopra*

## ■ INTRODUCTION

### Incidence and Prevalence of Peripheral Vascular Disease

- In clinical practice, atherosclerosis is the most common cause of lower limb peripheral artery disease (PAD).
- Early PAD is asymptomatic and gradually progresses to intermittent claudication.
- Cardiovascular mortality is independent of stage of atherosclerosis.
- Using ankle-brachial index (ABI) as the criterion, prevalence was 20% after 75 years of age.
- Around 3–6% of the population after 60 years of age suffers from intermittent claudication. According to an Edinburg Artery study (*Leng GC et al. 1995*), 4% over 55 years of age were symptomatic, though atherosclerosis was present in 25% of the asymptomatic people.
- PAD was more prevalent in males.

### Risk Factors for Claudication

As we see Figure 1, all the risk factors have a direct relationship to the progression except high-density lipoprotein (HDL) cholesterol, which has an inverse relationship. As atherosclerosis is a systemic disease, it is closely related to coronary artery disease (CAD) and cerebrovascular disease.

## ■ CLINICAL FEATURES

### Presenting Features

- Intermittent claudication (IC) is pain in one or both legs on walking or exertion, worsening on continued activity, and relieved by rest (2–3 min) or reducing the pace of the activity (Fig. 2).

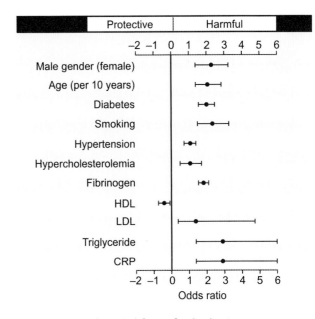

**Fig. 1** Risk factors for claudication
*Abbreviations:* HDL, high-density lipoprotein; LDL, low-density lipoprotein; CRP; C-reactive protein.

- The claudication distance varies with the severity of the disease.
- The pain is cramp like with or without muscle weakness.
- It may present atypically—not classically claudication.

### Pathophysiology

Regardless of the site of PAD, calf muscles are always involved because of the greater metabolic demand of this group of muscles. The most common site of PAD in the lower extremity is the superficial femoral artery (SFA) at the adductor canal.

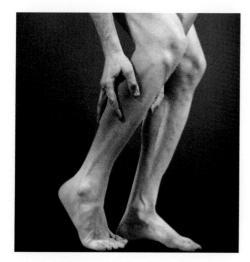

**Fig. 2** Intermittent claudication

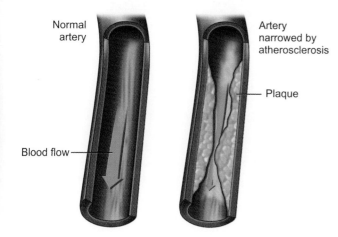

**Fig. 3** Normal arterial flow and flow in an atherosclerotic artery

The pathophysiology of IC is multifactorial and includes:
- Hemodynamic causes—at rest, even a 70% stenosis may not produce symptoms but may be flow limiting on exercise
- Deconditioning
- Metabolic changes such as accumulation of acylcarnitines and ADP or impaired synthesis of phosphocreatine
- Skeletal muscle injury—distal axonal denervation leading to muscle fiber loss and atrophy of the affected muscles.

As deposition of cholesterol and calcium occurs within the arterial wall (atherosclerosis), it leads to narrowing or blockage of the artery. This reduces the blood supply to the leg. This process is aggravated in diabetic individuals, smokers, or people with high levels of blood cholesterol (Fig. 3).

At rest, as the oxygen demand of the leg muscles is minimal, even the reduced blood flow is adequate and the patient remains asymptomatic. On walking, the calf muscles need more oxygen, which is not available due to reduced blood flow, and cramps occur. This is made better by resting a few moments or reducing the pace of exercise. Greater the demand (walking uphill or upstairs or running), quicker the symptoms appear.

Intermittent claudication is a manifestation of chronic PAD that has taken years to develop.

As the disease progresses, the blood supply to the limb reduces proportionately. A time comes when the blood supply is so poor that there is hardly any oxygen to the muscles even at rest. These patients start getting pain at night. The patients use gravity to improve the blood supply by hanging their legs out of the bed at night or sleep on the chair. The patient has developed critical leg ischemia and is in danger of amputation.

## Natural History of the Disease During the First 5 Years after Detection

Around 70% remain static and only 25% worsen. This deterioration is more during the first year (7–9%) and thereafter only 2–3% per annum. The worsening leads to critical limb ischemia (CLI).

Around 1–3% need a major amputation over 5 years.
- The progression to CLI is much faster in: Diabetic individuals
- Smoking
- ABI less than 0.5 or ankle pressure less than 70 mm Hg (progression rate to CLI of 7–9% per year).

## ■ DIAGNOSIS

## History and Physical Examination

The history of pain must include:
1. Site of pain or discomfort and its duration (Fig. 4)
2. Distance of walking before
   a. Experiencing the discomfort (initial claudication discomfort)
   b. Being forced to stop (absolute claudication discomfort)
   c. Time elapsed between stoppage and the relief from symptoms
   d. Type of rest or position (standing at rest, sitting, or lying) to relieve the symptoms.

Examination of the entire vascular system:
- Palpation of the carotid, radial, femoral, popliteal, dorsalis pedis, and posterior tibial pulses
- The pulses are graded as: 0 (absent); 1 (diminished); 2 (normal); 3 (bounding)
- Auscultation for carotid or abdominal bruit is a must
- In 10% ankle, pulses (dorsalis pedis [DP] and posterior tibial [PT]) are absent. The lateral tibial branch must be palpated medial to the bony prominence of the fibula
- In the presence of palpable ankle pulses, severe foot ischemia may be present if foot arteries are occluded from cholesterol embolization syndrome or in diabetic individuals.

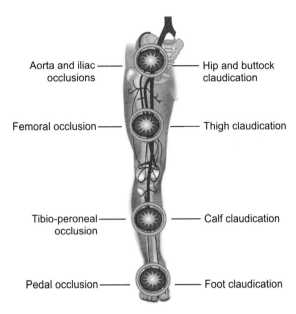

**Fig. 4** Site of occlusion or stenosis correlated with pain

## Differential Diagnosis

Although PAD is the most common cause of IC, some other arterial conditions may present with IC and given in Table 1.

## Pseudoclaudication

In this, claudication takes place in the absence of any arterial disease. It generally involves the nerve and veins.

### Nerve Claudication

It is generally due to lumbar canal stenosis. The pain is sharp and associated with paresthesia, coming on at variable walking distances and relieved by sitting or leaning forward (Fig. 5).

### Venous Claudication

In this, there is swelling and bursting type of pain progressively increasing on walking and relieved by elevation of feet over 1–2 h (Fig. 6).

## Investigations: Laboratory Testing

Routine tests include:
- Blood tests—CBC with platelets; blood sugar; HbA1c levels; renal functions (BUN and creatinine); fasting lipid profile; coagulation profile and blood grouping
- Urine test—for microalbuminuria
- 12-lead ECG
- Carotid artery ultrasound if indicated
- Coronary artery investigations if indicated
- In patients with premature disease, family history of thrombosis or early graft thrombosis—hypercoagulability workup is indicated in Table 2.

Ankle-brachial index (ABI) is the first screening test in suspected PAD and if between 0.4 and 0.9, it is considered severe.

↓

Segmental limb pressure (SLP) and waveform analysis are then performed to localize the lesion in patient with abnormal ABI.

**Table 1** Differential diagnosis of intermittent claudication

| Diagnosis | Clinical features |
| --- | --- |
| Buerger's disease | Typically presents with ulcers and foot claudication but may involve calf vessels causing IC |
| Hypoplasia and acquired coarctation of abdominal aorta (mid-aortic syndrome) | It is acquired disease and is associated with renal artery involvement |
| Vasculitis (Takayasu's) | May involve abdominal aorta and iliacs |
| Collagen vascular disease (giant cell arteritis—GCA), systemic lupus erythematosus (SLE), pseudoxanthoma elasticum (PXE) | GCA involves femorals and subclavians bilaterally >50 years. SLE involves smaller vessels but may cause IC. PXE also causes IC |
| Remote trauma or irradiation injury | Due to radiation treatment of pelvic and abdominal cancers with iliofemoral lesions |
| Peripheral embolization from proximal aneurysm (popliteal, femoral, abdominal) | Distal embolization may cause foot claudication |
| Popliteal etiologies (adventitial cystic disease, entrapment) | Entrapment—due to abnormal origin of the medial gastrocnemius in young. Generally bilateral but may be unilateral |
| | Adventitial cystic disease—ganglion cyst involving the popliteal artery in young males |
| Fibrodysplasia (external iliac artery) | EIA third common vessel involved after renal and carotid |
| Persistent sciatic artery (thrombosed) | Rare congenital disease in which sciatic artery persists as major inflow artery |
| Iliac syndrome of the cyclist | Narrowing of iliac artery due to repeated trauma. Unilateral buttock symptoms provoked with cycling in male professional cyclists |

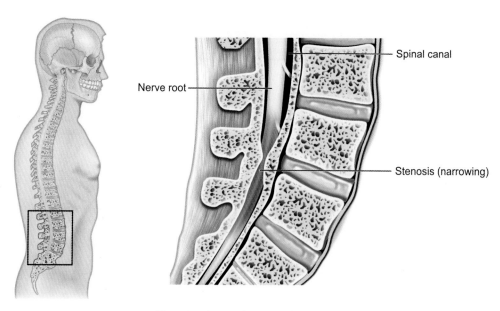

**Fig. 5** Lumbar canal stenosis of the spine

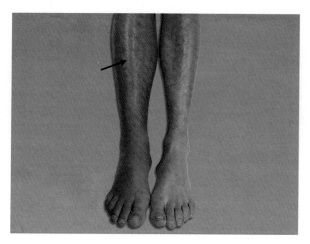

**Fig. 6** Swelling of one leg

**Table 2** Congenital risk factors for developing atherosclerosis and how to detect them

| Test | Condition |
|------|-----------|
| Homocysteine levels | Homocystinuria |
| Plasma fibrinogen levels | Dysfibrinogenemia |
| Antithrombin 111 levels | AT 111 deficiency |
| Plasma fibrinogen | Hyperfibrinogenemia |
| Protein C assay/activity | Protein C deficiency |
| Protein S antigen assay | Protein S deficiency (false positive results in presence of factor V Laden) |
| Antiphospholipid antibodies and lupus anticoagulant | Antiphospholipid antibody syndrome |
| Factor V laden PCR | Resistance of activated protein C |
| Prothrombin G20210A PCR | Prothrombin G20210A mutation |

↓

Exercise ABI may also be obtained when the diagnosis is uncertain.

↓

Magnetic resonance angiography (MRA) and conventional angiograms are performed only when surgery is must.

↓

A false high ABI of more than 1.2 is mostly associated with diabetes wherein calcification prevents compression. Here, toe-brachial index less than 0.7 confirms PAD (Flow chart 1).

## ■ MANAGEMENT

The aims of treatment are:
- Reduction of cardiovascular risk
- Relieve lower limb symptoms
- Better walking capacity
- Improving quality of life.

## Risk Factor Modification (Table 3)

This must be aggressive.

### Smoking Cessation

This is important for the following reasons:
- Slows the progression of IC to CLI
- Reduces need for revascularization
- Improves graft patency
- Reduces cardiovascular events.
  They all must be referred for nicotine replacement therapy (NRT) in form of gum, spray, or patch and/or bupropion

**Flow chart 1** Algorithm for diagnostic modalities and approach to IC

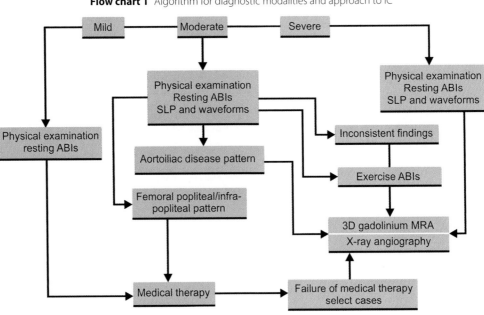

**Table 3** Risk factor modification in PAD

| Risk factor | Goals | Therapy |
|---|---|---|
| Tobacco smoking | Complete cessation | Counseling and drugs |
| Lipoproteins | LDL-C <100 mg/dL | Statin first line but if goal not achieved then add Ezetimibe or BAR (bar acid resin) |
| Antiplatelet therapy | Mandatory | Aspirin and/or Clopidogrel |
| Blood pressure | <140/90 mm Hg | ACEI (angiotensin converting enzyme inhibitor) first line. If CAD then beta-blockers |
| Diabetes mellitus | HbA1c <7% to reduce microvascular complications | Metformin first line in obese |
| Emerging risk factors | Homocysteine, Lp(a) (lipoprotein-a), apoE genotype CRP (C-reactive protein) | Other drugs are needed. Treatment as indicated |

(Wellbutrin) starting with 150 mg 6 hourly for 3 days and then 12 hourly for 6–10 weeks. NRT and Wellbutrin show higher rates of smoking cessation than when either is used alone.

## Correction of Hyperlipidemia

This prevents progression of PAD, though there is not much improvement in IC. Statins are mandatory in patients with IC with reduction in cardiovascular events even when low-density lipoprotein (LDL) cholesterol is within normal limits (<100 mg/dL). Statins also improve IC. Additional medication may be needed to get the LDL cholesterol within normal range. Insulin resistance and high triglycerides with low LDL cholesterol are common in PAD. One must try to achieve the target of total cholesterol minus non-HDL cholesterol less than 130 mg/dL. The addition of niacin or fibric acid therapy may be needed with monitoring of LFT.

## Hypertension Control

Peripheral artery disease (PAD) points to the involvement of target organs such as heart and brain and calls for blood pressure (BP) control using antihypertensive drugs aiming to keep the BP below 140/90 mm Hg in nondiabetic individuals and less than 130/80 mm Hg in diabetic individuals. It is not certain whether BP control is helpful to reduce progression of PAD and improve IC.

Beta-blockers should be used for control of BP in patients with PAD along with coronary artery disease (CAD) or angina.

Angiotensin-converting enzyme inhibitors (ACEI) are used for BP control in PAD cases with diabetes and CAD.

## Glycemic Control

Diabetic individuals with IC have a 20% risk of amputation and a 5-year mortality of 50%. Aggressive blood sugar control

**Table 4** Anticoagulation regimen recommended for peripheral bypasses

| Site of proximal anastomosis | Site of distal anastomosis | Graft material | Thrombotic potential | Prophylactic agent of choice |
| --- | --- | --- | --- | --- |
| Aorta | Iliac or Femoral | Prosthetic | Low | Aspirin or Clopidogrel |
| Femoral | Popliteal (AK) | Vein | Low | Aspirin or Clopidogrel |
| Femoral | Popliteal (BK) | Prosthetic (good flow >100 mL/min and good run off) | Medium | Clopidogrel + Aspirin 75 mg |
| Femoral | Popliteal (BK) | Prosthetic (flow <100 mL/min) and poor runoff | High | Warfarin |
| Femoral | Distal | Vein | Medium - high | Clopidogrel and aspirin 75 mg. Consider warfarin |
| Femoral | Distal | Prosthetic | High | Warfarin |
| Femoral | Femoral | Prosthetic | Low to medium | Clopidogrel and aspirin 75 mg |
| Axillary | Femoral | Prosthetic | Medium to high | Clopidogrel and aspirin 75 mg consider warfarin |

reduces microvascular complications such as neuropathy and retinopathy. Intensive control of atherosclerotic risk factors along with control of BP to less than 130/80 mm Hg and LDL-C less than 100 mg/dL should be done.

### Antiplatelet Therapy for Cardiovascular Risk Reduction

Aspirin should be used in doses of 75–325 mg in PAD cases to reduce cardiovascular risk. It helps reduce the need for peripheral revascularization and increases postsurgical graft patency. Clopidogrel reduces the vascular deaths, myocardial infarction (MI), and CVA by 24%. Whether both aspirin and clopidogrel be given alone or in combination is still not proven.

### Antithrombotic/Anticoagulation Postlower Extremity Bypass Grafting

Aspirin must be given postoperatively to reduce risk of graft occlusion and for its cardioprotective effects. Warfarin may be given to patients to prevent graft thrombosis (Table 4).

## Nonpharmacological Therapy for IC

### Exercise Rehabilitation (Fig. 7)

This improves functional capacity, symptoms, and quality of life for PAD patients. There is an increase of 140 m on pain-free walking and the total walking distance increases by 180 m. Supervised walking programs are much superior to home walking programs. The improvement is by:
• Better oxygen utilization and metabolism by leg muscles
• Improved collateral blood flow

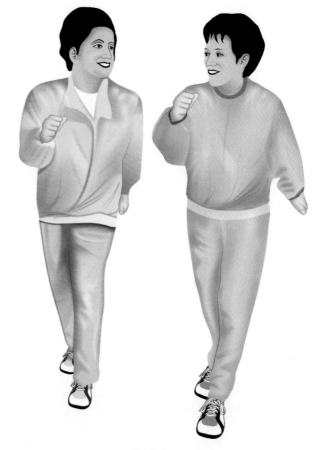

**Fig. 7** Exercise

• Decreased blood viscosity
• Enhanced walking efficiency
• Increased pain threshold.

Exercise therapy is carried out as follows:

- Type of exercise—treadmill or track walking are most effective in IC
- Walk till moderate claudication pain and then rest till no pain and walk again. Total session 35 minutes.
- Maintenance goals are:
  - Increase duration of walking by 5 minutes in every visit
  - Increase in treadmill incline if patient walks 10 minutes at a previous setting
  - Double the speed from 1.5 mph to 3 mph
- Exercise regimen at three to five times per week.

## Pharmacological Therapy for IC (Table 5)

These give symptomatic relief and improve functional capacity. They are as follows:

### Cilostazol

- Type III phosphodiesterase inhibitor that increases the intracellular cyclic AMP levels
- Releases prostaglandin $I_2$
- Inhibits platelet and vascular smooth muscle proliferation
- Improves serum lipoproteins—10% decrease in triglycerides and 4% increase in HDL
- 100 mg bd over 6 months results in 130-m maximal walking distance
- Contraindicated in patients with congestive heart failure (CHF) and ejection fraction (EF) less than 40%

### Pentoxifylline

Pentoxifylline marginally improves symptoms and walking ability (27 m in peak walking distance).

### Oral Prostaglandin Analogs

They are potent vasodilators with antiplatelet effect. Recent trials have not shown encouraging results.

L-carnitine—improves skeletal muscle metabolism and bioenergetics by replenishing deficient levels in ischemic tissue. This drug is more effective in severely impaired patients who walk less than 250 m. Patients with mild disability do not respond.

L-arginine—these increase the vascular endothelial nitric oxide, a vasodilatory molecule with potent antiatherosclerotic properties. Initial studies suggest good efficacy.

## Percutaneous Treatment of IC

It is indicated in lifestyle-limiting claudication interfering with the quality of life and vasculogenic impotence. This includes:

- Percutaneous transluminal angioplasty (PTA)
- Stenting
- Stent grafting.

The first two procedures are for short focal lesions, while the stent grafting is for:

- Long occlusions
- Aneurysmal dilatation of the artery or
- Lesions causing atheromatous embolization needing surgical approach.

The TASC (Trans-Atlantic Inter-Society Consensus) classification is helpful in guiding therapy (Table 6).

Endovascular procedure is the treatment of choice in type A and surgery is the procedure of choice in type D. In type B, endovascular treatment is mostly recommended, while in type C, surgery is recommended. Types B and C are gray areas where there is nothing clear-cut on the nature of treatment.

## Perprocedural Antithrombotic Use

Three hundred milligrams clopidogrel is given 12 hours prior to procedure as a loading dose. Along with this, glycoprotein IIb/IIIa is used to prevent distal embolization if:

- Patient is diabetic
- Thrombus or ulceration seen on angiography
- Poor outflow with one vessel runoff or no vessel visible.

The glycoprotein used is abciximab—loading bolus 0.25 mg/kg IV over 5 minutes followed by 0.125 µg/kg/min IV infusion for 12 h Or

Integrilin—loading bolus 180 µg/kg × 2 separate by 10 minutes followed by 18-h IV infusion of 2 µg/kg/min.

**Table 5** Pharmacological therapy of intermittent claudication

| Drug | Dose | Mechanism of action | Side effects | Interactions |
|---|---|---|---|---|
| Cilostazol | 50–100 mg bd | Inhibition of phosphodiesterase III | Headache, diarrhea, flatulence, palpitation, and dizziness | Macrolide antibiotics, ketoconazole, grapefruit juice, omeprazole |
| Pentoxifylline (trental) | 400 mg tds | | Nausea, bloating, dizziness | Theophylline |
| Beraprost | 40 µg tds | Oral prostaglandin I2 analog | Headache, flushing | |

**Table 6** The Trans-Atlantic Inter-Society Consensus (TASC) guidelines helping management of intermittent claudication

| | Iliac disease | Femoral lesions |
|---|---|---|
| **TASC-A** | Single <3 cm of CIA or EIA (unilateral or bilateral) | Single <3 cm not involving the SFA or popliteal |
| **TASC-B** | • Single 3–10 cm not extending into the CFA<br>• 2 stenoses <5 cm long in CIA and/or EIA not extending into CFA<br>• Unilateral CIA occlusion | • Single stenosis 3–5 cm long not involving distal popliteal artery<br>• Heavily calcified <3 cm or multiple stenosis or occlusion each <3 cm<br>• Single or multiple lesions in absence of continuous tibial run-off |
| **TASC-C** | • Bilateral 5–10 cm stenosis of CIA and/or EIA not extending to CFA<br>• Bilateral EIA stenosis or occlusion not extending onto CFA<br>• Bilateral CIA occluison | • Single stenosis or occlusion >5 cm<br>• Multiple stenosis or occlusions 3–5 cm long with or without heavy calcification |
| **TASC-D** | • >10 cm lesion or diffuse multiple unilateral stenosis involving CIA, EIA, and CFA.<br>• Unilateral occlusion involving both CIA and EIA<br>• Bilateral EIA occlusion<br>• Diffuse disease involving both aorta and iliac arteries or lesion in a patient needing aortic or iliac surgery (AAA) | Complete CIA or SFA occlusion |

# Percutaneous Treatment of Aortoiliac Disease

Percutaneous transluminal angioplasty and/or stenting is the procedure of choice for focal stenosis involving the distal abdominal aorta, CIA, or EIA (<5 cm in the iliac arteries). Initial success is 95% with 70% at 2 years and 60% at 5 years. Complication rates are less than 5% and mortality less than 1%. Stenting improves the long-term patency rates of angioplasty (Fig. 8).

# Results of Percutaneous Interventions in IC (Table 7)

## Predictors of Failure

They are poor outflow and female gender.

## Hemodynamic Measurements

The resting pressure gradient across a stenosis is over 7 mm Hg and 10–15 mm Hg after vasodilatation is seen in a significant lesion.

## Percutaneous Treatment of Femoropopliteal Disease

In cases of severe IC due to femoropopliteal disease, the outcome is predicted by the following criteria:
• Absence of diabetes
• Short focal lesion
• Good distal runoff
• Lack of residual lesion.

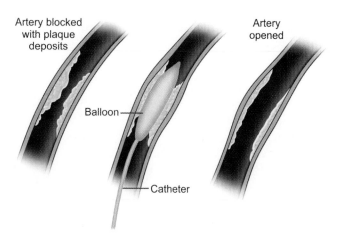

**Fig. 8** Balloon angioplasty in a stenotic vessel

**Table 7** Results of percutaneous interventions in IC

| Type of lesion and intervention | Initial technical success (%) | 1-year patency rate (%) | 3-year patency rate (%) | 5-year patency rate (%) |
|---|---|---|---|---|
| Iliac stenosis—PTA | 95 | 83 | 71 | 66 |
| Iliac occlusion—PTA | 83 | 85 | 77 | – |
| Iliac stenosis—stent | 99 | 91 | 75 | 73 |
| Iliac occlusion—stent | 82 | 90 | 82 | 71 |
| Femoropopliteal—PTA | 90 | 71 | 61 | 58 |
| Femoropopliteal—stent | 98 | 67 | 58 | 40 |

## Femoropopliteal PTA

Single stenosis less than 3 cm involving common or SFA may be ideal for PTA. The expense is lower than bypass surgery.

The long-term patency rates for occlusion (80–85%) are comparable to stenosis (90%).

### Stenting for Femoropopliteal Lesions

This is not indicated as a primary approach. It is indicated as a complication of PTA wherein dissection has taken place or there is thrombus formation.

### Predictors of Success or Failure

The most important predictor is the outflow status (number of vessels in direct continuity).

### Prevention of Restenosis after Femoropopliteal Stenting

This is by vascular brachytherapy (γ or β radiation) delivered to the site through catheter-based strategies directed at reducing restenosis in poststenting. There is a 50% reduction in incidence of restenosis without late stenosis or thrombosis (Figs 9A to C).

### Drug-eluting Stents in Femoropopliteal Lesions

This has shown encouraging results in SFA lesions with 0% restenosis compared with 36% in ordinary stents at 6 months (Fig. 10).

## Surgical Revascularization Approaches in IC

Absolute indications:
- Acute arterial obstruction
- Progression to rest pain
- Relief from disabling symptoms that interfere with the quality of life and vasculogenic impotence.
  The decision making is dependent on the following considerations:
- Long-term patency rates of aortoiliac bypass are superior to femoropopliteal bypass, which are superior to femoro-distal bypasses.
- Proximal reconstruction surgery such as aortoiliac has higher mortality than the distal procedures.
- Vein bypasses are preferred in below knee bypasses, whereas prosthetic bypasses are acceptable in above knee bypasses.
- Establishing good inflow to the affected area is critical for achieving good results.

### Surgical Bypass for Aortolliac Disease

The results are excellent with mortality of less than 3%, long-term patency of over 90% at 5 years, and 70% at 10 years for aorto-femoral bypass and aortic endarterectomy (Fig. 11).

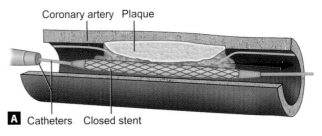
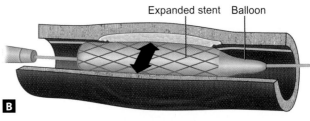
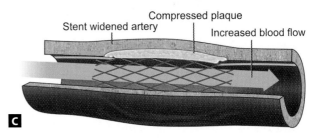

**Figs 9A to C** Angioplasty and stenting in a atherosclerotic artery

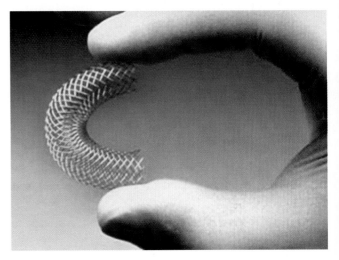

**Fig. 10** Stent

### Aorto-bifemoral Bypass

Aorto-bifemoral bypass (ABB) uses polytetrafluoroethylene (PTFE) grafts and has a mortality less than 3% and a morbidity of 8%. Patency rates at 5 years were 91% compared with 87% at 10 years.

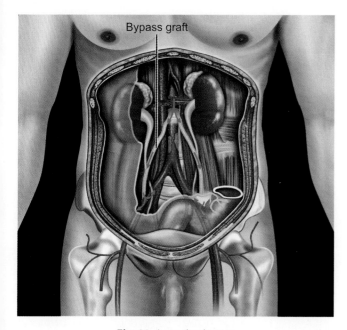

**Fig. 11** Aorto-iliac bypass

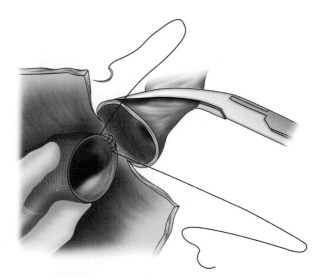

**Fig. 12** End to end anastomosis at the proximal end in an aorta-femoral bypass

## The Choice of Graft

Mostly, PTFE is used because of the easy handling, no preclotting, and no blood loss due to seepage from the graft. The most important predictor of success is:
- Good inflow and outflow
- Proper operating technique
- Choice of correct size of prosthesis (avoiding graft-outflow vessel mismatch). A 16 mm × 8 mm graft is put with a 14 mm × 7 mm in females.

## Proximal Anastomotic Considerations

Proximal anastomosis in the ABF could be either end to end or end to side. The advantages of end to end (Fig. 12) are:
- Direct flow into the graft without native aorta competing for the blood flow
- Due to resection of a portion of the aorta, the anastomosis is higher and in a less diseased vessel
- Applying tangential clamps to occlude the blood supply can mobilize the thrombus and create a risk of clot dislodgement to the pelvis and lower limb arteries.

The end to side anastomosis (Fig. 13) is favored:
- When end to end will affect the renal, mesenteric, or pelvic flow
- When a patent and enlarged IMA or aberrant renal arises from the distal aorta
- When only the EIA is involved with preserved CIA and IIA (the most common indication as sexual function is preserved due to perfusion into the IIA)
- Proximal graft protrudes anteriorly and prevents intestines from coming in contact with the anastomotic site, thus reducing the chances or aorto-enteric fistula

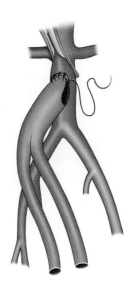

**Fig. 13** End to side anastomosis at the upper aortic end

- Absence of good pelvic circulation increases risk of hip claudication, colonic ischemia, and paraplegia secondary to spinal ischemia
- Collaterals arising from distal aorta are preserved.

## The Distal Anastomotic Considerations

There are five types of distal anastomosis (Fig. 14):
1. If the profunda femoris artery (PFA) and the superficial femoral artery (SFA) are widely patent, then they are preferred to the CFA.
2. The hood of the graft extends to the SFA where there is stenosis of the proximal SFA, and beyond this, the SFA is widely patent and so is PFA.

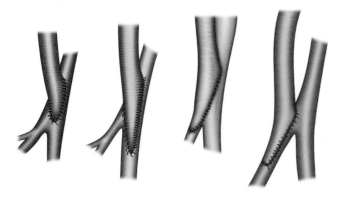

**Fig. 14** End to side anastomosis to the common femoral, superficial femoral or the profunda femoris arteries

3. The hood of the graft extends onto the PFA provided, it is more than 3 mm diameter and the length is more than 15 cm.
4. The graft is put onto the PFA, as CFA and SFA are occluded.
5. The hood is split to patch proximal stenosis involving SFA and PFA.

## Long-term Results of Patency of Stents and Grafts (Fig. 15)

### Rare Situations in Aorto-bifemoral Bypass Grafting

*Totally occluded aorta*
This occurs in 5–10% that may extend to the levels of the renals proximally and distally to the aortic bifurcation. Collaterals are supplied by the lumbars and the IMA. There is a fear of dislodging thrombus into the renal and mesenteric arteries, but surveys have shown that the risk is minimal. This generally is composed of clot that is removed easily by thrombectomy leaving space for the graft to be inserted. In short, segment occlusion stent may be indicated.

*Hypoplastic aorta syndrome*
Small aorta is seen occasionally in female, with the aorta 13.2 mm just below the renal and 10.3 mm at the bifurcation. The disease is localized and endarterectomy is done with a smaller graft to prevent mismatch.

*Aortoiliac endarterectomy*
This is very rarely performed and is for localized lesions. However, the results are good with 92% at 5 years and no prosthesis bypass grafts or their risk of infection.

*Associated renal and visceral artery lesions*
The assessment is mandatory to avoid catastrophic post-operative complications such as colonic ischemia, renal failure, and impotence. One should avoid end to end anastomosis at the aorta in patients with significant SMA or celiac artery disease, as perfusion is maintained to these structures via the IMA collaterals. Renal disease may lead to hypertension and renal failure and should be addressed.

### Postoperative Complications

*Early complications* account for 1–3% and include:
- *Major bleed* from aortic anastomotic site presents with hypotension and tachycardia leading to hypovolemic shock. If there is bleeding from the femoral anastomotic

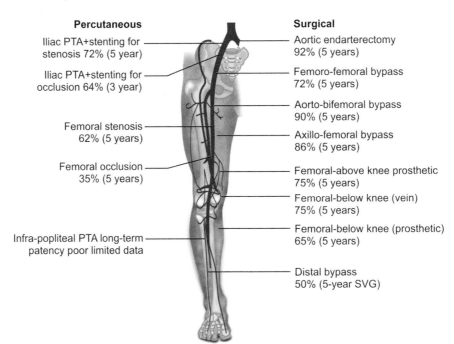

**Fig. 15** Patency rates of various endovascular and surgical procedures performed in the lower limbs

Percutaneous
- Iliac PTA+stenting for stenosis 72% (5 year)
- Iliac PTA+stenting for occlusion 64% (3 year)
- Femoral stenosis 62% (5 years)
- Femoral occlusion 35% (5 years)
- Infra-popliteal PTA long-term patency poor limited data

Surgical
- Aortic endarterectomy 92% (5 years)
- Femoro-femoral bypass 72% (5 years)
- Aorto-bifemoral bypass 90% (5 years)
- Axillo-femoral bypass 86% (5 years)
- Femoral-above knee prosthetic 75% (5 years)
- Femoral-below knee (vein) 75% (5 years)
- Femoral-below knee (prosthetic) 65% (5 years)
- Distal bypass 50% (5-year SVG)

site, groin hematoma is present. Prompt recognition is needed and corrective surgery performed. Generalized ooze due to dilution of coagulation factors with transfusion of crystalloids and banked blood are corrected by fresh frozen plasma (FFP).

- *Limb ischemia*—occurs due to acute graft occlusion or distal embolization. It is recognized by signs of acute ischemia of the limb, disappearance of the pulses, or absent Doppler signals distally. Immediate embolectomy is needed for graft thrombosis or major artery embolus. The distal arterial emboli in the digital vessels are treated with heparin infusion or intra-arterially infused thrombolytics along with glycoproteins IIb/IIIa inhibitors.
- *Renal failure*—is rare in elective surgery with no pre-operative renal compromise. The precautions are avoidance of postoperative hypotension or declamping hypotension. The removal of clamp may dislodge emboli distally. Therefore, it may be acceptable to clamp the aorta above the celiac trunk and accept the small risk of renal ischemia.
- *Colonic ischemia*—mostly involves the rectosigmoid and is more common in aneurismal surgery than in occlusive aortic disease. The cause is interruption of collateral or primary flow to the bowel, atheromatous embolization, or prolonged perioperative hypotension. There may be significant celiac and SMA disease, and if a large patent IMA is occluded by end to end anastomosis, it would lead to colonic ischemia. Arterial reconstruction by reimplanting of IMA or bypass of the SMA or celiac axis may be needed. Colonic ischemia is recognized postoperatively by (i) liquid brown diarrhea, (ii) abdominal distension, (iii) signs of peritonitis, and (iv) unexplained metabolic acidosis. Mild cases may need supportive care and major one's bowel resection.

*Late complications*
- *Anastomotic pseudoaneurysm*—2–5% and commonly at the femoral anastomosis where it presents as a pulsatile mass. The abdominal mass is mostly asymptomatic and is diagnosed on routine computed tomography (CT) scan of the abdomen in the late follow-up.
- *Sexual dysfunction*—in 25% with proximal aortic surgery. It presents as impotence or lack of ejaculation after normal coitus. Make a special note of the preoperative status and take written consent of this complication. At surgery, minimize dissection of the aortic bifurcation and avoid nerve fibers along the left lateral wall of aorta. Try to preserve hypogastric arterial flow.
- *Infection*—is less than 1% and is mostly at the femoral site. *Staphylococcus* is the most offending pathogen. The only treatment is graft removal.

*Femoral artery occlusion*—here an iliopopliteal bypass is performed as shown in Figure 16.

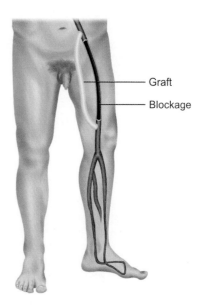

**Fig. 16** Iliofemoral bypass

# ■ SURGICAL TREATMENT OF INFRA-INGUINAL DISEASE

Even if extensive rarely justifies surgical treatment of IC. If it is confined to SFA in disabling claudication and endovascular treatment is not possible, then bypass grafting is indicated.

*Femoropopliteal bypass grafting*—vein and synthetic grafts have almost equal patency rates being 65–70% at 5 years. Below knee bypasses should have veins used. Besides femoro-femoral or axillo-femoral bypasses are advocated.

*Complications of infra-inguinal bypasses*—postoperative morbidity is 1–5% due to CAD.

Local complications are bleeding, infection, graft thrombosis, lymphatic leaks, wound infection, and delayed healing. Early graft thrombosis is due to poor outflow, small caliber vein, or technical faults such as venous kinks, intimal flaps, and idiopathic thrombosis of vein.

Hypercoagulable states such as heparin-induced thrombocytopenia (HIT), antiphospholipid syndrome, and protein C and S deficiency may be present and cause thrombosis.

Wound infection is due to persistent lymph leaks that responds to immobility, leg elevation, and wound care. In resistant cases, re-exploration and lymphatic channel ligation may be needed.

## Extra-anatomic Bypass in IC

These are indicated in patients with threatened limb and those too sick for any other procedure, which is more durable

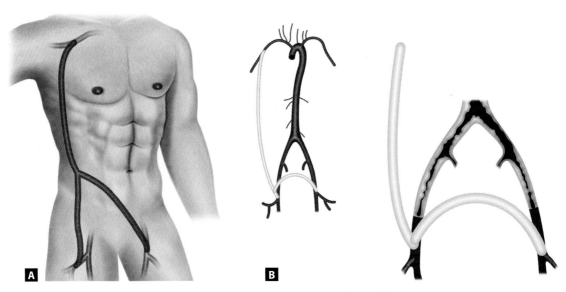

**Figs 17A and B** (A) Axillo-bifemoral bypass; (B) Femoro-femoral bypass

and lasting. Femoro-femoral bypass is only indicated in the elderly who are too sick for any other more aggressive procedure and have a long block in one iliac artery with other normal without any disease or stenosis. If there is a stenosis in the other iliac artery, then PTA with stenting must be done before the bypass. The SFA must be patent. Long-term patency rates are more than 70% (5 years) (Figs 17A and B).

*Axillo-femoral bypass*—should be performed only in very extreme cases and 5-year patency rates are 20–80%.

## ■ CONCLUSION

All PAD cases have a high cardiovascular risk. Aggressive management of all risk factors such as exercise rehabilitation and drugs have a future role in the long-term management of these patients. Percutaneous revascularization of aortoiliac disease is preferable to surgery, as it provides less risk and long patency results. Aorto-femoral and femoro-popliteal surgery is only indicated if percutaneous procedures are not possible. With newer stents and therapies present to prevent re-stenosis, endovascular approach may be superior to surgery.

## PRACTICAL POINTS

**Diagnosis**
- Normal ABI does not exclude PAD. Consider distal disease—diabetes or aortoiliac disease with good collaterals.
- Normal thigh pressures (SLP) may not exclude aortoiliac disease owing to overestimation of pressures.
- Exercise ABI provokes ischemia and is used in doubtful cases.

**Medical Treatment**
- Improvement with cilastazol take time (2–3 months). Patient education is important to improve compliance.
- Supervised exercise rehabilitation is superior to walking, which is superior to strength training.
- Warfarin is indicated for prosthetic bypass in high-risk cases as a prophylaxis—below knee bypass, distal bypasses, and axillofemoral bypass.

**Surgical Treatment**
- Vein bypass for below knee and prosthetic bypass above knee is recommended.
- Long-term patency of bypasses—aorto-iliac > femoro-popliteal > infrapopliteal bypass.

**Percutaneous Treatment**
- Pretreatment of clopidogrel prior to stenting.
- Limited role of infrapopliteal PTA in IC patients.

# 6

# Management of Acute Limb Ischemia

*Jaisom Chopra*

## ■ INTRODUCTION

- Acute limb ischemia (ALI) is one of the most common vascular problems and this is only likely to increase with the increasing population and as cardiac procedures increase (Fig. 1).
- According to the US statistics, in the year 2000 alone, 213,000 patients had lower limb acute ischemia due to embolism or thrombosis of the aorta and lower extremity.
- Around 85% of ALI occurs due to thrombosis and 15% due to embolism.
- This disease endangers loss of limb and life.
- It is vital to recognize and diagnose the condition and urgently restore the blood supply so as to:
  – Reduce the risk of amputation
  – Reduce the chances of reperfusion sepsis and multi-organ failure.

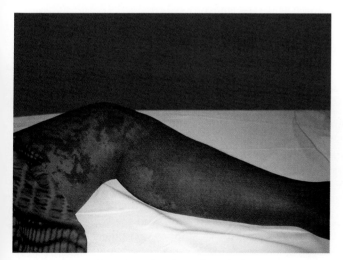

**Fig. 1** Acutely ischemic lower limb

- ALI occurs in aged with multiple other problems that can lead to their death even after successful revascularization of the limb.

## Dermatographic Profile

- Men and women are equally affected
- ALI is not the most common manifestation of PAD unless patients have had previous bypass graft surgery and the graft acutely occludes
- The average hospital stay is 10 days
- Amputation rates are 13%
- Mortality is 10%.

## ■ PATHOPHYSIOLOGY

Ischemia is a common clinical event leading to local and remote injury. ALI is due to the abrupt and complete blockage of the blood supply to the extremity. The tissues beyond the site of blockage become ischemic with energy metabolism shifting from aerobic to anaerobic phase. Prolonged ischemia leads to cell dysfunction and death. Nerve cells followed by muscle cells are most susceptible. A patient without any underlying vascular disease having acute arterial blockage has 6 hours (golden hours) for revascularization before irreversible functional damage occurs.

The injury is caused by activated neutrophils that accumulate after reperfusion. Initial production of reactive oxygen species on reperfusion leads to chemotactic activity for neutrophils. Once adherent to the endothelium, neutrophils damage by secretion of reactive oxygen species and proteolytic enzymes such as elastase.

The therapeutic options for reducing ischemic reperfusion injury are:
- Inhibition of oxygen radical formation
- Pharmacological prevention of neutrophils activation and chemotaxis

- Use of monoclonal antibodies that prevent neutrophil-endothelial adhesions.

Reperfusion injury causes secondary remote organ dysfunction due to factors released from the ischemic limb systemically leading to increased cell adhesion molecules and transmigration of neutrophils and monocytes into the lungs and kidneys. Experiments in animals using neutrophils depletion and anti-cell adhesion molecule therapy have shown encouraging results.

### Clinical Features—The 5 "Ps"

1. **P**ain
2. **P**aresthesia
3. **P**aresis to paralysis
4. **P**allor
5. **P**ulselessness.
   To this could be added—"Perishing with cold."

## Clinical Classification (Table 1)

- Class I is similar to chronic ischemic rest pain.
- Class IIb requires rapid revascularization.
- Class III is irreversible damage with major tissue loss, permanent nerve damage, profoundly anesthetic, and paralyzed limb. These patients normally land up with amputation.

## Etiology

- The most common source is the heart (75%) in which thromboemboli are thrown into the circulation. The thromboemboli form due to atrial fibrillation (AF) with the thrombus forming in the left atrial appendage. They may form after a myocardial infarction (MI) wherein the clot forms in the left ventricle.
- The common sites for the clot to lodge are the aortic bifurcation, femoral bifurcation or popliteal artery, and less commonly at other site. The thrombus may form in situ.
- Less commonly cardiac or septal tumor embolus.

**Table 1** Clinical classification of accute limb ischemia

| Category | Description | Neuromuscular findings | Doppler |
|---|---|---|---|
| I | Viable | No sensory or muscle weakness | Audible arterial and venous signals |
| IIa | Threatened (marginally) | Minimal | Often inaudible arterial but audible venous signal |
| IIb | Threatened (immediately) | Mild to moderate associated with pain | Inaudible arterial but audible venous signal |
| III | Irreversible | Profound deficit | No signals |

- Trauma—artery disruption.
- Dissection of a large vessel such as aorta and progression distally occluding the iliac artery.

## ■ DIAGNOSIS (TABLE 2)

### History

History and examination can be rapidly performed and guide us to the diagnosis and help in early and rapid reperfusion. One must look into the other problems such as cardiac. The patient may have had a cardiac event (anterior wall MI) followed by sudden pain in the limb with cyanosis and mottling and clear demarcation. This is one level below the site of occlusion. History of previous bypass surgery on the limb is usually absent and the severity falls in class IIb or III.

The classical 5 + 1 "p" apply—Pain, Pallor, Pulseless, Paralysis, Paresthesia, and Poikilothermia.

In situ thrombus has a vague onset of pain with no recent cardiac event, though CAD is present. There is always a history of PAD that may be very extensive. The limb is cooler and cyanosed with no distinct demarcation. Many times, there has been previous revascularization either surgically or endovascularly. These patients fall in class IIa.

### Physical Examination

Examine the pulses carefully. There is generally a contralateral pulse but absent pulse on the affected side (palpation and Doppler). There may be neurological deficit with numbness. Listen to the arterial and venous signals by handheld Doppler on the bedside but do not delay the treatment waiting for color Doppler study.

### Investigations: Laboratory Evaluation

- Determine potassium, creatinine phosphokinase (CPK), and acid–base status
- Echocardiography (ECG) to determine the rhythm and previous MI
- Prothrombin time and partial thromboplastin time (PT/APTT)
- Routine hematology and biochemistry screening
- Transfusion screening.

## ■ MANAGEMENT (TABLE 3)

After resuscitation and anticoagulation (if not contraindicated), the next step is to decide whether endovascular and thrombolytic therapy are indicated or surgical embolectomy. It is vital to confirm the limb viability at the outset because if the limb is in the class III, ischemia and nonviable primary amputation should be considered because revascularization of a nonviable limb could be fatal (Flow chart 1).

**Table 2**  Diagnosis of acute limb ischemia

|  | Embolism | Thrombosis in situ |
|---|---|---|
| History | Rapid onset. Prior cardiac event. No prior PAD history | Vague onset. No recent cardiac event. PAD present |
| Physical examination | Cold, mottled, paralyzed with clear demarcation Normal contralateral limb | Cool, bluish, and paresthesia with no demarcation. Abnormal contralateral pulse examination |
| Etiology | Cardiac thrombus, aortic arch plaque | Plaque rupture, hypercoagulation, pump failure |
| Prior vascular surgery | Usually no | Often yes |
| Rapid anticoagulation | Yes—heparin | Yes—heparin |
| Most common ischemic class | IIb | IIa |

**Table 3**  Management of acute limb ischemia

| Medication | Route | Dosage | Laboratory |
|---|---|---|---|
| Aspirin | PO/PR | 325 mg | None |
| Heparin | IV | 60 U/kg bolus and 12 U/kg/h infusion | APTT, platelets, Hct |
| Mannitol | IV | 12.5–25 g | Creatinine |
| Plasminogen activator | IA | Depends on agent | Hct, fibrinogen, FSP |
| UK | IA | 80–200,000 U/h tapered infusion | Hct, fibrinogen, FSP |

*Abbreviations:* APTT, activated partial thromboplastin time; IA, intra-arterially; IV, intravenous; PO, per oral; PR, per rectal; Hct, hematocrit; FSP, fibrinogen split products; UK, urokinase.

## General Measures

- Irrespective of the cause, initial resuscitation is done with IV fluids (normal saline without potassium till renal function is known) and oxygen.
- All patients are given aspirin orally or PR.
- IV mannitol to induce osmotic diuresis should be given, as it has free radical scavenging properties as well.
- Swan-Ganz catheter may be needed if the patient is very sick with multiple problems including a weak heart.
- Full-dose heparin infusion is started after giving bolus 60 U/kg with maintenance dose of 12–15 U/kg/h to keep APTT 2.5 times baseline levels.
- If the patient has a history of HIT (heparin-induced thrombocytopenia) or AT III deficiency, then direct thrombin inhibitors may be used. This is Hirudin given as a bolus 0.4 mg/kg slowly over 15 minutes and then infusion 0.15 mg/kg/h. There are no antagonists available for Hirudin and so fresh frozen plasma is given if needed.

## Approach to the Patient (Flow Chart 1)

If the patient has a clear embolic etiology and we can determine the site by examination, then embolectomy should be performed. If the embolic etiology is not clear,

then the angiogram (Fig. 2) must be performed after which the decision to do an embolectomy or endovascular approach is taken. If dissection is present, then it is dealt on an individual basis.

## Surgery versus Endovascular Therapy

Two major trials in the 1990s—Surgery or Thrombolysis In Lower Extremity ischemia (STILE) trial and Thrombolysis Or Peripheral Artery Surgery (TOPAS) trial. Both patients had angiography followed by thrombolytic therapy using urokinase or angiography followed by embolectomy or urgent bypass. Both trials suggested that the outcome was equivalent. However, in both trials, the patients mostly belonged to the class I or class IIa category and less than 25% belonged to the class IIb or class III. In reality, most patients belong to the latter two categories because most trials are conducted for 14 days after the onset of symptoms. Many of these patients had extensive PAD or occluded grafts wherein thrombolysis or endovascular procedures are anyway indicated. A large database hospital trial showed that amputation rates after embolectomy were lower than after thrombolysis. Thus, the choice must be made very carefully depending on the cause. Poor outcome in both procedures also depends upon other factors such as—old age, history of malignancy, central nervous system (CNS) disease, and low body weight. Age should not be a factor relating to decision making.

## Surgical Therapy

The patient is always draped for a femorofemoral bypass or an axillofemoral bypass in case embolectomy fails to produce the desired result. Mostly embolectomy (Fig. 3) is performed from the femoral approach from where clots can be cleared from the aorta to the ankle. Many times below knee exposure of the popliteal may be needed to do embolectomy of the peroneal and the tibial arteries. In the same way, upper extremity is exposed at the bifurcation below the elbow so that the brachial, radial, and ulnar can all be cleared of clots.

Embolectomy may cause dissection or intimal damage if care is not taken while withdrawing the catheter with

**Flow chart 1** Treatment algorithm for patients with acute limb ischemia

```
┌─────────────────┐    History    ┌─────────────────┐    N    ┌─────────────┐
│ Patient with    │──────────────▶│ Acute and       │────────▶│ Elective    │
│ lower extremity │   Physical    │ limb-threatening│         │ work-up     │
│ ischemia        │               │ (class II, III) │         │             │
└─────────────────┘               └─────────────────┘         └─────────────┘
                                          │ Y
                                          ▼
                                   ┌─────────────────┐
                                   │ Heparinization  │
                                   │ ±               │
                                   │ antiplatelet Rx │
                                   └─────────────────┘
                                          │
          ┌─────────────┐    N            ▼
          │ Amputation  │◀──────── ┌─────────────────┐
          └─────────────┘          │ Viable limb?    │
                                   └─────────────────┘
                                          │ Y
                                          ▼
  ┌──────────────────┐     ┌──────────────────────┐  Y  ┌─────────────────┐
  │ • Work-up of     │     │ • Maximize           │◀────│ Clear embolic   │
  │   etiology       │◀────│   resuscitation      │     │ etiology?       │
  │ • Postoperative  │     │ • To OR, surgical    │     └─────────────────┘
  │   anticoagulation│     │   thromboembolectomy │            │ N
  │ • Risk factor    │     │ • Bypass             │            ▼
  │   modifications  │     └──────────────────────┘     ┌─────────────────┐
  └──────────────────┘                                  │ Arteriography   │
          ▲                                             └─────────────────┘
        Y │        ┌─────────────┐    N                        │
          └────────│ Successful? │─────┐                       │
                   └─────────────┘     │                       ▼
                                       │              ┌─────────────────┐
  ┌──────────────────┐                 │         Y    │ Thrombosis in   │
  │ • Lytic therapy  │◀────────────────┴──────────────│ situ or Bypass  │
  │ • Catheter suction│                               │ graft occulusion│
  │   embolectomy    │                                └─────────────────┘
  │ • Antiplatelet   │                                         │ N
  │   antagonist     │                                         ▼
  └──────────────────┘                                ┌─────────────────┐
                                                      │ Dissection,     │
                                                      │ other           │
                                                      └─────────────────┘
```

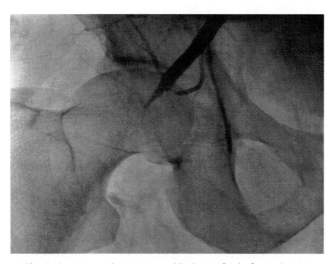

**Fig. 2** Angiogram showing acute blockage of right femoral artery with no collaterals

correct insufflations. If signals at the ankle are not present at the end of the procedure, an on-table angiogram is done to document any residual emboli or native arterial lesion. Intra-arterial thrombolysis during the procedure using 10 mg tPA (tissue plasminogen activator) in 100 mL saline and blocking the inflow and outflow for several minutes has shown mixed results in terms of improved limb salvage. Critically ill may undergo embolectomy under local anesthesia (LA) if needed. Postoperatively, the patient is maintained on heparin and other medications as required.

## Endovascular Therapy

Angiography and thrombolysis are considered in patients with uncertain etiology or history and examination suggest thrombosis in situ. Still, surgery is the procedure of choice, as the time for lysis to be effective is 18–24 h, which may be too long for the survival of the limb. Endovascular therapy is appropriate in most cases of nonembolic ALI. Here, tPA

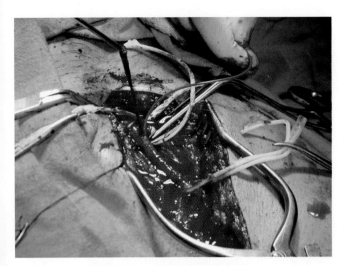

**Fig. 3** Femoral artery embolectomy

or urokinase is used and works by agent-activating plasmin, which is the active enzyme that breaks down fibrin, allowing the thrombus to dissolve.

## Procedure of Thrombolysis

A catheter is passed from the contralateral femoral. An angiogram is performed and the clot located. A multisided port catheter positioned within the clot and thrombolysis started as an infusion for 18–24 h using tPA (reteplase 0.2–1 U/h or alteplase 0.2–1 U/h) or urokinase (80–200,000 U/h tapered infusion). Low-dose heparin is given through side port of sheath to prevent catheter-induced thrombus formation.

A re-look angiogram is done after 12 hours to see the effectiveness of thrombolysis. Also clinically assess the patient for improvement of symptoms, capillary filling, and warmth of the leg.

## Hazards Associated with Thrombolysis

- The patient's symptoms may get temporarily worse as clots break and travel distally.
- Infusions longer than 48 hours may be hazardous and lead to bleeding. Fibrinogen levels are checked every 6 hourly and levels less than 100 mL/dL are associated with risk of systemic fibrinolysis and bleeding.

On completion of thrombolysis, the catheter and sheath are removed and the heparin continued for 4 more hours in full dose.

## Contraindications for Thrombolysis

*Absolute contraindications* to thrombolysis are bleeding tendency, CNS injury, or recent major surgery.

*Relative contraindications* include uncontrolled hypertension, recent eye surgery, pregnancy, and intracranial neoplasm.

## ■ OCCLUDED GRAFT

Thrombolytic therapy has been extensively used in this setting in the follow circumstances:
- Good operative risk
- Biological graft is used
- Ischemic class I or IIa
- It is a secondary or tertiary bypass
- Lacks good autologous couduit
- Extensive collaterals (Fig. 4).

# Thrombolysis

### Factors Predicting Successful Lysis

- Graft occlusion less than 14 days
- Guidewire passes through the thrombosed graft
- Graft has been in place for over 1 year
- If the cause for the failure is known.

### Poor Outcome with Thrombolysis

- Diabetes
- Continued smoking
- Prosthetic graft material.

The graft patency rates at 2 years are 10–40%, which are so poor that it may be better to replace the graft to improve long-term patency.

### Newer Thrombolytic Protocols

Tissue plasminogen activator has replaced urokinase largely but has more bleeding complications. Low doses of tPA and heparin are used to reduce complications. Adjunctive therapy with GIIb/IIIa antagonists allows faster thrombolysis without increasing the bleeding complications. Platelet counts are regularly checked and thrombolysis shortened

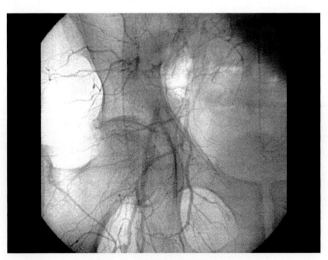

**Fig. 4** Extensive collaterals seen in thrombotic occlusive disease

by 50% saving both patient time and expenses and speeding re-establishment of blood flow.

### Mechanical Catheter-based Devices

This includes:
- Catheter suction thrombectomy
- Thrombus fragmentation
- Thrombus fragmentation and aspiration (rheolytic).

These have shown promising results in native arteries, pulmonary artery, and arteriovenous (AV) prosthetic access grafts. Many of these catheters allow concurrent pulse spray of lytic agents. These agents need further evaluation but have the potential to minimize the two main drawbacks of lytic therapy—long duration of lytic infusion needed for full arterial perfusion and hemorrhagic complications.

### Special Issues and Complications

Complications of embolectomy include infection, hemorrhage, and cardiac events. Endovascular therapy reduces the risk of general anesthesia (GA) and operative risk, though the risk of hemorrhage is 6–12%. The most feared complication of thrombolysis is intracranial bleed, which could be fatal. Computed tomography (CT) scan of the head is done if the patient complains of severe headache, vomiting, and neurological deficit and thrombolysis is immediately stopped.

Four-compartment fasciotomy is recommended in reperfusion edema of the extremity to prevent compartment syndrome in class IIb and IIIa ischemia. This compartment syndrome is associated with limb loss and mortality.

## ■ REPERFUSION INJURY

Following the re-establishment of blood flow to the ischemic tissue or organ, a group of complications can be seen that are collectively known as Reperfusion Syndrome.

Reperfusion syndrome is seen:
- Blood flow established to ischemic muscles in extremities—embolic, thrombotic, and traumatic
- Following heart surgery
- Following organ transplant
- Revascularization of ischemic intestines.

There are two components to this injury:
1. Local response
2. Systemic response.

In local response, there is limb swelling aggravating the tissue injury. The systemic response leads to multiple organ failure and death.

Irreversible muscle cell damage starts within 3 h and is nearly complete at 6 h (only 3% of the functional muscular activity left). The intensity of ischemia will depend upon:
- Nature of the tissue involved
  - Muscle—4 h
  - Nerve—8 h

- Fat—12 h
- Skin—24 h
- Bone—4 days
- Severity of ischemia
- Presence of collaterals
- Duration of ischemia
- Bulk of the tissue involved
- Ambient temperature.

## Assessing the Viability of the Muscles

It is practically impossible to assess the extent of viability of the muscles for the following reasons:
- There are two types of skeletal muscles depending on the amount of myoglobin content of the muscle. Most muscles have mixed fibers of varying quantities from these two types. Type 1 is the muscles of the anterior compartment of the leg while type II is the gastrocnemius. Type I uses oxidative metabolism as the source of energy, while type II uses anaerobic metabolism of glycogen as the energy source. Thus, duration of ischemia is different in the two groups of muscles.
- Another theory points to usage of ATP by the muscles, and at 6 h of ischemia, 20% ATP of the pre-ischemic levels is left.
- It is also observed that central portions of the muscles showed more necrosis than superficial portions making on-table assessment difficult and unreliable.

Thus, the treatment offered will vary from patient to patient and there are no hard and fast rules to be followed.

## Clinical Criteria for Determining Muscle Viability

- Nonviable muscles are identified on table by the 4 "Cs"- Color, Consistency, Contraction, and Circulation.
- The best indicator for viability is bleeding during debridement.
- Nonviable muscles are recognized by:
  - Dark color
  - Mushy consistency
  - Failure to contract when pinched with forceps
  - Absence of bleeding from cut surface.
- IV fluorescein dye to identify dead tissue.
- Consider second look at 24–48 h.

Microvascular damage is present with muscle cell damage. There was first damage to the capillaries where there was aggregation of the red blood cells (RBCs) plugging the capillaries and also breaks in the capillary intima. Later, leukocytes and platelets also invaded the area. These microvascular changes lead to increased vascular permeability to plasma proteins and interstitial edema.

It is observed that there continues to be focal malperfusion despite restoration of the blood supply and palpable pulsating large arteries—"the no reflow phenomenon". This is due to the intravascular hemoconcentration and thrombosis, swelling of the capillary endothelial cells, plugging the capillaries with leukocytes, and increased extravascular pressure from interstitial edema.

Muscle death probably takes place before the no reflow phenomenon sets in. It is the duration of ischemia and not reperfusion that kills the muscle. Distal to the occlusion of the arterial supply, there is a tapering zone of ischemia ranging from partial proximally becoming progressively more severe until a zone of absolute ischemia is reached.

Reperfusion takes place to devitalized tissue along with injured viable tissue. It is in this injured viable tissue zone that inflammatory mediators are generated and are responsible for the local and systemic effects of reperfusion. It is the amount of reperfused damaged but viable tissue that determines the morbidity of the patient. This inflammatory response is probably the breakdown products of the ischemic muscle cells that are procoagulants and these trigger the intrinsic clotting system that is responsible for progression of venous thrombosis and arteriolar vascular spasm in the arteriolar collateral. This causes the damage of the capillaries leading to interstitial edema. These factors further reduce the blood supply to the tissue. At this stage, high doses of heparin may improve the situation by preventing clot propagation. But the right dose of heparin has not yet been determined.

Depending on the bulk of the muscle involved, the inflammatory response may be entirely local or local and systemic. Renal failure is due to myoglobin released from ischemic muscles. The mortality from reperfusion injury could be due to renal, pulmonary, or cardiopulmonary involvement—either separately or in combination.

The inflammatory process leads to release of toxic products causing increased permeability of capillaries leading to third space loss resulting in multiple organ failure.

## Treatment of Local Consequences of Reperfusion

Re-establish circulation within 4–6 hours. These ischemic tolerance times can be increased by systemic anticoagulation and cooling of the extremity. It is likely that in the future, the use of anti-inflammatory agents could be of some benefit.

In areas in which there is collateral flow, the ischemic muscular damage is delayed. In such patients, therapy such as fasciotomy (Figs 5 and 6) or anticoagulation will prevent further thrombosis and be of any benefit.

The purpose of fasciotomy is to decompress the compartment and therefore must be complete—four-compartment.

Fasciotomy is beneficial where there is increased compartmental pressure (compartmental syndrome) due to:
- Bleeding
- Cellular swelling
- Interstitial edema
- External compression.

Thus, fasciotomy is indicated in arterial embolic and thrombotic occlusion; arterial and venous injury; following

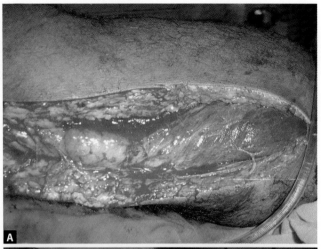

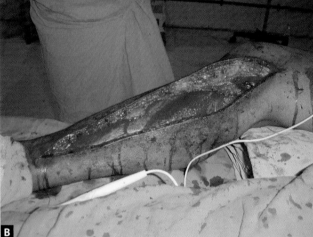

**Figs 5A and B** (A) Unhealthy pale edematous muscles which are non-viable; (B) Healthy muscles at fasciotomy

fractures; crush injury; venous thrombosis; drug injection; snake bite; tight fitting casts, burns, etc.

If the muscle is dead, then fasciotomy will not bring the muscle back to life.

Heparin anticoagulation helps in:
- Reducing thrombosis
- Lessens chances of venous thromboembolism
- Reduces microvascular permeability and interstitial edema
- Shuts down the local inflammatory response
- Improves collateral blood flow
- Lowers the level of demarcation in limbs with irreversible damage.

To have an effect in poorly perfused tissue, very large doses of heparin are used—the same as for cardiopulmonary bypass. By this, there will be:
- Drop in the level of skin demarcation
- Reduction of pain

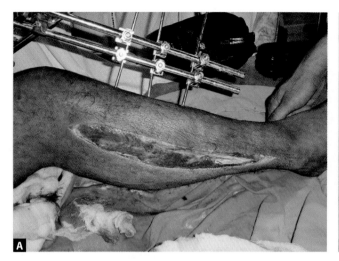

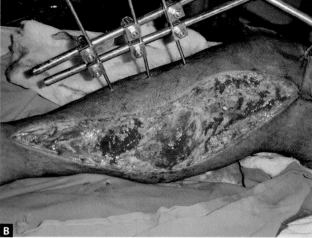

**Figs 6A and B** (A) Lateral compartment fasciotomy; (B) Medial compartment fasciotomy

- Once the vascular spasm is controlled by high heparin dose within 24–48 h, more conventional doses may be used.

  These high heparin doses may not be possible if fasciotomy or revascularization is contemplated.

## Treatment of Systemic Complications of Reperfusion

More than 4 hours of ischemia affecting a large area of the muscle presents potential for development of life-threatening complications following reperfusion. There is large amount of toxic substances released from the ischemic muscles responsible for the local and systemic life-threatening complications.

Limbs subjected to life-threatening ischemia for 6–8 h should have amputation to avoid exposing the body to life-threatening complications. As amputation is a major decision, ischemia was further classified as follows:

- *Mild ischemia*—cool pale limb with no impairment of loss of sensation or impaired muscle function—all tissues are viable and reperfusion is safe with little to no problems.
- *Moderate ischemia*—painful and cold limb, which is soft or slightly firm. The impaired sensation is limited to toes and distal foot. On dependency, the skin capillaries that fill are pink. Here, the extensive tissue necrosis is unlikely. Anticoagulation or operative revascularization is possible. This is because the toxic substances are minimal and the arteriolar vasospasm will soon reverse to allow collaterals to open and improve the blood supply. The risk of systemic complications following surgical reperfusion is 15–25%.
- *Severe ischemia*—the limb has severe pain, loss of sensation, and muscular paralysis. Muscle rigidity and blue mottled skin develops in 6–8 h following onset

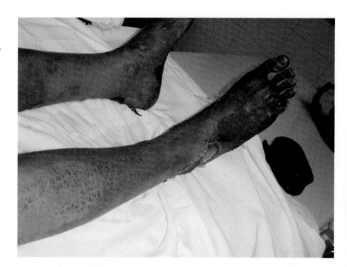

**Fig. 7** Progressive increasing ischemia as we go distally

of symptoms and are signs of irreversibility. Severe ischemia is mostly associated with embolic occlusion of traumatic injury where there is little chance for collaterals to develop—the risk of reperfusion is only acceptable if the limb is reperfused within 4–6 h of ischemia. Beyond this time, the surgery may or may not be successful but is associated with high mortality (Fig. 7).

### Practical Points

- If the bulk of the muscle is involved, it may be wiser to amputate the leg rather than risk toxins from entering the circulation and promoting sepsis and possible death.

- Anticoagulation is the best method to prevent progressive thrombosis of collaterals that supply ischemic but viable muscles—mild and moderate ischemia patients. By this technique, there may be a higher rate of limb loss but much lower mortality.
- If amputation is necessary, it is essential to allow maximum collaterals to develop, as it provides the best chance to stump healing at the level selected (Fig. 8).

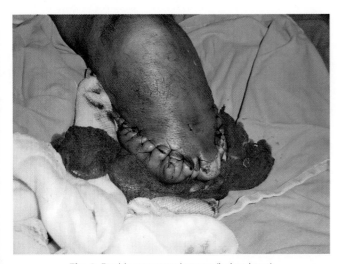

**Fig. 8**  Freshly amputated stump (below knee)

### Recent Advances

- Newer inflammatory mediators' antagonists are being produced in an attempt to reduce the toxic effects of reperfusion.
- There are agents capable of modifying inflammation—antioxidants, antithromboxanes, antileukotrienes, and antiplatelet activating factors. They have shown promise in experiments but not clinically.

### ■ CONCLUSION

- Favorable outcome is to establish quick and complete blood flow
- The greater the magnitude of ischemic tissue, the worse the prognosis
- Embolectomy is the procedure of choice in class IIb and III ischemias
- The general approaches to ischemic limb are:
  - Rapid diagnosis and establishing the ischemic class and prompt anticoagulation therapy (aspirin and IV heparin)
  - Determining the therapeutic approach—embolectomy or emergency bypass versus angiogram and thrombolysis
  - Remember to save life over limb—emergency primary amputation to save life
  - Adjunctive therapy GIIb/IIIa antagonists, use of thrombin inhibitors, and newer devices for percutaneous mechanical revascularization are being tested and appear promising.

## PRACTICAL POINTS

- History and examination help determine the cause and plan the therapy.
- Pulse examination is a must—especially femoral pulse status and Doppler examination.
- Immediate aspirin and therapeutic heparin and careful hydration are a must for all ALI cases.
- Surgical embolectomy is best for embolic ALI in most cases.
- Endovascular therapy is good for thrombosis in situ of native vessel or bypass graft and cases in which etiology of ALI is unclear.

# 7

# Management of Chronic Critical Limb Ischemia

*Jaisom Chopra*

## ■ INTRODUCTION

Peripheral vascular disease progresses through various stages starting from asymptomatic, leading to intermittent claudication (IC) and finally landing up as limb-threatening ischemia with severe rest pain, ulceration, and possibly gangrene. This limb-threatening ischemia is referred to as critical limb ischemia (CLI). 15–20% of the IC patients progress onto CLI, and 3–10% of the population over 50 years are suffering from CLI globally.

The sequence of events is as below:

> Atherosclerosis > Ischemia > Limb pain > Functional loss > Gangrene > Amputation

Critical limb ischemia is characterized by:
- Persistent rest pain with or without tissue loss. Burning pain in the arch or distal foot occurs at night with the patient lying and relieved by dependency
- Ankle-brachial index (ABI) of 0.4 or less
- Ankle pressures <40 mm Hg (systolic) and
- Toe pressures <30 mm Hg
- The transcutaneous tissue oxygen concentration ($TCPO_2$) is <50 mm Hg.

## Natural History

Critical limb ischemia almost exclusively involved atherosclerotic lower limb. The disease is always multilevel and multisegmental.

## Risk Factors

- Smoking
- Diabetes—10 times more likely to have amputation than nondiabetics at a younger age. 40% of the diabetic CLI patients get gangrene compared with 9% nondiabetics

- Smoking + diabetes worsens the risk even further
- Increasing age
- Male gender
- Hyperlipidemia
- Hyperhomocysteinemia.

## Prognosis in CLI

- The prognosis is poor due to the diffuse nature of the disease and the additional factors like cardiac, pulmonary, cerebrovascular, and renal disease involvement.
- The mortality rate is 10% per year.
- Primary amputation rates are 25% and rise even further at the end of 6 months.
- Those unsuitable for reconstructive surgery—20% had amputation at 1 month, 30% at 3 months, and 46% at 1 year.
- The perioperative mortality of amputation in CLI is 10% for below knee amputation.
- The quality of life is considered like that of a terminally ill patient.
- The cost incurred by patient with CLI is very high (about $ 47,000 in US).

## ■ CLINICAL FEATURES

- The main clinical features are rest pain, ulceration, and gangrene (Fig. 1).
- Skin changes—dry skin with loss of hair, thickened nails, and loss of subcutaneous fat (Fig. 2).
- The pain is burning in nature in distal foot and toes and severe at night. The patient dangles his foot for relief.
- Over time there is pedal edema due to dependency and dependent rubor (Fig. 3).
- Ischemic ulcers occur on the sole at the head of the first and fifth metatarsal heads. They do not bleed and are very painful. They heal very poorly. They are considered

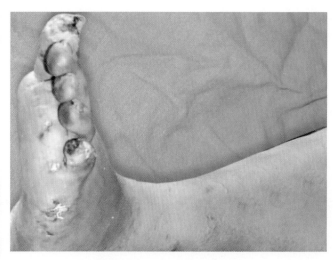

**Fig. 1** Ulceration and gangrene

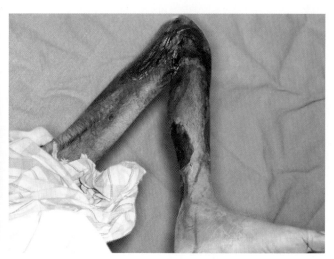

**Fig. 2** Dry skin with loss of subcutaneous fat

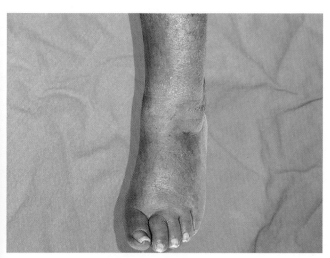

**Fig. 3** Dependency rubor

nonhealing as they persist from 4 to 12 weeks despite regular dressings, treatment of infection, avoidance of trauma, and regular debridement.

Gangrene finally occurs due to tissue necrosis.

## Differential Diagnosis

- Night cramps—awaken the patient from sleep and present in the calf muscles relieved by massaging, walking, or antispasmodic medication.
- Arthritis of the metatarsal bones—occurs at night and relieved by standing. It occurs intermittently and sporadically.
- Diabetic neuropathy—reduced pulses with trophic skin changes. It may or may not come on with decumbency. Then there is loss of light touch (monofilament test) and reduced vibratory sense.

## ◼ DIAGNOSTIC EVALUATION

The accurate diagnosis is reached by examination and appropriate investigation to predict the extent of arterial disease and prognosis for limb survival. Pulse status tells us about the nature of treatment required. If the femoral pulse is absent then we know the patient has aortoiliac disease and percutaneous transluminal angioplasty (PTA) or aortofemoral bypass may be needed.

## Investigations

### Evaluation of CLI Prior to Imaging

This is routine in CLI and includes:
- Ankle-brachial index (ABI)
- Segmental limb pressures (SLP)

  Advantages of SLP—assess the severity and level of peripherical artery disease (PAD).

  Disadvantages of SLP—inaccurate in stiff arteries. One cannot differentiate between stenosis and occlusion.

  Significant occlusion—if the pressure between two segments falls by >20 mm Hg in the same leg or the same segment on the other leg.

  Localization (by where reduction in pressure is seen):
  - Thigh—aortoiliac or SFA disease
  - Calf—distal SFA disease or popliteal disease
  - Ankle—infrapopliteal disease.
- Plethysmography—pulse volume recording or Doppler waveform analysis. Waveforms change from triphasic > biphasic > monophasic > stenotic waveform and are typical of CLI (Fig. 4).

  Advantages—useful in patients with noncompressible vessels.

  Disadvantages—qualitative and not quantitative. It is inaccurate in low stroke volume.

  Segmental Doppler and plethysmography—95% accuracy in localizing and identifying significant occlusions.

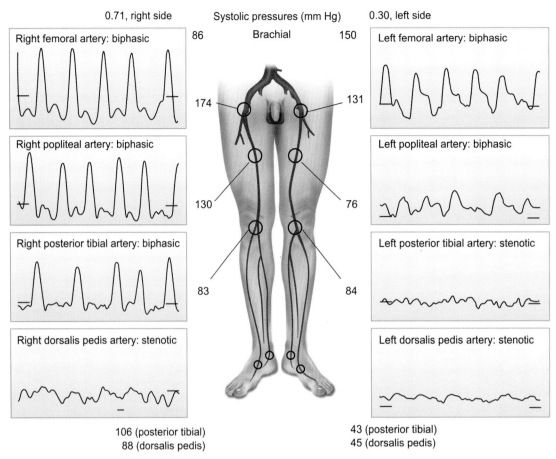

0.71, right side           Systolic pressures (mm Hg)           0.30, left side

Right femoral artery: biphasic        86        Brachial        150        Left femoral artery: biphasic

174        131

Right popliteal artery: biphasic        Left popliteal artery: biphasic

130        76

Right posterior tibial artery: biphasic        Left posterior tibial artery: stenotic

83        84

Right dorsalis pedis artery: stenotic        Left dorsalis pedis artery: stenotic

106 (posterior tibial)        43 (posterior tibial)
88 (dorsalis pedis)        45 (dorsalis pedis)

**Fig. 4** Segmental pressures and ABI in a patient. The right brachial pressure is 86 mm Hg due to subclavian artery stenosis. Therefore, the left arm pressure is taken which is 150 mm Hg. The left ABI is 0.30 with stenotic nonpulsatile waveform in PT and DP arteries

Stenosis causes flattening and widening of waveform seen in PAD.
- Toe-brachial index and waveform.
- Treadmill exercise testing in ambulatory patients and assessing recovery of ankle pressures (Fig. 5).

### Noninvasive Imaging: Duplex Doppler Ultrasound

Critical limb ischemia usually reveals multilevel disease with ankle pressures <50 mm Hg and toe pressures <30 mm Hg.

*Advantages*
- Differentiates occlusions from stenosis
- Assessing severity and location
- Sensitivity and specificity of stenosis >50% is 88–96%.

*Disadvantages*
- Takes a long time
- Dense calcification limits evaluation
- Proximal stenosis limits evaluation
- Operator dependent
- Cannot be used for preoperative mapping.

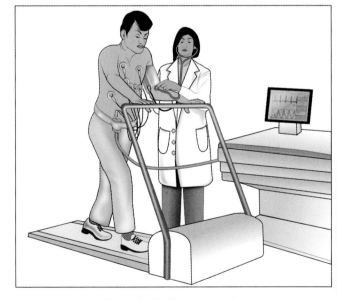

**Fig. 5** Treadmill exercise testing

# Imaging in CLI

## Purpose of Imaging in CLI

- Confirmation of diagnosis
- Localizing and severity of lesion
- Assessment of hemodynamic requirement for successful revascularization
- Assessment of patient's endovascular/operative risk.

This is only carried out once the decision is made to revascularize the limb, otherwise not. Routinely angiogram along with digital subtraction angiography (DSA) is done. Though this is presently considered the gold standard but new modalities are becoming popular like 3-D gadolinium-based magnetic resonance angiography (MRA). However, MRA is not very effective for pedal arteries in distal bypasses because of delayed contrast arrival, motion artifacts, and rapid arterial venous transit. For pedal bypass, DSA is currently the best. Then, there is computerized tomographic angiogram (CTA) (Table 1).

## Assessment for Other Conditions

Because atherosclerosis is a generalized disease, one must examine for coronary artery disease, cerebrovascular disease, and abdominal vascular disease (renal artery, mesenteric artery, and aneurismal disease).

- Carotid and abdominal ultrasound
- Venous ultrasound if necessary.

## ◼ MANAGEMENT (FLOW CHART 1)

## Conservative Management

This includes risk factor modification including:

- Smoking cessation
- Blood pressure control
- Good glycemic control
- Reduction of lipid levels.

Aspirin reduces the risk of MI, CVA, and death in patients with PAD and also reduces the risk of arterial reocclusion after angioplasty or bypass grafting.

## Ischemic Rest Pain

Give the patient pain medication as needed and correct the cause of inadequate blood flow like cardiac failure. This treatment is given for 4–8 weeks and if pain still persists then one must consider operative intervention. The patient must be told of all the risks and the benefits.

Operative intervention consists of revascularization and amputation. If revascularization is considered then angiography is done to assist further planning. MRA is a good acceptable alternative.

## Nonhealing Wounds

These patients should be evaluated for infection and if present, need antibiotics, surgical debridement, or both. The patient is taught to avoid trauma and ill-fitting shoes.

We consider surgical intervention if:

- Conservative treatment does not lead to improvement as shown by:
  - Increasing wound size
  - Persisting or spreading infection
  - No evidence of healing after 4–8 weeks
  - Progressive gangrene
  - Continuous severe rest pain unrelieved by dependency.

About 40% of the patients with CLI have limb loss in 3 years but 60% are spared.

## Medical and Pharmacological Approach to CLI (Flow chart 2)

Mostly the treatment of CLI is either surgical or endovascular but conservative treatment is justified under the following circumstances:

- Intermittent rest pain with minor skin loss
- Awaiting more definite measures
- Revascularization measures are too risky or not possible.

**Table 1** Magnetic resonance angiography versus computerized tomographic angiogram

| MRA | CTA |
| --- | --- |
| **Advantages** | **Advantages** |
| Assesses location and degree of stenosis and selects cases for intervention | Fast scan times |
| More accurate for detecting stenosis and preoperative planning than US | Works in those with contra-indication to MRA |
| Sensitivity and specificity are 95% and 97% for stenosis >50% | Sensitivity and specificity are 91% and 91% for stenosis >50% |
| More accurate in heavily calcified vessels and thus better in patients >84 years and diabetics | Images soft tissue surrounding vessels |
| | Localizes PAD and selects cases for intervention |
| **Disadvantages** | **Disadvantages** |
| Costly | Requires contrast and ionization radiation |
| Motion artifact | |
| Overestimates degree of stenosis | |
| Loss of signals in arterial segments with metal clips and stents | |
| Usual MRI contraindications apply | |
| Small risk of nephrogenic systemic fibrosis (NSF) | |

**Flow chart 1** Plan of managing critical limb ischemia

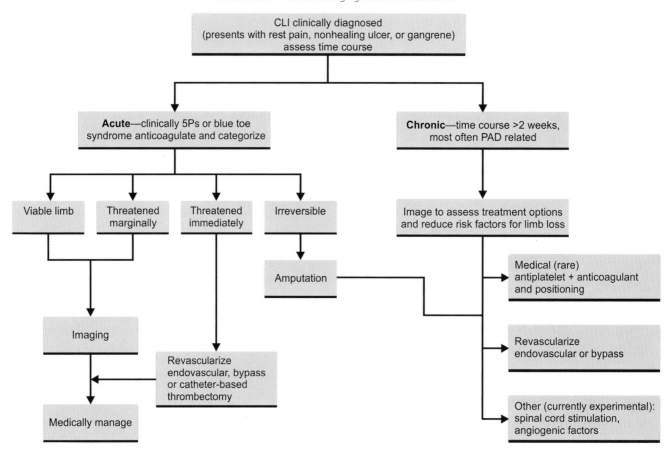

*Medical treatment includes:*

1. Pain control—assess it at every visit and record on a scale of 1–10. The only relief from pain is by revascularization or amputation but pain relief is needed during the planning of these measures. Narcotics are often needed for total pain relief.
2. Footwear and ulcer care—proper footwear avoids trauma to an ischemic limb. The guidelines of ischemic ulcer care include:
   - Keep area very clean
   - Saline dressings three to four times a day with weeping ulcers
   - Dry dressings once the ulcer is dry
   - No excessive debridement or topical antibiotics
   - May need recombinant human platelet-derived growth factor BB (rhPDGF-BB) at night time, if ulcer is not infected.
- Antibiotics—this is indicated for cellulitis or superadded infection when the area surrounding the wound is red and tender. Wound infection is mostly polymicrobial, especially in diabetics. Its use should not delay definitive treatment.

- Specific pharmacotherapy in CLI—no drug has shown promising results in reducing the morbidity and mortality or limb loss in CLI.
  - Prostanoids—this is prostaglandin E1, which is a potent vasodilator. The results are better if administered for 4 weeks rather than a short time. Iloprost, a derivative of prostacyclin, showed reduction of amputation rate from 39% in those on placebo to 23% in those on iloprost, justifying its use in those with failed revascularization or those unsuitable for revascularization.
  - Angiogenic growth factor in CLI has shown promising results.
  - Adenoviral gene therapy.
  - Vascular endothelial growth factor.
  - Hypoxia inducible growth factor.

## Adjunctive Measures

Since the most common cause of CLI is atherosclerosis, which puts these patients at high risk of cardiovascular

**Flow chart 2** Plan of managing long standing critical limb ischemia

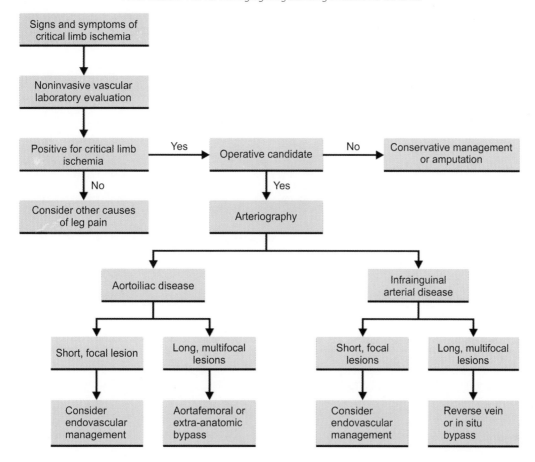

events, they should be put on antiplatelet drugs and statins unless contraindicated.

- Antiplatelets—they are aspirin and clopidogrel groups, and no trial has been conducted in CLI to compare the efficacy of these two drugs.
- Statins—trials suggest they reduce the amputation rate in PAD. Their role in CLI is not proven as yet.
- Anticoagulation—no trials have tested the use of anticoagulation in CLI. Anticoagulation for 3 months following bypass grafting is acceptable to prevent acute graft thrombosis and thromboembolic complications. Long-term anticoagulation is indicated in problematic surgeries like below knee grafting or patients who have atrial fibrillation or low ejection fraction. There is some evidence that low molecular weight heparin (LMWH) at 2500 U/day for 3 months is better than aspirin and dipyridamole in maintaining femoropopliteal graft patency in CLI patients undergoing salvage surgery.
- Vasoactive drugs—like cilostazol—no trials to show the efficacy of this drug in CLI.

## Percutaneous Therapy in CLI

Since CLI is a multilevel and multisegmental disease, it is difficult to generalize the optimal therapy and revascularization decision needs to be tailored according to the patient's findings. Both percutaneous and surgical treatment has roles in CLI. Whatever treatment is chosen, one must strike a balance between maximum durability and minimal risk. Very high-risk patients may require primary amputation. CLI mostly involves both the inflow and outflow vessels.

## Aortoiliac Percutaneous Transluminal Angioplasty with or without Stenting (Figs 6A and B)

This is the treatment of choice for localized stenotic lesions <3 cm long (TASC type A) in the iliac segment. CLI is very unlikely to occur because of a solitary lesion in the iliac segment and is almost always multifocal (TASC type C or D)

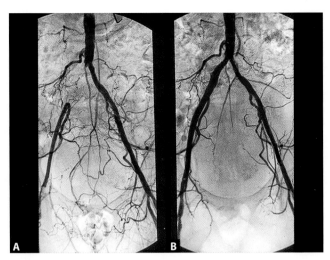

**Figs 6A and B** (A) Occlusion of right iliac artery; (B) Right iliac artery patent after insertion of stent

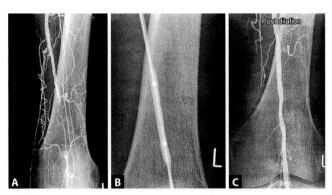

**Figs 7A to C** (A) Short occlusion Left popliteal artery; (B) Balloon catheter passed through occlusion; (C) Final result—artery patent with normal flow through it

**Table 2** Primary patency rates for angioplasty and stenting of iliac artery stenosis and occlusion

|  | Patients | Percent with IC | Technical success % | 1 year | 3 years | 5 years |
|---|---|---|---|---|---|---|
| PTA iliac stenosis | 1,264 | 77 | 95 | 78 | 66 | 61 |
| PTA iliac occlusion | 291 | 82 | 83 | 68 | 60 | – |
| Stent iliac stenosis | 1,365 | 78 | 99 | 90 | 74 | 72 |
| Stent iliac occlusion | 187 | 86 | 82 | 72 | 64 | – |

**Table 3** Primary patency rates for angioplasty and stenting of femoropopliteal stenosis and stenting

|  | Patients | Percent with IC | Technical success (%) | 1 year | 3 years | 5 years |
|---|---|---|---|---|---|---|
| PTA femoropopliteal stenosis and occlusion | 1241 | 72 | 90 | 61 | 51 | 48 |
| Stents femoropopliteal stenosis and occlusion | 585 | 80 | 98 | 67 | 58 | – |

along with infrapopliteal disease. TPA alone leads to elastic recoil and dissection and is preferable to do stenting along with PTA. The technical success rate was 95% with patency rates at 1 and 5 years of 80% and 60%, respectively. Short distance iliac occlusions are dealt with by TPA with 82% technical success rate and 60% patency at 3 years (Table 2).

## Femoropopliteal PTA and Stenting (Figs 7A to C)

Since CLI is a multilevel and multifactorial disease, the PTA results are not very encouraging. In patients with IC undergoing PTA, the initial technical success rate is 90%, whereas the 1 and 5-year primary patency rates are 60% and <50%, respectively. In CLI, they are much worse. The primary patency rates are listed (Table 3).

Several factors alter the success of PTA in femoropopliteal artery:
- Lesion length <3 cm (TASC A lesions) have much better results than longer ones.
- Occlusions have a poorer technical success rate compared with stenosis. However, once the occlusion is opened then it has the same long-term success rate as a stenosis.
- Eccentric and heavily calcified lesions have poor chances of success.
- The runoff is one of the most important predictors of long-term patency. Patients with two to three vessel runoff have far greater success in the long-term than those with one or no vessel runoff at 2–3 years (71–78% vs. 25–37%).
- Patient with associated disease like diabetes and renal failure adversely affect the outcome of intervention.

## Infrapopliteal PTA

This is not recommended as a standard stratagy because of the multilevel and multifactorial nature with occlusions and stenoses along with a poor runoff in CLI. There are occasional studies that claim an 80% limb salvage rate at 2 years.

## Surgical Therapy in CLI

### Aortoiliac Revascularization in CLI (Fig. 8)

The most frequently performed procedures are aorto-bifemoral bypasses or extra-anatomic (axillobifemoral or

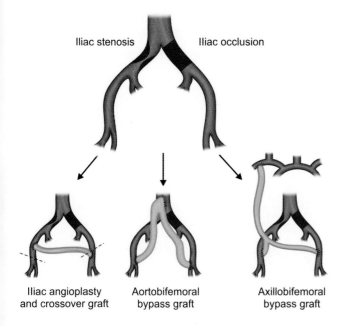

**Fig. 8** Various options in the surgical treatment of iliac occlusive disease

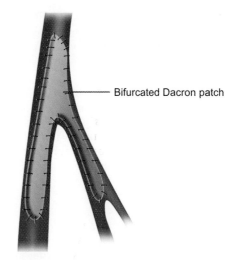

**Fig. 9** A vein patch of synthetic Dacron patch to prevent narrowing of the vessel

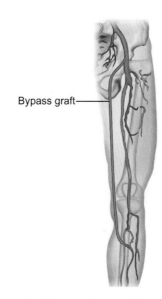

**Fig. 10** Femoropopliteal bypass with the graft inserted below the knee

femorofemoral) bypasses. The 5-year patency rates for aortobifemoral bypass are 80–90%.

Generally, an end-to-side approach is preferred as it maintains the blood to the IMA and to the IIA. However, if the aorta is aneurysmal or source of emboli then and end-to-end anastomosis is preferable. Is retroperitoneal or transperitoneal approach better? No patency differences have been demonstrated by either retroperitoneal or transperitoneal approach. Nor has any patency differences been shown between end-to-end and end-to-side anastomosis. The morbidity in aortobifemoral bypass is 5–10%, whereas the mortality is 1–5%. For the very sick who cannot undergo aortobifemoral bypass, extra-anatomic bypass is advised. An axillobifemoral bypass is for bilateral disease and femorofemoral bypass for unilateral disease. With improved techniques and improved grafts, the 5-year patency rates of axillofemoral bypass are 50–75%.

### Adjunctive Profundoplasty (Fig. 9)

The profunda femoris artery and its collaterals are a major source of blood supply to the leg in patients with occluded SFA. About 49% of CLI cases have occluded SFA arteries. One must look for stenosis of the profunda femoris by taking oblique views at angiography as the profunda arises postero-laterally from the femoral artery.

Profundoplasty is a low morbidity procedure performed:
- When there is a stenosis in the presence of SFA occlusion and CLI.
- Aortoiliac disease needing AFB.
- Failure of distal bypass to improve limb salvage.

## Infrainguinal Revascularization in CLI (Fig. 10)

Most CLI cases have critical infrainguinal disease. The most important factor determining the long-term patency in CLI is the type of conduit used. Autogenous vein is always the preferred conduit whenever possible. Reverse autogenous vein and in situ vein have same patency rates. The long saphenous vein (LSV) is always the first choice. If not available then the other veins that can be used are discussed further.
- Basilic vein
- Cephalic vein
- Short saphenous vein
- Superficial femoral vein.

Synthetic *conduits* are very inferior to veins and are only used when veins are not available. Always perform a duplex scan to assess the vein to be used for conduit. We are looking for:

- The veins of 4 mm diameter are preferable but up to 3 mm are acceptable.
- Thick walled and poorly distensible—give unsatisfactory results.

The site of *proximal anastomosis* is chosen depending on the length of vein available. The only requirement for this is unimpeded pulsatile flow. The most common site is common femoral artery though SFA and profunda femoris are equally effective. The inflow must be uncompromised. Even minor stenosis proximally must be corrected to prevent eventual graft failure.

The choice of the *distal anastomosis* is based on angiographic findings done preoperatively. It is dependent on the quality of the artery and the distal runoff. Femoral to below knee bypass and distal bypasses yield similar results being dependent on the quality of the artery and its distal runoff. It is not dependent on the length of the graft. Popliteal artery is chosen if it is minimally diseased and there is good tibial runoff. However, if popliteal artery is diseased then the tibial artery is chosen, which is minimally diseased and the runoff beyond the site is good. Bypass to an isolated popliteal artery segment is not recommended unless the distal runoff is very poor or the venous graft is limited. If bypass is to be performed to the tibial arteries then which tibial artery is to be used depends on the angiographic findings? Intraoperatively finding calcification should not make one. Abandon the procedure if the angiographic findings suggest a satisfactory lumen and there is good distal runoff (Table 4). If popliteal artery is diseased then the tibial artery is chosen which is minimally diseased and the run-off is good (Table 5).

*In reverse vein bypass grafting*, the vein is used as a conduit. It is harvested by directly incising the skin over it. It is important to find out the length of the usable vein as it would dictate the levels of the proximal and the distal anastomosis (Table 6). The common femoral artery and its bifurcation are exposed and if needed the inguinal ligament is divided to gain access to the external iliac artery. A median knee incision is made to expose the above knee and below knee popliteal artery. The posterior tibial and peroneal arteries are exposed from the medial approach. The anterior tibial artery is approached through calf lateral to the tibia. The foot arteries are approached by an incision directly over the artery—posterior tibial and dorsalis pedis. The vein is reversed so that the flow is not hampered.

*In situ vein bypass grafting* is always done from the same side LSV. The proximal end is anastomosed to the femoral artery and the distal end to the popliteal or tibial artery. The vein match is superior to the reversed technique. A special valve cutter is used to divide all the valves without damaging the vein wall. An operative completion angiogram is done to see any residual vein valves and AV fistulas.

**Table 4** Patency and limb salvage rates for femorodistal (infrapopliteal) bypass

| | 1 year | 2 years | 4 years |
|---|---|---|---|
| **Patency rates** | | | |
| Reverse LSV graft | 77% | 70% | 62% |
| In situ vein graft | 82% | 76% | 68% |
| Arm vein | 73% | 62% | - |
| Human umbilical vein | 52% | 46% | 37% |
| Synthetic PTFE graft | 46% | 32% | 21% |
| **Limb salvage rates** | | | |
| Reverse LSV graft | 85% | 83% | 82% |
| In situ vein graft | 91% | 88% | 83% |
| Synthetic PTFE graft | 68% | 60% | 48% |

**Table 5** Patency and limb salvage rates for below knee femoropopliteal bypass in critical limb ischemia

| | 1 year | 2 years | 4 years |
|---|---|---|---|
| **Patency rates** | | | |
| Reverse LSV graft | 84% | 79% | 77% |
| In situ vein | 80% | 76% | 68% |
| Arm vein | 83% | 83% | 70% |
| Human umbilical vein | 77% | 70% | 60% |
| Synthetic PTFE graft | 68% | 61% | 40% |
| **Limb salvage rates** | | | |
| Reverse LSV graft | 90% | 88% | 75% |
| In situ vein graft | 94% | 84% | – |

**Table 6** Patency rates for above knee femoropopliteal grafts in critical limb ischemia

| | 1 year | 2 years | 5 years |
|---|---|---|---|
| Reverse LSV graft | 84% | 82% | 69% |
| Arm vein graft | 82% | 65% | 60% |
| Human umbilical vein graft | 82% | 82% | 70% |
| Synthetic polytetrafluoroethylene (PTFE) graft | 79% | 74% | 60% |

Human umbilical vein grafts may be used if LSV is unavailable and it is risky to use synthetic graft due to high chances of infection.

*Patency and limb salvage with infrainguinal revascularization* mainly depends on length of the graft and the distal anastomosis.

## Postoperative Follow-up

Diligent follow-up is mandatory as these patients have recurrent limb specific and cardiovascular problems. The patient is seen 3 monthly for the first year and then 6 monthly. At each visit:

- Palpate peripheral pulses
- Rest and exercise ABIs. Fall in ABI by 0.15 is an indication for graft revision
- Color Doppler study to identify areas of stenosis within the graft or the native vessel proximal or distal to the graft. A focal peak systolic velocity over 300 cm/s or a pre to intrastenotic velocity greater than 3.5 is an indication for revision of the graft.

Graft stenosis occurs because of fibrointimal hyperplasia, fibrosis of the valve site, or atherosclerosis may cause graft thrombosis or failure. Once the vein graft has thrombosed, it rarely can be salvaged. Sometimes, the graft occlusion leaves the patient with ischemia worse than before the insertion of the graft. To find another vein graft also becomes a problem. Thus, early detection of graft stenosis is an indication for graft revision. Using all these measures including diligent follow-up, the limb salvage rate at 5 years is 91% and 94% for synthetic graft and vein.

### Management of Failing Grafts

Routine and diligent follow-up of CLI patients is done:

- Using palpation of pulses
- Resting and exercise ABI
- Color Doppler study helps to detect patients with lesions within the graft and in the native vessel
- These patients should have diagnostic angiography followed by intervention.

The successful surgical techniques are:

- PTA
- Patch angioplasty
- Segmental vein resection and interposition of vein graft
- Since synthetic grafts produce suboptimal images on color Doppler study, a fall in ABI is sufficient criteria to ask for diagnostic angiography. Stenosis of the inflow or outflow vessels can be treated by PTA or surgery but if there is stenosis within the graft, it is best to revise the graft surgically.

### Primary Amputation (Fig. 11)

Indications in CLI:

- No possibility of revascularization and there is tissue loss and gangrene.
- Ulceration and necrosis of plantar aspect of digits, metatarsophalangeal joints and heel account for 75% of primary amputations.
- Nonambulatory elderly with multiple crippling diseases and rest pain with tissue loss.

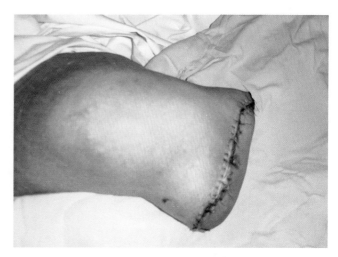

**Fig. 11** Below knee amputation

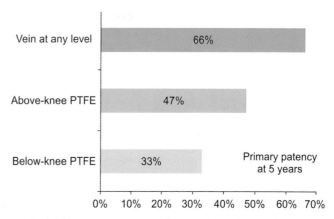

**Fig. 12** Five-year patency rates for vein and synthetic grafts in CLI

Revascularization and debridement of necrotic muscles and tissue followed by myocutaneous flaps involves multiple procedures over a period of 6 months. Despite these aggressive efforts a functional foot is obtained in 50–86% cases at a very high cost. Thus, aggressive vascular reconstruction efforts are not recommended.

## Functional Outcomes

### Following Revascularization (Fig. 12)

Almost all the studies so far used graft patency, limb salvage, and patient survival parameters to review the outcome. These parameters only record the functional outcome and do not tell us about the patient satisfaction. It is now seen that 50% of the patient feel that they are completely cured and achieve ideal surgical results (uncomplicated operation with elimination of symptoms, maintenance of functional status, no recurrence of ischemia, or need for further surgery). The rest 50% have perioperative complications needing repeated hospitalization for wound care, redo vascularization, and poor recovery of functional status.

## Following Amputation

Postoperative ambulation following below knee amputation (BKA) is higher than above knee amputation (AKA). Mobility after any amputation (BKA or AKA) remains poor and only one-third were ambulatory at 17 months follow-up.

## ■ SUMMARY

Critical limb ischemia is an infrequent complication of atherosclerosis and may present with severe rest pain and a threatened limb. The severity of the disease is determined by color Doppler study with angiography reserved for planning treatment options. Surgical revascularization and endovascular techniques remain the mainstay of the treatment options and are possible in a majority of the patients. The use of autogenous conduit is preferred over synthetic bypass whenever possible. Although bypass graft patency and limb salvage are achievable as goals, the impact of procedures on pateint's quality of life is less defined.

## PRACTICAL POINTS

- Critical limb ischemia is a multilevel and multisegmental disease needing multimodality approach to successful management.
- Femoropopliteal and infrapopliteal PTA have high failure rates in CLI and not recommended.
- Good autogenous vein conduit has shown best patency results for femoropopliteal and femorodistal bypasses. A good vein with less optimal anastomotic sites is more likely to succeed than optimal anastomotic sites and poor venous conduit.
- Preoperative color Doppler vein marking is indicated to find a suitable vein for grafting. By this, unneccessary incisions are avoided.
- Long saphenous vein is the preferred conduit but if not available then basilic or cephalic vein from the arm is used or the short saphenous vein from the leg.
- Prosthetic bypasses are used only when veins are unavailable.
- The site of proximal anastomosis is chosen depending on the length of available vein.
- Profunda femoris is an excellent site when:
  - Common femoral artery is not available.
  - It is less frequently affected by arterial calcification.
  - It is easier to find in complicated reoperative surgery.
  - Allows a more distal proximal anastomotic site when the vein site is suboptimal.

The choice of distal anastomosis is based on preoperative angiographic findings.

The peroneal artery is the least affected tibial vessel by atherosclerosis and graft patency and limb salvage are comparable to those in the more distal pedal bypasses.

# 8

# Buerger's Disease (Thromboangiitis Obliterans)

*Jaisom Chopra*

*The true story of my life. I have Buerger's Disease. Cigarettes didn't do this to me. I did it myself. Smoking Got Me. I lost.*

## ■ INTRODUCTION

It goes after the name of the New York Surgeon, Leo Buerger, who described 11 cases in 1908 with highly cellular nature of thrombus and perivascular inflammation that made him suggest thromboangiitis obliterans (TAO).

It is a rare disease of the arteries and the veins in the arms and the legs. The blood vessels swell and block by thrombi. This damages the skin tissue leading to infection and gangrene (Fig. 1).

Everyone with Buerger's disease either smokes cigarettes or chews tobaccos. Quitting all forms of tobacco is the only way to stop Buerger's disease. For those who do not quit, amputation of part of the limb or whole of it is the final result.

Buerger's disease or thromboangiitis obliterans is a:
- Nonatherosclerotic inflammatory vasculitis
- It involves the medium and small arteries, veins, and nerves
- It involves both the upper and lower extremities
- It is most commonly seen in young male smokers
- Recently, there is an increasing incidence in young females
- Patients present with distal digital ischemia involving multiple extremities and need amputation.

The etiology remains elusive and there is a very high degree of association with smoking. It is a chronic and progressive disease with little treatment options except giving up smoking. Despite the poor prognosis, the life expectancy is not affected in this disease.

## ■ EPIDEMIOLOGY

It affects people all over the world, though it is more common in the Asian community and less so in blacks.

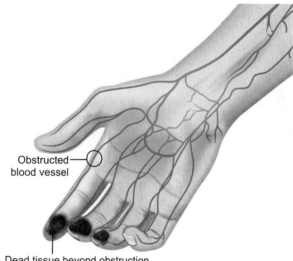

**Fig. 1** Diminished blood supply causes damage and death of tissue

Although considered a disease of the young male smokers, the involvement of females has progressively increased over the years due to smoking and now accounts for 8–23%. The incidence of Buerger's disease has progressively fallen over the years that could be due to the improvement in diagnostic techniques and also declining incidence of smokers.

## ■ ETIOLOGY

The cause of Buerger's remains unknown, though there is a direct association with tobacco use even in casual and passive smokers. Measurement of urine cotinine, a nicotine metabolite, monitors tobacco exposure in uncertain cases and correlates with recurrence of disease.

How tobacco causes Buerger's disease is not known but is thought to damage the vascular endothelium and develop autoantibodies to the endothelium.

It is considered an autoimmune disease because of:
- Deposition of autoantibodies, complement C3, has been demonstrated within the vessel wall in Buerger's disease patients.
- T3 lymphocytes showing cellular sensitivity to type II and type III collagens.

## ■ CLINICAL PRESENTATION (TABLE 1)

- Involves young male smokers 20–40 years of age
- There is an increasing incidence in females
- Exposure to tobacco is universal, most being heavy smokers
- Pain and weakness in feet and legs and hands and arms
- Swelling in the hands and feet
- Fingers and toes turn pale when exposed to cold (Raynaud's phenomenon)
- Open sores on toes and fingers
- Claudication, rest pain, and ulceration are often the initial presentation of the disease
- The small vessels are often involved causing distal ischemia that spreads proximally and there is super-infection present
- Involvement of multiple limbs including the upper limbs is often seen
- Venous involvement may be present before the arterial involvement with migratory phlebitis.

**Table 1** Clinical presentation in three large clinical trials

| | Olin et al. | Sasaki et al. | Shionoya |
|---|---|---|---|
| **Demographic data** | | | |
| Mean age at presentation (years) | 42 | 40 | 36 |
| Gender | | | |
| Male (%) | 77 | 91 | 98 |
| Female (%) | 23 | 9 | 2 |
| Clinical presentation | | | |
| Raynaud's phenomenon (%) | 44 | – | 37 |
| Claudication (%) | 62 | 38 | 31 |
| Rest pain (%) | 81 | 24 | 16 |
| Gangrene or Ulceration (%) | 76 | 45 | 18–72 |
| Superficial thrombophlebitis (%) | 38 | 16 | 3–43 |
| Upper extremity involvement (%) | 54 | 25 | 90 |

## ■ CLINICAL COURSE

- With continued tobacco use, the disease progresses proximally
- Smoking cessation ensures a benign course
- About 25% undergo amputation
- Rarely, it involves the visceral, coronary, and cerebral arteries with a fatal outcome
- Most patients with Buerger's have a normal life expectancy.

## ■ DIAGNOSIS

This is based on clinical findings. Five criteria are recommended:
1. Smoking
2. Onset before 50 years
3. Infrapopliteal arterial occlusive disease
4. Upper or lower extremity involved or phlebitis migrans
5. Absence of atherosclerotic risk factors other than smoking.

The criteria that make the diagnosis doubtful:
- Ischemic heart disease
- Cerebrovascular disease
- Hypercoagulable states
- Collagen vascular disease.

## Investigations

Angiographic findings in Buerger's disease:
- Severe segmental occlusive disease involving distal lower and upper limb arteries
- Iliacs and femorals are involved in 10% of advanced cases
- Areas of stenosis or occlusion with normal arteries in between
- Abundant collaterals—corkscrew or tree-root in appearance
- Distal vessels are thin with abrupt occlusions
- No aneurysms or atherosclerosis that leads to distal emboli.

Laboratory tests have a limited role. Other vasculopathies and hypercoagulable states are ruled out by serological tests and coagulation profiles.

Biopsy has a limited role and when available shows highly inflammatory thrombus in arteries and veins, inflammation of all three layers of the arteries, and the veins and preservation of the integrity of the internal elastic lamina. In advanced cases, there is extensive fibrosis of the vessel and perivascular areas.

## ■ GENERAL TREATMENT

No treatment can cure Buerger's disease and all treatment is directed reducing the signs and symptoms.

Treatment options are:
- Counseling or medications to help stop smoking and the swelling in the blood vessels

- Medications to improve the blood flow or stop clot formation
- Surgery to cut the nerves in the affected areas (surgical sympathectomy) to control the pain
- Amputation if infection or gangrene occurs.

The cessation of smoking tobacco or tobacco products is a must otherwise all medical or surgical treatment is bound to fail. Even passive smoking and usage of smokeless tobacco will help progression of disease and therefore must be avoided. In a study from Cleveland Clinic, 89 Buerger's patients were followed up. Forty-three of them (48%) stopped smoking and only two of these patients who gave up smoking (5%) underwent amputation, while 46 continued to smoke and of these 22 (42%) had amputation due to progression of disease. Thus, every effort should be made to discourage patients from smoking.

## Lifestyle and Home Remedies

Take care of fingers and toes and check arms and legs daily for cuts and bruises. As sensation is lost in Buerger's, you may not feel the pain of cuts. The low blood flow in this disease prevents cuts from healing and leads to infection. Keep cuts clean and cover with dressings. Be sure that they are healing otherwise see a doctor.

Buerger's disease patients must be asked to avoid injury to the extremities by wearing protective footwear to heels and soles.

Avoid cold and medications that lead to vasoconstriction.

## ■ PREVENTION

## Quit Smoking in Any Form

Smoking in any form is dangerous and helps worsen the disease by swelling the vessels and preventing blood from reaching the tissues. By giving up smoking, the likelihood of amputation reduces markedly. But with continued smoking, the chances of amputation are greatly enhanced.

It is hard to give up smoking. There are medications to ease craving for cigarettes that do not have nicotine, as nicotine patches or gum will only worsen the disease.

A urine test may be ordered to test whether the patient is not smoking.

## ■ MEDICAL THERAPY

## Analgesics

Pain is generally very severe and not controllable till the patient stops smoking and is given narcotic analgesics on a long-term basis. If this is not adequate, then epidural anesthesia is given allowing the patient to elevate the limb and improve the healing as edema lessens. This also allows us to know how the patient will respond to lumbar sympathectomy, if the disease persists. Spinal cord stimulators are used with benefit, as they relieve pain and improve circulation resulting in pain control, wound healing, and limb salvage.

## Immunosuppression

If Buerger's disease is an autoimmune disease, then immunosuppression should be beneficial. Although corticosteroids are of little benefits, but more potent immunosuppressive agents such as cyclophosphamide showed a marked improvement in claudication, rest pain, and ulcer healing. It is not clear how these changes are brought about because parameters such as pulse volume, angiography, and skin temperature remain unaltered. However, there is a reduction in the inflammatory cells within the vessel wall and autoantibody formation, thus helping further immune mediated injury.

## Antiplatelet Therapy

Aspirin has not shown to have much benefit. Prostaglandins are potent vasodilators and antiplatelet agents. Trials were conducted comparing iloprost, a stable prostaglandin analog with low-dose aspirin. Either 6-h IV iloprost was used daily or low-dose aspirin for 28 days. Of the 152 patients present in the study—85% of the iloprost patients had pain relief and healing of the ischemic ulcer compared with 28% of those receiving aspirin. Around 38% of iloprost patients had complete healing of ulcer compared with only 13% in aspirin group. The effect of iloprost lasts 6 months and the amputation rate was 6% compared with aspirin group of 18%. The oral version of iloprost has not been very effective and so only IV version is seen.

## Thrombolytic Therapy

As the basic pathology is inflammatory thrombolysis has no role but in acute exacerbation due to thrombus, thrombolytic therapy may be helpful. Around 58% of the 11 patients with acute exacerbation who underwent thrombolysis with streptokinase showed a reduction in ischemic symptoms, limb salvage, and less extensive amputation.

## Gene Transfer Approaches

Injection of vascular endothelial growth factor, which contains plasmid (ph VEGF 165) is given intramuscularly. The injection is supposed to increase the collateral flow. The increased flow was manifest in patients with ulcers which healed and there was relief of rest pain.

Magnetic Resonance Angiography (MRA) showed an increase in collateral circulation with ph VEGF 165.

# ■ SURGICAL THERAPY

Revascularization—as this is a diffuse segmental occlusive arterial disease affecting the distal vessels, revascularization is rarely an option. If there is proximal occlusion with good runoff, then revascularization may be possible provided the patient has given up smoking. Thromboendarterectomy has no role and is never used. Endovascular techniques are also rarely indicated. Autogenous vein is the conduit of choice. Due to the venous involvement, the long and short saphenous veins may be diseased. The key to success is cessation of smoking. In a study, Sasajima and colleagues used vein bypass in patients who had stopped smoking. Their study contained 71 patients who had bypass for claudication (41%) and rest pain with gangrene (59%). The patency rates at 5 years were 49 and 53%, respectively, achieving 85% limb salvage. The patency in smokers was 35% compared with 67% in nonsmokers.

Sympathectomy—as Buerger's disease has poor options, sympathectomy remains a viable option. The sympathetic nerves are divided to provide vasodilatation to the desired area by removal of the vasoconstrictor tone. By this, the flow increases to the cutaneous vascular beds but not to the muscles. Thus, sympathectomy has no role in claudication but is reserved for those with superficial ulcers and vasospastic disease. The effect of sympathectomy lasts few months to 1–2 years allowing sufficient time for wounds to heal. For upper extremity, cervical sympathectomy is indicated where T2, T3, and lower half of the stellate ganglion are removed. It may be performed via a surgical approach—supraclavicular or axillary or may be performed thoracoscopically. The latter approach has given fewer complications and good results and is fast becoming a procedure of choice for cervical sympathectomy.

In lumbar sympathectomy, entry into the retroperitoneal space and division of L2–L4 lumbar ganglion are done. The complication for cervical approach is Horner's syndrome, while for lumbar sympathectomy, it is retrograde ejaculation.

## Amputation (Table 2)

Early diagnosis and cessation of smoking gives a good prognosis with little limb loss. In continued smoking and disease progression, amputations are common. Although

**Table 2** Amputation distribution in 24 patients (39 limbs) with Buerger's disease

| Part amputated | Number and percentage |
| --- | --- |
| Finger | 6 (15%) |
| Toe | 13 (33%) |
| Transmetatarsal | 4 (10%) |
| Below knee | 14 (36%) |
| Above knee | 2 (5%) |

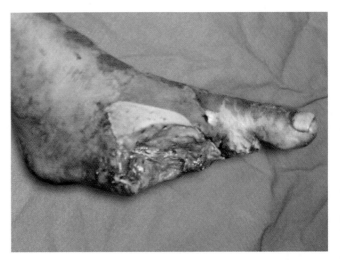

**Fig. 2** Amputated toes in Buerger's disease with skin grafting

most amputations are distal, over 40% needed major amputations (Fig. 2).

# ■ CONCLUSION

Buerger's disease is a nonatherosclerotic inflammatory vasculitis involving the small and medium size arteries, veins, and nerves in the upper and the lower extremity in young male smokers. The cause is unknown, though there is very close correlation to smoking. Although surgical and medical options exist, the main stay of treatment is cessation of smoking. If smoking is not stopped, the prognosis is poor.

# PRACTICAL POINTS

- Buerger's disease (TAO) is nonatherosclerotic inflammatory vasculitis involving the small and medium sized arteries, veins, and nerves of the upper and lower limbs.
- There is a strong and well-established association with smoking.
- Venous involvement is variable and may be present before arterial involvement with migratory phlebitis.
- Angiography shows severe occlusive segmental disease involving the distal vessels in the two extremities. Collaterals are abundant.
- The only effective treatment is to stop smoking.

# 9

# Aortic Dissections

VS Bedi, Anand Chandrasekar, Ajay Yadav, Ambarish Satwik, Kamran Ali Khan

## ■ INTRODUCTION

Acute aortic dissection is one of the most common catastrophic events affecting the aorta like a ruptured abdominal aortic aneurysm. The first report of aortic dissection and the concept of a true and a false lumen are attributed to Shekelton in the early 1800s.[1] Acute dissections can occur in both dilated diseased aortas and aortas of normal diameter in seemingly healthy individuals. Accordingly, the terms *dissection* and *aneurysm* should not be used interchangeably. Dissections can occur in a pre-existing degenerative aneurysm and aneurysms can complicate chronic dissections. The overall mortality associated with acute dissection remains significant despite improvements in both medical and surgical therapeutic options. The annual age-adjusted and sex-adjusted incidences were 3.5 per 100,000 persons (95% confidence interval, 2.4–4.6) for acute aortic dissections in which 85% of cases had ascending aortic involvement.[2] Data from Swedish national healthcare register had shown that the incidence of thoracic aortic disease is 16.3/1,00,000 per year for men and 9.1/1,00,000 per year for women.[3] Death from acute dissection of the ascending aorta is usually secondary to the central cardioaortic complications like aortic rupture into the pericardium, acute aortic regurgitation, and coronary ostial compromise,[4] whereas descending aortic dissections are more commonly associated with death from end-organ compromise secondary to obstruction of visceral or extremity vessels.[5] Meszaros et al. in his series of 86 aortic dissections have described that 21% of patients died before admission itself, whereas 22.7% of the hospitalized patients died within the first 6 h, 33.3% within 12 h, 50% within 24 h, and 68.2% within the first 2 days after admission.[6] This substantial mortality rate in undiagnosed patients underscores the importance of early diagnosis and initiation of appropriate therapy. Only six patients were operated on, with a perioperative mortality of two of six patients.[6] In this chapter, we will review the classification, pathology, clinical findings, and diagnostic and treatment modalities for acute aortic dissection, with an emphasis on the role of the vascular/endovascular surgeon.

## ■ CLASSIFICATION

### Temporal

Any tear occurring in the intima of the aorta causes surging of blood through the tear, creating a new false channel and separating (dissecting) the media from the adventitia of the aorta. A dissection is considered acute when the diagnosis is made within 2 weeks of the initial onset of symptoms and thereafter becomes chronic.

### Anatomical Classification

The anatomic classification of aortic dissection is based on:
- Location of the intimal tear
- Extent of the dissection along the aorta.

Two classification schemes are used to describe aortic dissections. The initial classification was proposed by DeBakey and colleagues in 1965, which delineates both the origin of the entry tear and the extent of the descending aortic dissection (Fig. 1).

- *Type I:* The dissection originates in the ascending aorta and extends through the aortic arch and into the descending aorta or abdominal aorta (or both) for a varying distance.
- *Type II:* The dissection originates in the ascending aorta and is confined to the ascending aorta
- *Type IIIa:* The dissection originates in the descending aorta and is limited to the same.
- *Type IIIb:* The dissection involves the descending and variable extents of the abdominal aorta.

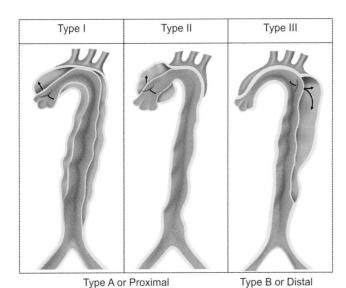

| Type I | Type II | Type III |
|--------|---------|----------|

Type A or Proximal                    Type B or Distal

**Fig. 1** Anatomical classification of aortic dissections

**Table 1** Demography and risk factors of patients (N = 464) with acute aortic dissection (IRAD series)[9]

| Variable | Type A | Type B | p value |
|----------|--------|--------|---------|
| Male sex | 63% | 69.1% | 0.18 |
| Marfan syndrome | 6.7% | 1.8% | 0.02 |
| Hypertension | 69.3% | 76.7% | 0.08 |
| Atherosclerosis | 24.4% | 42% | <0.001 |
| Known aortic aneurysm | 12.4% | 2.2% | 0.006 |
| Prior cardiac surgery | 15.9% | 21.1% | 0.16 |
| Iatrogenic (post-PTCA, cardiac surgery) | 4.8% | 3.4% | 0.47 |
| Prior aortic dissection | 3.9% | 10.6% | 0.005 |

This was subsequently modified by Daily and his associates in 1970 (Stanford classification), which was based on entry tear location only (Fig. 1).[7]

- A Stanford type A dissection originates in the ascending aorta (therefore encompasses DeBakey types I and II dissections).
- A Stanford type B dissection originates in the descending aorta distal to the origin of the left subclavian artery.

As the origin of the entry tear is the key predictor of early outcomes, most patients are now stratified into Stanford type A or B at diagnosis to direct initial therapy.

## ■ INCIDENCE AND RISK FACTORS FOR DEVELOPING AORTIC DISSECTION

As the presenting clinical features are diverse and serious complications occur rapidly, antemortem has proven difficult. The International Registry of Acute Aortic Dissection (IRAD) was established in 1996 enrolling patients from large referral centers, to assess the presentation, management, and outcomes of acute aortic dissections. All patients with acute aortic dissection either confirmed by diagnostic imaging studies or at autopsy are included in the registry. Recent population-based studies have estimated the incidence of acute aortic dissection to range from 2.9 to 3.5 per 100,000 person-years.[8] Men are more frequently affected, with a male-female ratio of 4:1 reported in a recent IRAD series (Table 1).

## ■ PATHOGENESIS

Aortic dissection occurs by separation of aortic media with the presence of extraluminal blood within the layers of the aortic wall. There are two possible mechanisms regarding the initial event in the formation of aortic dissection.

- Primary intimal tear (caused by atherosclerosis, connective tissue disorders, penetrating aortic ulcers, iatrogenic intimal injury, systemic hypertension, and so on)
- Intramural hemorrhage causing delamination of tunica media (caused by rupture of vasa vasorum).

Ultimately, the weakening of aortic wall (especially the media) occurs, leading to higher wall stress causing aortic dilatation, intramural hemorrhage, aortic dissection, and rupture. Deterioration and loss collagen and elastin in the media appear to be the major predisposing factors for the development of spontaneous dissections.

## ■ MALPERFUSION SYNDROME

Malperfusion syndrome is a complication of aortic dissection caused by branch-vessel involvement and resulting in end-organ ischemic damage (Fig. 2). Clinical diagnosis is mandatory, and imaging plays a critical role in confirmation and treatment planning. It can involve one or more vascular beds simultaneously. Virtually, any aortic branch can be affected.

The incidence of aortic branch vessel compromise in association with aortic dissection ranges from 25% to 50%.[10] Ischemic complications can arise when the dissection compromises blood flow, by either extrinsic compression of the true lumen by the false channel or an intimal flap occluding the orifice of a branch artery. This can also lead to secondary distal thrombosis inside the aortic branch vessel. Obstruction may be static (extension of the dissection flap directly into a visceral or lower limb artery, thus narrowing its lumen) or dynamic (obstruction of the vessel by means of the dissection flap prolapsing into the vessel origin).

## ■ CLINICAL FEATURES (TABLE 2)

### Pain

Aortic dissection symptoms may be similar to those of other cardiac problems, such as a myocardial infarction. It is not

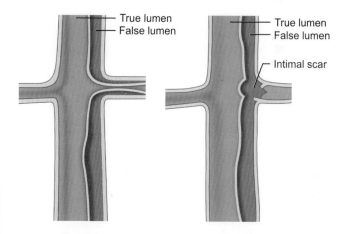

**Fig. 2** Malperfusion phenomena in aortic dissection

**Table 2** Presenting symptoms and clinical findings of patients with acute aortic dissections (IRAD series)[9]

| Symptoms and signs | Incidence | Type A | Type B | p value |
|---|---|---|---|---|
| Chest pain | 72.7% | 78.9% | 62.9% | <0.001 |
| Abdominal pain | 29.6% | 21.6 % | 42.7 % | <0.001 |
| Syncope | 9.4% | 12.7 % | 4.1 % | 0.002 |
| Hypertension | 49% | 35.7% | 70.1% | <0.001 |
| Hypotension | 8% | 11.6% | 2.3% | <0.001 |
| Shock | 8.4% | 13% | 1.5% | <0.001 |
| Murmur due to aortic insufficiency | 31.6% | 44% | 12% | <0.001 |
| Pulse deficit | 15.1% | 18.7% | 9.2% | 0.006 |
| Cerebrovascular accident | 4.7% | 6.1% | 2.3% | 0.07 |
| Congestive cardiac failure | 6.6% | 8.8% | 3% | 0.02 |

uncommon for the patient to pinpoint the exact time at which the dissection occurred. Typical signs and symptoms include sudden severe chest or upper back pain, often described as a tearing, ripping, or shearing sensation, which radiates to the neck or down the back. The pain is typically (in 78% of patients) described as anterior in location in type A dissections, whereas for type B dissections, the pain is more often experienced in the back (in 64% of patients).[11] The location of the pain depends on the location of the dissection and the pain may travel as the dissection propagates. Pain is localized to the anterior, midline chest with involvement of the ascending aorta. The patient may have jaw and neck pain if the dissection involves the aortic arch and its branches. Intrascapular, back, and abdominal pain are common with dissections of the descending aorta. Pain has been localized to the abdomen in up to 43% with type B dissection.[9] In such patients, a high index of suspicion for mesenteric vascular compromise is warranted.

## Neurologic Symptoms

Neurological symptoms may occur because of occlusion of supplying vessels or general hypotension. Gaul et al. in his series of 102 patients with aortic dissections had found that the incidence of neurological symptoms was 29%.[12] Neurological symptoms were attributable to ischemic stroke (16%), spinal cord ischemia (1%), ischemic neuropathy (11%), and hypoxic encephalopathy (2%).[12] Aortic dissections might be missed in patients with neurological symptoms but without pain. Neurological findings in elderly hypertensive patients with asymmetrical pulses or cardiac murmur suggest dissection. Especially in patients considered for thrombolytic therapy in acute stroke further diagnostics is essential.

Spinal cord ischemia from the interruption of intercostal vessels is clearly more common with type B aortic dissections and occurs in 2–10% of all patients.[13]

## Hypertension

Most of the patients with type B dissections are hypertensive (Table 1).

## Hypotension

Sometimes, patients with type A dissections presents with normotension or hypotension. Hypotension in acute aortic dissection is usually related to cardiac tamponade, aortic rupture, or congestive cardiac failure associated with severe aortic regurgitation. Type A dissection has to be suspected in patients presenting with sudden onset of chest or back pain accompanied by pulse deficits, aortic regurgitation, or neurological manifestations.

## Peripheral Vascular Involvement

It is not uncommon to miss the diagnosis of acute aortic dissection presenting as acute limb ischemia. The mortality is clearly linked to the number of pulse deficits at initial evaluation. Lower limb ischemia caused by acute dissection remains a marker for extensive dissection and may be accompanied by other compromised vascular territories. The clinical course of lower extremity ischemia can be variable in that up to one-third of this group may demonstrate spontaneous return of pulses.[14]

## ■ DIFFERENTIAL DIAGNOSIS

- Acute coronary syndrome
- Aortic regurgitation
- Aortic aneurysms
- Musculoskeletal pain
- Pericarditis
- Pleuritis
- Pulmonary embolism
- Cholecystitis.

## Factors Predicting Death in Acute Aortic Dissection[15]

- Age at least 70 years (OR, 1.70; 95% CI, 1.05–2.77; $p = 0.03$)
- Abrupt onset of chest pain (OR 2.60; 95% CI, 1.22–5.54; $p = 0.01$)
- Hypotension/shock/tamponade (OR, 2.97; 95% CI, 1.83–4.81; $p < 0.0001$)
- Kidney failure (OR, 4.77; 95% CI, 1.80–12.6; $p = 0.002$)
- Pulse deficit (OR, 2.03; 95% CI, 1.25–3.29, $p = 0.004$)
- Abnormal ECG (OR, 1.77; 95% CI, 1.06–2.95; $p = 0.03$).

## ■ DIAGNOSTIC EVALUATION

About 20% of patients with type A dissection have ECG evidence of acute ischemia or acute myocardial infarction.[16] An ECG must be acquired in all patients. This test helps distinguish acute myocardial infarction, for which thrombolytic therapy may be life-saving, from aortic dissection, in which thrombolytic therapy may be detrimental.[16]

## Plain Radiography

The findings of aortic dissection on chest radiography are nonspecific and never diagnostic. Such findings include widening of the cardiac or aortic silhouette, displacement of aortic calcifications, and effusions. Widening of the mediastinum is the most common finding. As these findings are not diagnostic, additional imaging is required.

## Computed Tomographic Angiography

Computed tomographic (CT) scanning is readily available, is noninvasive, and has a reported sensitivity of 83–95% and a specificity of 87–100% for the diagnosis of acute aortic dissection (Fig. 3).[17] The ability to view vessels in multiple projections helps in evaluating the complex three-dimensional (3D) anatomy of the aorta. The main advantages of multidetector computed tomography (MD-CT) scan include rapid image acquisition, postprocessing flexibility, and also for planning purpose. A noncontrast scan through the chest is useful to screen for acute hemorrhage particularly in the aortic wall (intramural hematoma) or intimal vascular calcifications. Arterial phase imaging is timed to coincide with arterial contrast opacification; delayed venous phase imaging is also useful to evaluate solid organs for mass lesions or for endoleaks in patients with stent grafts.

In most cases, the true lumen may be localized by its continuity with an undissected segment of the aorta.[18] The presence of intraluminal thrombus is a fairly good marker of the false lumen, but in patients with a concomitant degenerative aneurysm, thrombus may be present in the true lumen. In descending thoracic aorta, the false lumen is larger than the true lumen in more than 90% of

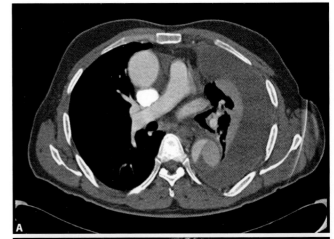
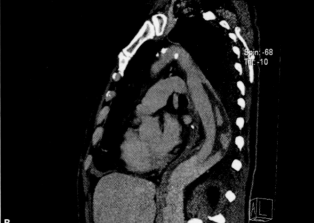
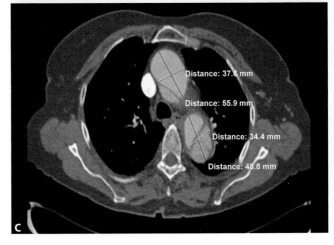

**Figs 3A to C** (A) CTA picture of a patient with type B aortic dissection showing expanded false lumen and compressed true lumen; (B) CTA picture of type B aortic dissection with aneurysmal degeneration of DTA following EVAR for AAA (iatrogenic aortic dissection); (C) CTA of 70 years old lady with type A aortic dissecting aneurysm. She underwent successful two stage hybrid surgery

cases ($p < 0.05$).[18] Axial imaging affords the best opportunity to detect topographic relationships of the true and false lumina and potential aortic branch compromise.

Computed tomography (CT) artifacts occur in obese or uncooperative patients with noise and motion, causing image distortion. In aortic side branches such as coronaries or renal arteries, CTA tends to overestimate calcified stenoses and underestimate luminal narrowing by noncalcific plaque.[19]

## Magnetic Resonance Imaging

Magnetic resonance angiography (MRA) is a complementary rather than competing imaging modality for the thoracic aorta. MRI has an overall sensitivity and specificity for the diagnosis of aortic dissection in the range of 95–100%.[20] Whereas MRA methods without contrast enhancement have been available for some time, gadolinium-enhanced MRA has dramatically shortened examination time and emerged as preferred MR modality for aortic disease; adequate images result from only 15 mL of gadolinium.[20] Discovery of nephrogenic systemic fibrosis in patients with renal dysfunction receiving gadolinium has tempered enthusiasm.[21] The chief limitations of MRI include the lack of immediate availability, long examination times, and lack of monitoring for critically ill patients. In addition, patients who have pacemakers, aneurysm clippings, or ocular implants are not candidates for MRI.

## Echocardiography

Advantages of TEE for detection of acute aortic syndromes result from close proximity of the esophagus to the thoracic aorta and its ability to visualize both ascending and descending aorta and parts of the arch with high spatial resolution in real time (which is the chief limitation of transthoracic echocardiography). Aortic dissection is confirmed when two lumens are separated by an intimal flap visualized within the aorta. Tears can be identified and differentiation between true and false lumen is often easy and diagnostic with optional color Doppler flow mapping; intimal tear(s) can be localized in the majority of patients.[22] The sensitivity of TEE has been reported to be as high as 98%, and its specificity ranges from 63% to 96%.[23] An experienced operator is needed for image acquisition and interpretation.

## ■ TREATMENT

### Medical Management

Although waiting for diagnostic imaging, it is necessary to control pain and reduce systolic blood pressure to values between 100 and 120 mm Hg.

The cornerstone of the management of all dissections is strict, lifelong blood pressure control, regardless of any surgical, endovascular, or other interventions. For most patients, this control requires pharmacologic treatment, closely monitored by the patient's primary care physician and by specialists. Antihypertensives to lower systemic blood pressure and pulse (dP/dt) are a key element of initial therapy for all patients. The main aim is to stabilize the extent of the dissection, reducing intimal flap mobility, relieving dynamic aortic branch obstruction, and decreasing the risk for rupture. Mortality in the acute phase of a proximal dissection may exceed 1% per hour[24] as a result of the central cardioaortic complications such as cardiac tamponade, acute aortic valvular insufficiency, and coronary obstruction.

Beta-blockers are considered first-line therapy; they reduce the dP/dt (the rate of rise of the blood pressure), in addition to the heart rate and the mean and peak systolic pressures. Commonly used IV beta blockers are esmolol and labetalol. Labetalol has also got alpha-blocking property. In contemporary practice, the combination of a beta-blocker and a vasodilator is standard medical therapy. If the target blood pressure cannot be achieved with beta blockade alone, a second agent may be added, such as nitroprusside or nicardipine.

Although angiotensin receptor blockers (ARBs) and angiotensin converting enzyme (ACE) inhibitors remain second-line choices for the treatment of hypertension in the absence of other compelling indications, drugs in these classes have been of particular interest as potential treatments for patients with Marfan syndrome because of their antagonism of transforming growth factor-beta (TGF-β) activity.

Pain management is equally important, as it relieves the anxiety. Opiates are often required for these cases unless strongly contraindicated.

Once the patient's blood pressure has been controlled to a systolic pressure of 105–120 mm Hg (or a mean arterial pressure of 60–70 mm Hg) and the pain has resolved, oral antihypertensives can be started.

### Indications for Surgery

- Acute type A aortic dissections (considered a surgical emergency)
- Aneurysmal dilation (the most common indication for chronic dissections)
- Malperfusion syndrome
- Rupture or leak
- Intractable pain.

Prompt surgical intervention for the acutely dissected ascending aorta is only rarely contraindicated. Complications, such as rupture of the distal aorta and mesenteric malperfusion syndrome, may need to be addressed first by surgical intervention. Severe neurologic impairment from stroke is considered grounds for delaying and reconsidering surgery (as opposed to paralysis or paraparesis from spinal ischemia, which may improve with surgery).

## Open Surgery

### Open Surgical Treatment of Ascending Aortic Dissection

Optimal surgical management of these complex patients depends on the coordinated efforts of a skilled team. The patient is expeditiously transported to the operating room, wherein endotracheal intubation, intravenous access for rapid infusion, and monitoring—including blood pressure monitoring via left radial and femoral arterial lines—are instituted. TEE is performed before and even during the procedure. Electroencephalogram has to be monitored throughout the initial stages of the procedure. After median sternotomy, the right axillary artery is cannulated with an interposition 8-mm Dacron graft anastomosed end-to-side to the vessel (Fig. 4A); because the aortic dissection rarely extends far enough to involve the axillary artery, this technique almost always ensures perfusion of the true lumen and causes fewer complications than femoral cannulation might. In case of aortic valve incompetence, retrograde cardioplegia is used. Systemic cooling is then started. Once the ventricle

fibrillates, an aortic cross-clamp may need to be applied. When the aorta is clamped, the ascending aorta can be opened, and antegrade cardioplegia can be administered directly via ostial cannulae. The patient is cooled for at least 20 minutes, usually down to 16°–18°C, until electroencephalographic silence is achieved. Under circulatory arrest, the aorta is opened, and the dissection membrane is excised from the ascending aorta, as well as from the arch if an aneurysm or intimal tear there necessitates its replacement also. Thus, the intimal tear is usually excised unless it is located in the descending thoracic aorta. During circulatory arrest, antegrade or retrograde cerebral perfusion maintains the cerebral metabolism.

Antegrade flow into the right carotid artery is easily accomplished by snaring the innominate artery and perfusing through the right axillary artery (Fig. 4A). Alternatively, it is possible to use balloon-tipped perfusion catheters inserted directly into the innominate and left carotid arteries (Fig. 4B) from within the open aorta or, less commonly, an end-to-side, 8-mm graft anastomosed to the carotid through a neck incision.

To accomplish retrograde cerebral perfusion, the superior vena cava must be encircled and cannulated and serves as

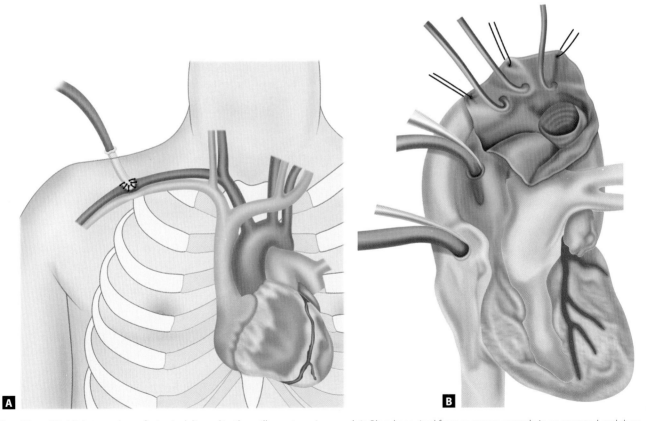

**A**    **B**

**Figs 4A and B**  (A) Antegrade perfusion is delivered to the axillary artery via a conduit. Blood acquired from a venous cannula is oxygenated and then recirculated into the arterial system via a femoral arterial line and, if desired, an axillary line. The axillary line is typically inserted through a conduit; (B) Antegrade cerebral perfusion can also be given by cannulating the origin of innominate and left common carotid artery

the means to deliver flow in a retrograde manner into the cerebrovascular system (Fig. 5).

Intraoperative decisions regarding the root are often difficult. Typically, the root is replaced if it is aneurysmal. Root replacement is commonly required in all patients with Marfan syndrome or Loeys-Dietz syndrome, regardless of the root diameter.[25]

Finally, the coronary artery bypasses are rarely necessary and should be reserved for patients with evidence of segmental wall motion dysfunction (Table 3).

## Open Surgical Treatment Type B Aortic Dissection

The aim of the surgical treatment is to prevent death and irreversible ischemic damage of the involved organs of the abdomen, as well as of the lower limbs. Despite the success of medical therapy in the acute management of uncomplicated aortic dissection, long-term morbidity and mortality are high.

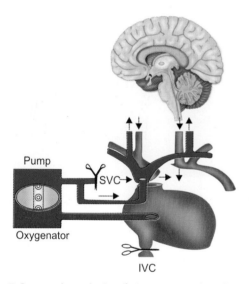

**Fig. 5** Retrograde cerebral perfusion via internal jugular veins

## Indications for Surgical Treatment

- *Distal ischemia:* Visceral vessels, renal vessels, and lower limbs
- Continuous chest pain not responding to medical management
- Drug-resistant hypertension
- Rupture/imminent rupture
- Increase in diameter >5 cm
- Pseudoaneurysm
- Aortic arch involvement
- Relatively younger patients without severe comorbidities
- Marfan syndrome.

Similar to the open repair of descending thoracic aortic aneurysm (DTAA), spinal cord and visceral protection is maintained during the open repair of type B aortic dissections. They are as follows:

- Distal perfusion of the aorta
- Systemic hypothermia
- Cerebrospinal fluid drainage.

Full cardiopulmonary bypass combined with deep hypothermia, with or without circulatory arrest, is used if the distal aortic arch is replaced or if extensive resection of the descending thoracic or thoracoabdominal aorta is required. After proximal and distal occlusion of the affected aorta, it is opened longitudinally and the true lumen is entered. Intercostal or segmental arteries below the level of the sixth intercostal space (from which the artery of Adamkiewicz is generated) are crucial for the adequate perfusion of the spinal cord. These arteries should be selectively perfused until their implantation into the graft. Rest of the procedures such as transection of proximal neck, separation from the esophagus, proximal anastomosis, reimplantation of spinal arteries, and other visceral arteries followed by distal anastomosis are done as described previously in the surgery for descending thoracoabdominal aortic aneurysms (DTAAA). The results of open repair of type B aortic dissection are summarized in Table 4.

## Endovascular Repair

In both complicated acute and chronic type B aortic dissections, endovascular therapy may emerge as an attractive

**Table 3** Results of surgical repair of type A aortic dissection

| Author | No of patients | 30 day mortality | Stroke/ any focal neurological deficits | Paraplegia | Visceral damage | Follow-up |
|---|---|---|---|---|---|---|
| Sun et al.[27] | 257 | 4.67% | 5/257 | 2/257 | 2[ω], 2[€], 1[∞], 1[π] | 35 months |
| Biancari et al.[28] | 308[μ] | 36.7% | 11.9 % | NA | NA | NA |
| Mehta[29] | 550 (32%[£]/ 68 %[¥]) | 43%[£]/28%[¥] | 18%[£]/26%[¥] | NA | NA | NA |
| Ehrlich[30] | 124 | 15.3% | NA | NA | NA | 41 months |

ω, Number of patients with renal ischemia; €, Number of patients with paraparesis; ∞, Number of patients with hepatic failure; π, Number of patients with MODS; μ, age >80 years; NA, not available; £, age >70 years; ¥, age <70 years.

**Table 4** Results of open repair of type B aortic dissection

| Author | No. of patients | Medical management | Surgery (open/TEVAR) | Inhospital mortality | Paraplegia (or any neurological complications) | Visceral damage | Follow-up |
|---|---|---|---|---|---|---|---|
| Safi H J et al.[31] | 206 | 92 | 114/Nil | 12/114 (11%) | 15/114 (13%) | NA | NA |
| Verdant A et al.[32] | 366 | Nil | 336/Nil | 12 % | Nil | 0.2%π | NA |
| Lansman SL et al.[33] | 34 | Nil | 34€/Nil | Nil | 1/34µ | 4/34π | 5.8 years |
| Sasaki S et al.[34] | 22 | Nil | 22/Nil | 2/22 | 3/22µ | NA | NA |

π, Renal failure; NA, Not available; €, Emergency surgery; µ, Paraplegia.

alternative to open surgery. Stenting aortic dissections may alter the course of this disease by sealing the tear in the short-term and inducing thrombosis of the false lumen over the longer term. Ideally, all fenestrations should be covered, although in practice this may not be a prerequisite for success, because a blind-ended false lumen with a single uncovered fenestration and no flow may still thrombose. Nevertheless, many dissections are accompanied by multiple fenestrations, because these fenestrations are not always covered, they may permit persistent patency and pressurization of the false lumen with risk of expansion and rupture. This risk may be exacerbated by endoleaks of various origins.

### Advantages of Endovascular Treatment

- The endovascular technique is minimally invasive, safe, shorter, and effective
- All the complications related to extracorporeal circulation and thoracotomy are avoided
- The reduced blood loss
- The shorter hospitalization
- The avoidance of any clamping in the friable thoracic aortic wall.

## ■ THORACIC ENDOVASCULAR AORTIC REPAIR

The goals of thoracic endovascular aortic repair (TEVAR) for acute type B dissection include coverage of the proximal entry tear, expansion of the true lumen with restoration of flow to the visceral vessels, and obliteration of false lumen flow with subsequent complete thrombosis. To date, the application of available endovascular devices for acute dissection constitutes off-label use because such devices are currently FDA approved in the United States only for the treatment of degenerative thoracic aneurysms.

### Definition of Treatment Success

"Technical" success is defined as closure of the primary entry tear (i.e. absence of type I A or I B endoleak) and induction of false lumen thrombosis.

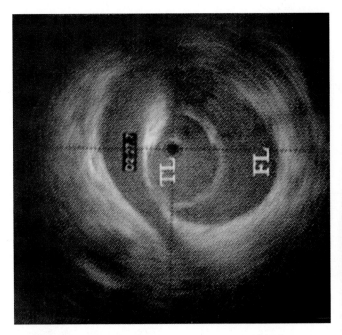

**Fig. 6** Intravascular ultrasound showing true and false lumen

Preoperative planning, choosing the device, selection of access sites are almost identical to that of TEVAR for thoracic aortic aneurysms. Once selected, stent-graft repair of acute aortic dissection should be performed in an operating room with adequate fluoroscopic imaging.

The focus is the occlusion of the primary entry tear. The size of the selected stent graft should be based on the diameter of the aorta proximal to the dissected segment, applying almost no oversizing (<10%). The technical challenge, especially in complicated type B dissections, may be to cannulate the narrowed, sometimes collapsed true lumen. To assure access to the true lumen, transesophageal echocardiogram (TEE) or intravascular ultrasound (IVUS) (Fig. 6) may often be necessary. Because the tear in type B dissection is distal to the left subclavian artery, rapid true lumen access is easily obtained through a right transbrachial approach. Procedure-related difficulties may be overcome by an antegrade approach via the brachial artery with the guidewire being snared in the aorta. After deployment, ballooning is not recommended, because retrograde dissection and rupture of the dissection membrane has been reported due to ballooning. In case if the device has not opened completely, a compliant, large-diameter (33–40 mm) aortic occlusion balloon is used to ensure adequate apposition of the device to the aortic wall (it should be used cautiously within the stent-graft not the native aorta). Induction of hypotension or bradycardia by pharmacologic means may increase the accuracy of entry tear sealing during deployment (Fig. 7).

## Complications of Endovascular Treatment

A recent meta-analysis of all published series of stent-graft repair for aortic dissection before 2005 identified 609 patients with a procedural success rate of 98.2%. Thirty-day mortality was 5.3% (it was three-fold higher in patients with acute dissection).[35] Cerebral vascular accident, owing to catheter manipulation in the ascending aorta and/or aortic arch, affected by atherosclerosis. Stroke is the most serious and commonly experienced complication after endovascular stent-grafting, with an incidence of 3–10%.[36] Type 2 endoleaks are very common in TEVAR mainly from the intercostal vessels and are frequently observed (Fig. 7C), whereas type 1 and 3 endoleaks should not occur. The exact incidence of these endoleaks grossly varies with each case series as they are less reported. Delayed type 1 endoleaks are common following TEVAR in aortic dissections due to

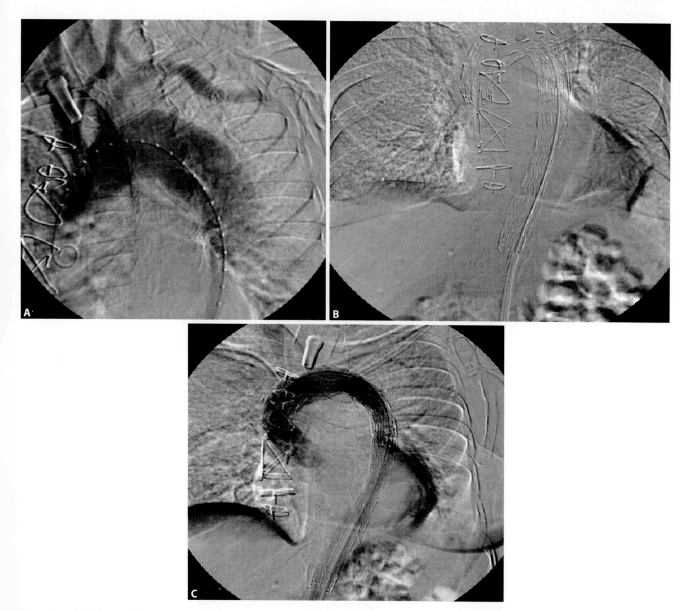

**Figs 7A to C** (A) A case of type A aortic dissection who had already underwent arch debranching and replacement of ascending aorta, showing patent aorto-bi-carotid and Lt CCA to LSA grafts; (B) Same case where the main device has been deployed; (C) Completion angiography showing type 2 endoleak

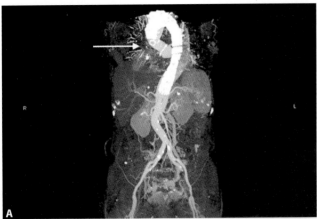
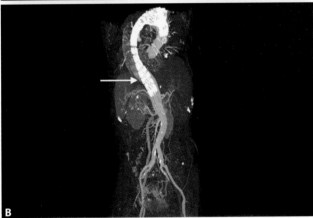

**Figs 8A and B** (A) Post-TEVAR type 1A endoleak due to aneurysmal degeneration of the aorta at the proximal landing site; (B) Post-TEVAR type 1B endoleak due to aneurysmal degeneration of the aorta at the distal landing site

aneurysmal degeneration at the site where stent graft is attached (Fig. 8).

## Investigation of STEnt Grafts in Aortic Dissection (INSTEAD) Trial

This trial represents the first prospective randomized study of elective stent graft placement in survivors of uncomplicated chronic type B aortic dissection.[37] In a prospective trial, 140 patients with clinically stable type B dissection were randomly subjected to elective stent-graft placement in addition to optimal medical therapy ($n$ = 72) or to optimal medical therapy ($n$ = 68) with surveillance and recurrent computed tomography imaging. Primary endpoint was 2-year all-cause mortality, while aorta-related mortality, progression of disease (with need for crossover to stent-graft or additional endovascular or open surgery), and

aortic remodeling were secondary endpoints. There was no difference in all-cause mortality at 2 years, with cumulative survival of 95.6 ± 2.5% with optimal medical therapy versus 88.9 ± 3.7% with thoracic endovascular aortic repair (TEVAR) ($p$ = 0.15). The INSTEAD trial demonstrates that thoracic stent graft (TEVAR) placement failed to improve the rates of 2-year survival and adverse events when compared with optimal medical therapy, despite favorable aortic remodeling.

## Endovascular Treatment of Malperfusion Syndrome

Malperfusion syndrome is a complication of aortic dissection caused by branch-vessel involvement and resulting in end-organ dysfunction. Clinical diagnosis is mandatory, and imaging plays a critical role in confirmation and treatment planning. Stent-graft repair of type B dissection is an attractive alternative to surgical repair for correcting ischemic complications. Usually, stent-graft occlusion of the entry site in the descending thoracic aorta results in thrombosis of the false channel and flow increase in the true lumen, normalizing the vessel perfusion and restoring branch vessels patency. Therefore, immediate relief of malperfusion syndrome may be the first result of endovascular stent graft treatment of aortic dissection. Endovascular stent grafting can be a challenge when aortic branches are totally supplied by the false lumen. If multiple vessels require treatment, the most sensitive areas should be addressed first with selective stent placement. For this reason, priority should be given to the superior mesenteric artery (SMA) or celiac artery obstruction, followed by at least one kidney; this is because the gut has the least tolerance for underperfusion.

Fenestration of the intimal flap may be performed by several techniques under the combined guidance of ultrasound and fluoroscopy.

A fenestration is created close to the compromised aortic branch. After the needle and a stiff wire are advanced from the true to the false lumen, a 5 Fr catheter is advanced into the alternate lumen. Confirmation of position across the membrane is performed by injection of contrast material. Subsequently, an angioplasty balloon at least 12–15 mm in diameter and 20–40 mm in length is used to create a fenestration tear.

Stiff guidewires are placed in each lumen from a single femoral access, and a single long sheath is advanced over the two wires, thus dividing the membrane over this distance, the "scissors technique" have reported both clean longitudinal tears (the ideal result) and circumferential separation of the flap from the aortic wall (not ideal).

Midulla et al. in his series of 35 cases of aortic dissection with malperfusion had 100% technical success rate and concluded that fenestration is the procedure of choice in acute dissections with malperfusion syndrome.[38]

# ■ CONCLUSION

1. Acute aortic dissection has a high mortality rate. Hence, early diagnosis and initiation of appropriate treatment is important.
2. The cornerstone of the management of all dissections is strict lifelong blood pressure control.
3. In both complicated acute and chronic type B aortic dissections, endovascular therapy is set to emerge as an attractive alternative to open surgery.

# ■ REFERENCES

1. Shekelton J. Healed dissecting aneurysm. Dublin Hosp Rep. 1922;3:231-2.
2. Clouse WD, Hallett JW Jr, Schaff HV, Spittell PC, Rowland CM, Ilstrup DM, Melton LJ 3rd. Acute aortic dissection: population-based incidence compared with degenerative aortic aneurysm rupture. Mayo Clin Proc. 2004;79(2):176-80.
3. Olsson C, Thelin S, Ståhle E, Ekbom A, Granath F. Thoracic aortic aneurysm and dissection: increasing prevalence and improved outcomes reported in a nationwide population-based study of more than 14,000 cases from 1987 to 2002. Circulation. 2006;12; 114(24):2611-8. Epub 2006 Dec 4.
4. Cambria RP. Surgical treatment of complicated distal aortic dissection. Semin Vasc Surg. 2002;15:97-107.
5. Cambria RP, Brewster DC, Gertler J, et al. Vascular complications associated with spontaneous aortic dissection. J Vasc Surg. 1988; 7:199-209.
6. Mészáros I, Mórocz J, Szlávi J, Schmidt J, Tornóci L, Nagy L, Szép L. Epidemiology and clinicopathology of aortic dissection. Chest. 2000;117(5):1271-8.
7. Daily PO, Trueblood HW, Stinson EB, et al. Management of acute aortic dissection. Ann Thorac Surg. 1970;10:237-46.
8. Clouse WD, Hallett Jr JW, Schaff HV, et al. Acute aortic dissection: population-based incidence compared with degenerative aortic aneurysm rupture. Mayo Clin Proc. 2004;79:176-80.
9. Hagan PG, Nienaber CA, Isselbacher EM. The International Registry of Acute Aortic Dissection (IRAD): New Insights Into an Old Disease. JAMA. 2000;283(7):897-903.
10. Panneton JM, Teh SH, Cherry KJ, et al. Aortic fenestration for acute or chronic aortic dissection: an uncommon but effective procedure. J Vasc Surg. 2000;32:711-21.
11. Spittell PC, Spittell Jr JA, Joyce JW, et al. Clinical features and differential diagnosis of aortic dissection: experience with 236 cases (1980 through 1990). Mayo Clin Proc 1993; 68:897-903.
12. Gaul C, Dietrich W, Friedrich I, Sirch J, Erbguth FJ. Neurological symptoms in type A aortic dissections. Stroke. 2007;38(2):292-7. Epub 2006 Dec 28.
13. Syed MA, Fiad TM. Transient paraplegia as a presenting feature of aortic dissection in a young man. Emerg Med J. 2002;19:174-5.
14. Cambria RP, Brewster DC, Gertler J, et al. Vascular complications associated with spontaneous aortic dissection. J Vasc Surg. 1988; 7:199-209.
15. Mehta RH, Suzuki T, Hagan PG, Bossone E, Gilon D, Llovet A, et al. Predicting death in patients with acute type A aortic dissection. Circulation. 2002;105:200-6.
16. Kamp TJ, Goldschmidt-Clermont PJ, Brinker JA, Resar JR. Myocardial infarction, aortic dissection, and thrombolytic therapy. Am Heart J. 1994;128:1234-7.
17. Fisher ER, Stern EJ, Godwin 2nd JD, et al. Acute aortic dissection: typical and atypical imaging features. Radiographics. 1994;14: 1263-71.
18. LePage MA, Quint LE, Sonnad SS, et al. Aortic dissection: CT features that distinguish true lumen from false lumen. AJR Am J Roentgenol. 2001;177:207-11.
19. Leber AW, Becker A, Knez A, von Ziegler F, Sirol M, Nikolaou K, et al. Accuracy of 64-slice computed tomography to classify and quantify plaque volumes in the proximal coronary system: a comparative study using intravascular ultrasound. J Am Coll Cardiol. 2006;47: 672-7.
20. Russo V, Renzulli M, Buttazzi K, Fattori R. Acquired diseases of the thoracic aorta: role of MRI and MRA. Eur Radiol. 2006;16: 852-65.
21. Kuo PH, Kanal E, Abu-Alfa AK, Cowper SE. Gadolinium-based MR contrast agents and nephrogenic systemic fibrosis. Radiology. 2007;242:647-9.
22. Penco M, Paparoni S, Dagianti A, Fusilli C, Vitarelli A, De Remigis F, et al. Usefulness of transesophageal echocardiography in the assessment of aortic dissection. Am J Cardiol. 2000;86:53G-6G.
23. Adachi H, Omoto R, Kyo S, et al. Diagnosis of acute aortic dissection with transesophageal echocardiography and results of surgical treatment.. Nippon Kyobu Geka Gakkai Zasshi. 1991; 39:1987-94.
24. Hirst AE, Jr, Johns VJ, Jr, Kime SW, Jr. Dissecting aneurysm of the aorta: A review of 505 cases. Medicine (Baltimore). 1958;37: 217-79.
25. LeMaire SA, Carter SA, Volguina IV, et al. Spectrum of aortic operations in 300 patients with confirmed or suspected Marfan syndrome. Ann Thorac Surg. 2006;81:2063-78.
26. Elefteriades JA, Lovoulos CJ, Coady MA, Tellides G, Kopf GS, Rizzo JA. Management of descending aortic dissection. Ann Thorac Surg. 1999;67:2002-5.
27. Sun L, Qi R, Zhu J, Liu Y, Chang Q, Zheng J. Repair of acute type A dissection: our experiences and results. Ann Thorac Surg. 2011; 91(4):1147-52.
28. Biancari F, Vasques F, Benenati V, Juvonen T. Contemporary results after surgical repair of type A aortic dissection in patients aged 80 years and older: a systematic review and meta-analysis. Eur J Cardiothorac Surg. 2011;40(5):1058-63.
29. Mehta RH, O'Gara PT, Bossone E, Nienaber CA, Myrmel T, Cooper JV, et al. International Registry of Acute Aortic Dissection (IRAD) Investigators. Acute type A aortic dissection in the elderly: clinical characteristics, management, and outcomes in the current era. J Am Coll Cardiol. 2002;40(4):685-92.
30. Ehrlich MP, Ergin MA, McCullough JN, Lansman SL, Galla JD, Bodian CA, et al. Results of immediate surgical treatment of all acute type A dissections. Circulation. 2000;102 (19 Suppl 3):III248-52.
31. Safi HJ, Miller 3rd CC, Reardon MJ, et al. Operation for acute and chronic aortic dissection: recent outcome with regard to neurologic deficit and early death. Ann Thorac Surg. 1998;66: 402-11.
32. Verdant A, Cossette R, Page A, et al. Aneurysms of the descending thoracic aorta: three hundred sixty-six consecutive cases resected without paraplegia. J Vasc Surg. 1995;21:385-90.
33. Lansman SL, Hagl C, Fink D, et al. Acute type B aortic dissection: surgical therapy. Ann Thorac Surg. 2002;74:S1833-S5.
34. Sasaki S, Yasuda K, Kunihara T, et al. Surgical results of Stanford type B aortic dissection. Comparisons between partial and subtotal replacement of the dissected aorta. J Cardiovasc Surg (Torino). 2000;41:227-32.

35. Eggebrecht H, Nienaber CA, Neuhauser M, et al. Endovascular stent-graft placement in aortic dissection: a meta-analysis. Eur Heart J. 2006;27:489-98.

36. Svensson LG, Kouchoukos NT, Miller DC, et al. Expert consensus document on the treatment of descending thoracic aortic disease using endovascular stent-grafts. Ann Thorac Surg. 2008; 85:S1-41.

37. Nienaber CA. Influence and critique of the INSTEAD Trial (TEVAR versus medical treatment for uncomplicated type B aortic dissection). Semin Vasc Surg. 2011;24(3):167-71.

38. Midulla M, Renaud A, Martinelli T, Koussa M, Mounier-Vehier C, Prat A, Beregi JP. Endovascular fenestration in aortic dissection with acute malperfusion syndrome: immediate and late follow-up. J Thorac Cardiovasc Surg. 2011;142(1):66-72.

## PRACTICAL POINTS

- Aortic dissections can be classified on temporal and anatomical basis. Stanford classification commonly used.
- Dissections are more frequent in males. Individuals with connective tissue disorders, hypertension and atherosclerosis are predisposed.
- Malperfusion syndrome results in end-organ ischemia and incidence range from 25% to 50%.
- Chest or upper back pain (tearing/shearing type) is the most common presentation.
- Imaging modalities—CT angiography, MRA, and TEE are used for definitive diagnosis.
- Treatment of all dissections involves control of hypertension and pain. A mean arterial pressure of 60–70 mm Hg should be targeted.
- Surgery is indicated for acute type A aortic dissections, aneurysmal dilation, malperfusion syndrome, rupture/leak, or intractable pain.
- Open surgical treatment involves use of circulatory arrest and antegrade or retrograde cerebral perfusion as required. Aortic root replacement is usually required in patients with connective tissue disorders.
- Endovascular treatment is an attractive option in type B dissections. INSTEAD trial found that at 5 years, the risk of all-cause mortality was lower with TEVAR than with medical therapy alone. TEVAR was also associated with decreased progression of disease at 5 years while medical management alone was unable to prevent late complications.
- Fenestration technique is advocated for endovascular treatment of malperfusion syndrome.

# 10

# Renovascular Hypertension

*VS Bedi, Ajay Yadav, Ambarish Satwik, Kamran Ali Khan*

## ■ BACKGROUND

Renovascular hypertension is a condition characterized by a rise of blood pressure, due to significant unilateral or bilateral renal arterial stenosis.[1] It has been a topic of controversy and debate in the medical community for many years. Many patients are now being diagnosed with this ailment due to the technological advances in imaging methods. It is one of the important causes of secondary hypertension and chronic renal disease, which is a consequence of renal ischemia.

The diagnosis can be easily missed, as it requires a high index of suspicion. As proven by studies, a 70% reduction in luminal diameter or a 15 mm Hg pressure gradient in the artery is required to induce this condition.[2] However, a radiological diagnosis of arterial stenosis may not always be sufficient enough to establish its causative role.

Renal artery stenosis causes release of rennin due to ischemia and it contributes to hypertension through a sequence of biochemical events. Angiotensin II is formed from angiotensin I, which causes vasoconstriction and release of aldosterone from the adrenal cortex. The presence of a normally functioning, non-ischemic kidney allows good handling of the aldosterone-mediated excess sodium and water retention, and thus prevents volume in contributing to the hypertension. On the contrary, a single ischemic kidney has no such capacity, and hence, volume happens to play a significant role in the elevated blood pressure.

Antihypertensive therapy should be instituted and optimal blood pressure control is of utmost importance. Control of smoking and modulation of other atherosclerotic risk factors needs to be addressed. The options for treatment of this condition (in recalcitrant cases, wherein medical options have failed) include percutaneous transluminal angioplasty (PTA), surgical revascularization, renal sympathetic denervation and nephrectomy. There is a significant difference of opinion regarding the effectiveness of renal revascularization. Some practitioners advocate endovascular procedures including the use of stents to improve the management of these patients, while others argue that there are no major benefits

and such interventions come with an inherent risk of surgical complications.

According to the recent randomized clinical trials on renovascular hypertension, revascularization procedures should be attempted in a small population of carefully selected patients. Patients with difficult to control hypertension (on best medical therapy), those with worsening renal function, and those presenting with unexplained pulmonary edema and unstable angina should be offered such therapy.

Patient education and counseling regarding this condition is also a neglected entity and should be tackled judiciously.

## ■ EPIDEMIOLOGY

Renovascular hypertension is the most common cause of atypical hypertension in the United States. It occurs due to a wide variety of clinically different disease conditions, such as atherosclerosis, fibromuscular dysplasia (FMD), vasculitis, congenital bands, radiation, extrinsic compression, and neurofibromatosis.[3] Atherosclerosis is the etiological factor in as much as 90% of the lesions, usually involving the proximal renal arteries. However, in younger individuals, FMD involving the distal renal artery and its branches is more common. Many cases present in childhood as well.[4]

## ■ ETIOLOGY

Atherosclerosis is responsible for about two-thirds of cases, whereas the remaining one-third may be caused by FMD, congenital disorders, or other clinical conditions.

### Causes of Renovascular Hypertension[5]

- Atherosclerotic disease of renal artery
- Fibromuscular disease
  - Medial fibroplasia
  - Perimedial fibroplasia
  - Intimal fibroplasia
  - Medial hyperplasia

- Extrinsic fibrous band
- Trauma
  - Arterial dissection
  - Segmental renal infarction
  - Page kidney (perirenal fibrosis)
- Aortic dissection
- Aortic endograft occluding the renal artery
- Arterial embolus
- Others
  - Hypercoagulable state with renal infarction
  - Takayasu's arteritis
  - Radiation-induced fibrosis
  - Tumor compressing the renal artery, for example, pheochromocytoma, *polyarteritis nodosa*, etc.

## ■ PATHOPHYSIOLOGY

The central pathophysiological mechanism behind renovascular hypertension is the activation of the rennin-angiotensin-aldosterone system and further events are dictated by the presence or absence of a normally functioning, nonischemic kidney. Renal artery stenosis causes release of rennin from the ischemic kidney, which further leads to the conversion of angiotensin I to angiotensin II and aldosterone secretion from the adrenal cortex. This results in systemic vasoconstriction and volume retention, which contribute to increased blood pressure.

In unilateral disease, the contralateral nonischemic kidney is capable of causing pressure diuresis and thus prevents volume overload in contributing to the hypertension. In these cases, increased plasma levels of angiotensin II and systemic vasoconstriction are responsible for the elevated blood pressures. However, in a solitary ischemic kidney, volume handling by the diseased kidney is not adequate and volume contributes to the hypertension, in addition to angiotensin-mediated vasoconstriction.

The hypertension in these patients evolves in stages. In the early period, increased plasma levels of rennin lead to immediate rise of blood pressure. When the contralateral kidney is well functioning, it excretes excess sodium and water and eventually, systemic hypertension is maintained by increased rennin and angiotensin levels.

In the second stage, when an ischemic solitary kidney is present, volume expansion occurs and rennin levels eventually fall. In these cases, hypertension is not primarily dependent on angiotensin-mediated vasoconstriction, instead, volume expansion is the predominant contributing factor.

If the blood flow to the diseased kidney(s) is restored within these two stages, normal blood pressure is restored. But if there is persistent renal ischemia, renovascular hypertension reaches an irreversible stage and restoration of blood flow to the kidneys may not lead to normalization of blood pressure. These patients are known to develop ischemic nephropathy.

## ■ COMPLICATIONS

Renovascular hypertension leads to chronically elevated blood pressure which causes end organ damage to the body. Patients may present with neurological symptoms such as headache or dizziness. Hypertensive stroke or retinopathy may be the initial presentation in some cases. Left ventricular hypertrophy and congestive cardiac failure are long-term consequences of this condition. Development of ischemic nephropathy may lead to renal failure. Patients may also present with malignant hypertension, which, if untreated, *may end up in coma or death.*

## ■ CLINICAL FEATURES

Renovascular hypertension is *not an easy diagnosis* as many patients are asymptomatic, or may present with nonspecific symptoms. At times, it may be impossible to distinguish it from essential hypertension. However, physicians should look for certain clinical clues to make them consider this diagnosis.

When to suspect renovascular hypertension?[6,7]
- New onset hypertension in young (less than 30 years of age) or elderly (more than 50 years of age)
- No history of hypertension in the family
- Accelerated hypertension
- Inadequate control despite multiple drugs
- Fundus showing hypertensive retinopathy of Grade III–IV
- Presence of abdominal bruit on examination
- Unequal kidney (discrepancy in renal sizes more than 1.5 cm)
- New onset azotemia on starting ACE inhibitor/ARB therapy
- Persistent hypokalemia
- Recurrent "flash" pulmonary edema.

Although there are no standard guidelines to screen patients for renovascular hypertension, the criteria proposed by Mann and Pickering are used on most occasions.[8]

## Clinical Risk Stratification for Renovascular Hypertension

- Low
  - Borderline and mild hypertension without hypertensive target-organ damage
- Moderate
  - Severe hypertension (diastolic blood pressure > 120 mm Hg)
  - Hypertension refractory to standard antihypertensive treatment
  - Hypertension with abdominal bruit
  - Moderate hypertension in patients with occlusive vascular disease (abdomen or legs)
  - Unexplained renal failure

- High
  - Severe hypertension, with either progressive renal insufficiency or refractoriness to combination therapy with three antihypertensive drugs
  - Accelerated or malignant hypertension (severe retinopathy)
  - Unexplained flash pulmonary edema
  - Hypertension with an angiotensin-converting enzyme (ACE) inhibitor or ARB-induced acute renal failure
  - Uncontrolled hypertension with asymmetry of renal size.

Patients are stratified into low-risk, moderate-risk, and high-risk profile for renovascular hypertension. Those with low risk do not require an initial diagnostic workup, but need to be started on antihypertensive medications and should be followed up. Patients with moderate and high-risk profile do benefit from further investigations.

## ■ DIAGNOSTIC TESTS

Diagnostic tests that are used to establish a diagnosis of renovascular hypertension can be categorized into anatomical tests (which essentially identify the vascular lesion and its hemodynamic consequences) and functional tests (which help us to assess the differential renal functioning).

### Doppler Ultrasonography

It is considered as an ideal first-line imaging method, as it is easily available, noninvasive, and affordable. It combines both anatomical and physiological and hemodynamic assessment of the renal arteries. The peak systolic velocity (PSV) at the point of arterial stenosis is considered as a measure of disease severity. In hemodynamically significant lesions, spectral broadening of waveform and markedly increased flow velocities are noted.[9-12] Moreover, the size of the kidneys can be assessed to note for shrinkage.

Duplex ultrasonography (DUS) is also utilized to check the vessel patency and follow-up patients who undergo endovascular treatment or surgical revascularization. However, it is observer dependent, the accessory renal arteries cannot be visualized properly, and it is not a good investigation in obese patients.

### Magnetic Resonance Angiography

Advances in MRI technology have made it a useful investigation in patients with renovascular hypertension. It is highly sensitive and specific (90–100%) for detecting renal arterial stenosis.[13,14] The use of iodinated contrast material or exposure to ionizing radiation are also avoided. However, it is expensive and cannot be used in patients who are claustrophobic or those with metallic implants. Earlier reports of gadolinium being a safe contrast agent are

no longer accepted after it was found to be associated with nephrogenic systemic fibrosis in few patients.

### Computed Tomography Angiography

It shows excellent images of renal artery stenosis with good spatial resolution and is comparable to MRA. It is faster to perform and can be used in patients with metallic implants. For detecting renal artery stenosis due to atherosclerosis, computed tomography angiography is highly sensitive (94%) and specific (60–90%).[13,14] The major drawbacks of this modality are the use of nephrotoxic contrast material and exposure of the patient to ionizing radiation.

### Intra-arterial Digital Subtraction Angiography

It is the gold standard investigation for anatomical delineation of the lesion. Apart from assessment of the severity of renal artery stenosis, digital subtraction angiography is also helpful in the categorization of intrarenal vascular anomalies and in the detection of any abnormalities of the aorta, renal arteries, or kidney. Intra-arterial pressure measurements and endovascular treatment options can be provided in the same sitting. In those patients with renal impairment, noniodinated and non-nephrotoxic contrast agents such as carbon dioxide can be utilized. It is a costly investigation and requires technical expertise.[15,16] Exposure to ionizing radiation and nephrotoxic contrast agent is highest in this modality.

### Blood Oxygen Level Dependent MRI

It is a newer technique in which there is no requirement of nephrotoxic contrast agents. It uses the properties of oxyhemoglobin and deoxyhemoglobin to depict tissue oxygenation and detect ischemia. Images are obtained at baseline and following administration of furosemide, which decreases renal oxygen consumption. More studies are required to establish its definitive role in being able to identify those patients who will need to undergo a revascularization procedure.[17]

### Captopril Renography

A renogram is instrumental in evaluating the total as well as differential renal function through the use of an isotope (DTPA–diethylene triamine penta-acetic acid). Use of ACE inhibitor Captopril leads to fall in the glomerular filtration rate (GFR) of the ischemic kidney (with arterial stenosis) and often causes an increase in the GFR of the normally functioning nonischemic kidney. The difference between the GFR of the two kidneys is appreciated on the renogram. Captopril (25–50 mg) is given orally about 1 h before injection of the isotope. Decrease in function after its administration is highly suggestive of renovascular stenosis. However, this test is no longer performed routinely because of its low predictive value and it does not visualize the renal vessels directly.

# ◼ MANAGEMENT

Definitive treatment for renovascular hypertension is essential in order to prevent permanent ischemic damage to the kidneys.[18] Both medical and surgical options are available and the therapy has to be tailored according to patient requirements. Hypertensive emergencies must be managed accordingly as and when they present. Whenever there is need for invasive procedures, a well-equipped medical facility with available expertise must be sought for.

## Pharmacological Therapy

All types of antihypertensive drugs are used to treat renovascular hypertension, but the most effective ones are angiotensin receptor blockers and ACE inhibitors. However, in solitary kidneys or cases of bilateral renal arterial stenosis, they markedly decrease blood flow to the stenotic kidney(s) and may cause a sudden decline in renal function. This is a reversible phenomenon and the kidneys recover spontaneously on discontinuation of the drug.

Beta blockers, diuretics, and calcium channel blockers are also used. Calcium channel blockers provide good blood pressure control and do not cause functional impairment of the ischemic kidneys as much as ACE inhibitors. Diuretics act by a mechanism causing sodium and water excretion by the kidneys, thereby counteracting the volume-mediated component of renovascular hypertension. In cases of malignant hypertension, phenoxybenzamine or nitroprusside may be used as an emergency drug. Eplerenone (a selective aldosterone inhibitor) is a newer drug that has shown some promise in the management of this condition.

Besides the pharmacological management of hypertension, control of cardiovascular risk factors that include lifestyle modification, control of blood cholesterol, and glycemic control are also essential.[19]

## Percutaneous Transluminal Angioplasty

Percutaneous transluminal angioplasty (PTA) is an invasive, therapeutic technique that involves the dilatation of a stenotic renal artery using a small balloon introduced through a special catheter. Multiple attempts of dilatation are required at times to achieve the desired therapeutic effect. In case there is a failure, the patient can always be taken up for surgical revascularization.

A large randomized trial that compared the efficacy of drug therapy versus PTA for renal artery stenosis was the Dutch Renal Artery Stenosis Intervention Cooperative (DRASTIC)

trial.[20] Herein, 106 patients were included in the study and randomized them into two groups. One group of patients received medical therapy alone, while the other group was treated with PTA and medical therapy. Patients who did not respond well to medical therapy alone were later shifted to the PTA group and underwent balloon angioplasty. The authors of this trial concluded that PTA, in combination with drug therapy, provided "little additional benefit" to patients with renal artery stenosis. However, it was noted during subsequent 12-month follow-up that patients undergoing PTA had better blood pressure control and were less likely to develop renal artery occlusion. This study had some major limitations as well, as many patients with insignificant atherosclerosis had been enrolled and stents were used in a very small fraction of patients (20%).

Another two prominent randomized controlled trials comparing renal artery stenting with medical therapy alone for the treatment of renal artery stenosis have been concluded—the Stent Placement in Patients with Atherosclerotic Renal Artery Stenosis and Impaired Renal Function (STAR) trial and the Angioplasty and Stenting for Renal Artery Lesions (ASTRAL) trial. In the STAR trial,[21] 140 patients were randomized into two groups—those who would undergo renal artery stenting and receive medical therapy and those who would receive medical therapy alone. The inclusion criteria were renal arterial stenosis greater than 50%, creatinine clearance less than 80 mL/min/m$^2$, and hypertension. The primary end point was a decline in creatinine clearance by 20% or more, although safety of the patient and cardiovascular outcomes were addressed in the secondary end points. The study pointed out that stent placement as compared with medical therapy alone did not seem to offer much benefit to the patients, while it increased the incidence of serious procedure-related complications.[22] This study also had its own drawbacks. As the primary end point was a decline in kidney function, it is understandable that patients with unilateral renal ischemia and a normally functioning contralateral kidney and patients with non-critical renal arterial stenosis of less than 70% did not benefit much from renal artery stenting.

Similarly, in the ASTRAL trial, 806 patients with atherosclerotic renal arterial stenosis were included and divided into two groups on the basis of therapeutic options—one group would receive medical therapy alone while the other group would undergo renal artery stenting along with medical therapy. The primary outcome was a change in kidney function as calculated by the reciprocal of serum creatinine level, while secondary outcomes included blood pressure control, renal events, major cardiovascular episodes, and mortality. Patients were followed up for an average of 34 months, and upon conclusion of the study, the authors found "substantial risks but no evidence of a worthwhile clinical benefit from revascularization in patients with atherosclerotic renal artery stenosis".[21] This study also had its own drawbacks. Selection bias was introduced in the study at the time of recruiting patients. Moreover, one-fourth of the patients had normal renal function, a large number had a normally functioning contralateral kidney and around two-fifths had less than 70% stenosis of the renal artery.

Another interesting fact concerning both the STAR and the ASTRAL trials is that creatinine clearance equations which were used to calculate glomerular filtration rate have not been validated in patients with atherosclerotic renal artery stenosis and both these trials recruited subjects with advanced nephropathy who were unlikely to benefit from renal revascularization.

Another important trial, which compares renal artery angioplasty and stenting with medical therapy alone is the CORAL (Cardiovascular Outcomes in Renal Atherosclerotic Lesions) trial, which is underway. It is a landmark trial of stent therapy for atherosclerotic renal artery stenosis.[23] The final results will take several years, but this trial is expected to clear up the debate concerning renal artery stenting.

The general consensus that has emerged currently is that outcomes after PTA and stenting are better in patients whose lesions occur due to FMD. Greater failure rate has been noted for arteries with narrowing at the ostia, or multiple stenotic areas within the same artery.[24]

The incidence of treatment failure in FMD lesions needing a second angioplasty due to restenosis has been noted in fewer than 10% patients, while around 8–30% patients with atherosclerotic disease. Other complications of this technique include arterial injury, dissection and thrombosis. Use of an intravascular stent during angioplasty is helpful in preventing restenosis and is advisable.

## Surgical Revascularization

With surgical revascularization, most patients derive benefit in terms of cure of disease or improvement in hypertension. But there is associated morbidity and mortality inherent with these procedures. The indications of surgical therapy for renovascular hypertension are given below.

### Indications for Renal Revascularization[25]

- Hypertension resistant to medical therapy
- Inadequate control despite full dose of three or more drugs (including one diuretic)
- Renal failure with salvageable kidneys
- Documented recent deterioration of renal function
- Reduction of GFR with ACE-inhibition and/or ARBs
- Recurrent "flash" pulmonary edema
- Congestive cardiac failure with bilaterally stenosed renal arteries.

Blood pressure control is of paramount importance before the surgical procedure. Preoperative abdominal aortography is essential for diagnosis as well as anatomical evaluation of the disease extent and to plan the surgical approach to intervention. A transperitoneal incision should be used to allow for adequate exposure and dissection of the kidneys is kept to a minimum to protect the collateral vessels which maintain renal perfusion while the main renal artery is clamped during the procedure. To protect these small vessels, dissection is commenced from the proximal portion of the renal arteries before proceeding to the distal part of the vessel. While constructing the renal artery anastomosis, interrupted monofilament sutures should be used in children to allow for their growth, while in adults with larger anastomoses, a continuous suture may be used.

*Renal autotransplantation* is a technique that involves bypassing the renal artery stenosis by disconnecting the renal artery distal to the point of stenosis and re-anastomosing it to the aorta. It requires extensive mobilization of the kidneys and may not always be feasible as dictated by the extent of arterial stenosis and spread of the disease.

*Aortorenal bypass*, which is the most commonly performed procedure, uses an interposition graft anastomosed to the aorta at one end and to the renal artery (after bypassing the stenosis) at the other end. Synthetic material may be used for the graft, but it increases the risk of infection. Some surgeons advocate the use of a hypogastric artery segment,[26,27] as it is much similar to the renal artery, suturing is easy, and there is low incidence of graft aneurysm. However, there is a future risk of potential arteritis in the graft and in those patients whose hypogastric arteries of both sides are used, there is a chance of impotence. Reversed saphenous vein grafts have also been used but there is a high chance of aneurysmal dilatation.[28]

*Aortoaortic bypass* is required in patients with midaortic syndrome wherein a Dacron or expanded polytetrafluoroethylene (ePTFE) graft is anastomosed to the thoracic aorta above and the aortic bifurcation below.

Postoperative follow-up by arteriography is recommended to detect any thrombosis, stricture, or anastomotic failure. A failure rate of 8–10% has been reported for most of these procedures and graft failure is associated with high mortality.

## Renal Sympathetic Denervation

Renal sympathetic denervation is being used as an effective modality for patients with resistant hypertension (those patients in whom we are unable to achieve target blood pressure despite the use of three antihypertensive drugs in full dosages, which includes a diuretic).[29] It blocks the sympathetic nervous system discharge to the kidneys and thereby results in decreased production of the hormone rennin and increased diuresis and natriuresis. It does not have any adverse effect on other functions of the kidney. It has been shown to cause a sustained decrease in blood pressure in short-term and medium-term.

Several studies with various follow-up periods have been conducted on this novel technique. Almost all studies noted a significant reduction in systolic as well as diastolic blood pressures. There have been no incidences of worsening of renal function. However, such techniques should be carried out in experienced centers with highly trained personnel.

Two different kinds of catheter are available for this technique—the PARADISE catheter and the SYMPLICITY catheter. The SYMPLICITY catheter has been used in most of these studies. The catheter is introduced through the femoral arteries and positioned into the distal portion of the renal artery. Renal sympathetic nerves, which travel in the adventitia of the arterial wall, are damaged by delivering low power radiofrequency energy (<8 W) to the endothelial layer of the vessel. The energy is applied for an average of about 2 minutes, after which the catheter is repositioned and the energy is reapplied at different points in the vessel, longitudinally and circumferentially. This is repeated on the other side.[30] The PARADISE catheter, in addition, allows circulation of cooled fluid through a balloon, which is incorporated in the catheter. This keeps the artery wall cool during the process of ablation and minimizes chances of collateral damage.[31]

This technique requires careful patient selection and has proven to be of benefit to many patients, however, more studies are required to establish its safety and efficacy in patients with renovascular hypertension.

## Nephrectomy

This is performed in cases of renovascular hypertension when all other treatment alternatives have been exhausted and no other options are available. It is indicated in patients with severe renal hypoplasia, where functional capacity of the kidney has severely declined. Nephrectomy may be unavoidable at times when surgical revascularization is attempted and complications occur, or if the disease is too extensive and bypass is technically impossible. Nowadays, it can be performed laparoscopically in most centers.

## ■ PROGNOSIS

The prognosis of patients with renovascular hypertension depends on various factors such as the extent of arterial stenosis, response to antihypertensive drug therapy and the effectiveness of surgical or endovascular intervention. Renal dysfunction in the presence of renovascular hypertension is a predictor of increased mortality.

Normal blood pressures are achieved in about one third of patients treated by angioplasty. In another one third, decrease in blood pressure levels have been noticed. Unfortunately, restenosis of the artery leading to recurrence of hypertension is common in these patients.

Surgical revascularization, on the contrary, has an excellent prognosis and 70% of patients achieve normal blood pressures without requiring additional medical therapy. In another 20%, hypertension is controlled with minimal drug therapy. Only about 5% of patients do not seem to benefit from revascularization.

## ■ CONCLUSION

Renovascular hypertension is one of the most common causes of atypical hypertension and requires a high index of clinical suspicion for diagnosis. These patients require multiple drugs for control of their blood pressure, along with lifestyle modifications. If there is associated significant renal artery stenosis, then transluminal angioplasty or surgical revascularization may be attempted, but these procedures require a high level of surgical expertise and should be performed only in centers of excellence. In short, the therapy has to be tailored according to the patient's requirements.

## ■ REFERENCES

1. Simon G. What is critical renal artery stenosis? Implications for treatment. Am J Hypertens. 2000;13:1189-93.
2. Krzesinski JM. Diagnostic criteria for renovascular hypertension. Acta Chir Belg. 2002;102:159-66.
3. Dubel GJ, Murphy TP. The role of percutaneous revascularization for renal artery stenosis. Vasc Med. 2008;13(2):141-56.
4. Tyagi S, Kaul UA, Satsangi DK, Arora R. Percutaneous transluminal angioplasty for renovascular hypertension in children: initial and long-term results. Pediatrics. 1997;99(1):44-9.
5. Textor SC. Current approaches to renovascular hypertension. Med Clin North Am. 2009;93:717-32.
6. American Heart Association. Hypertension prevalence and the status of awareness, treatment and control in the United States. Hypertension. 1985;7:457.
7. Simon N, Franklin SS, Bleifer KH, et al. Clinical characteristics of renovascular hypertension. J Am Med Assoc. 1972;220:1209.
8. Mann SJ, Pickering TG. Detection of renovascular hypertension. State of the art: 1992. Ann Intern Med. 1992;117:845.
9. Olin JW, Piedmonte MR, Young JR, et al. The utility of duplex ultrasound scanning of the renal arteries for diagnosing significant renal artery stenosis. Ann Intern Med. 1995;122(11):833-8.
10. Kohler TR, Zierler RE, Martin RL, et al. Noninvasive diagnosis of renal artery stenosis by ultrasonic duplex scanning. J Vasc Surg. 1986;4(5):450-6.
11. Taylor DC, Kettler MD, Moneta GL, et al. Duplex ultrasound scanning in the diagnosis of renal artery stenosis: a prospective evaluation. J Vasc Surg. 1988;7(2):363-9.
12. Helenon O, el Rody F, Correas JM, et al. Color Doppler US of renovascular disease in native kidneys. Radiographics. 1995;15(4):833-54.
13. Eklof H. A prospective comparison of duplex ultrasonography, captopril renography, MRA and CTA in assessing renal artery stenosis. Acta Radiol. 2006;47(8):764-74.
14. Rountas C, Vlychou M, Vassiou K, et al. Imaging modalities for renal artery stenosis in suspected renovascular hypertension: prospective intraindividual comparison of color Doppler US, CT angiography, GD-enhanced MR angiography, and digital substraction angiography. Ren Fail. 2007;29(3):295-302.
15. Zhang HL, Sos TA, Winchester PA, Gao J, Prince MR. Renal artery stenosis: imaging options, pitfalls, and concerns. Prog Cardiovasc Dis. 2009;52:209-19.
16. O'Connor JP, Ariyanagam-Baksh SM, Carroll LE. Nephrogenic systemic fibrosis: a clinical and pathologic perspective. J Lanc Gen Hosp. 2007;2:122-5.

17. Textor SC, Glockner JF, Lerman LO, et al. The use of magnetic resonance to evaluate tissue oxygenation in renal artery stenosis. J Am Soc Nephrol. 2008;19(4):780-8.

18. Textor SC, Lerman L. Renovascular hypertension and ischemic nephropathy. Am J Hypertens. 2010;23(11):1159-69.

19. Shafique S, Peixoto AJ. Renal artery stenosis and cardiovascular risk. J Clin Hypertens (Greenwich). 2007;9:201-8.

20. van Jaarsveld BC, Krijnen P, Pieterman H, et al. Dutch Renal Artery Stenosis Intervention Cooperative Study Group. The effect of balloon angioplasty on hypertension in atherosclerotic renal-artery stenosis. N Engl J Med. 2000;342(14):1007-14.

21. Wheatley K, Ives N, Gray R, et al. Revascularization versus medical therapy for renal-artery stenosis. N Engl J Med. 2009; 361(20):1953-62.

22. Bax L, Woittiez AJ, Kouwenberg HJ, et al. Stent placement in patients with atherosclerotic renal artery stenosis and impaired renal function: a randomized trial. Ann Intern Med. 2009;150(12):840-8, W150-W151.

23. Cooper CJ, Murphy TP, Matsumoto A, et al. Stent revascularization for the prevention of cardiovascular and renal events among patients with renal artery stenosis and systolic hypertension: rationale and design of the CORAL trial. Am Heart J. 2006;152(1):59-66.

24. White CJ. Catheter-based therapy for atherosclerotic renal artery stenosis. Circulation. 2006;113:1464-73.

25. Garovic VD, Textor SC. Renovascular hypertension and ischemic nephropathy. Circulation. 2005;112:1362-74.

26. Stanley JC, Zelenock GB, Messina LM, Wakefield TW. Pediatric renovascular hypertension: a thirty-year experience of operative treatment. J Vasc Surg. 1995;21(2):212-26; discussion 226-7.

27. Guzzetta PC, Potter BM, Ruley EJ, Majd M, Bock GH. Renovascular hypertension in children: current concepts in evaluation and treatment. J Pediatr Surg. 1989;24(12):1236-40.

28. O'Neill JA Jr. Renovascular hypertension. Semin Pediatr Surg. 1994;3(2):114-23.

29. Calhoun DA, Jones D, Textor S, et al. Resistant hypertension: diagnosis, evaluation, and treatment. A scientific statement from the American Heart Association Professional Education Committee of the Council for High Blood Pressure Research. Hypertension. 2008;51:1403-19.

30. Doumas M, Faselis C, Papademetriou V. Renal sympathetic denervation in hypertension. Curr Opin Nephrol Hypertens. 2011;20:647-53.

31. Mabin T, Sapoval M, Cabane V, et al. First experience with endovascular ultrasound renal denervation for the treatment of resistant hypertension. Eurointervention. 2012;8:57-61.

## PRACTICAL POINTS

- Renovascular hypertension is a condition characterized by a rise of blood pressure, due to significant unilateral or bilateral renal arterial stenosis.

- Renal artery stenosis causes release of rennin due to ischemia and it contributes to hypertension through a sequence of biochemical events.

- Atherosclerosis is the etiological factor in as much as 90% of the lesions, usually involving the proximal renal arteries.

- The central pathophysiological mechanism behind renovascular hypertension is the activation of the rennin-angiotensin-aldosterone system and further events are dictated by the presence or absence of a normally functioning, nonischemic kidney.

- Renovascular hypertension leads to chronically elevated blood pressure which causes end organ damage to the body. Development of ischemic nephropathy may lead to renal failure.

- Doppler ultrasonography is considered as an ideal first-line imaging method.

- Computed tomography angiography shows excellent images of renal artery stenosis with good spatial resolution and is comparable to MRA.

- Definitive treatment for renovascular hypertension is essential in order to prevent permanent ischemic damage to the kidneys.

- Antihypertensive therapy should be instituted and optimal blood pressure control is of utmost importance.

- All types of antihypertensive drugs are used to treat renovascular hypertension, but the most effective ones are angiotensin receptor blockers and ACE inhibitors.

- However, in solitary kidneys or cases of bilateral renal arterial stenosis, they may cause a sudden decline in renal function.

- The options for treatment of this condition (in recalcitrant cases, wherein medical options have failed) include PTA, surgical revascularization, renal sympathetic denervation and nephrectomy.

- PTA is an invasive, therapeutic technique that involves the dilatation of a stenotic renal artery using a small balloon introduced through a special catheter. Multiple attempts of dilatation are required at times to achieve the desired therapeutic effect.

- With surgical revascularization, most patients derive benefit in terms of cure of disease or improvement in hypertension. But there is associated morbidity and mortality inherent with these procedures.

- Renal sympathetic denervation is being used as an effective modality for patients with resistant hypertension.

- Nephrectomy is performed in cases of renovascular hypertension when all other treatment alternatives have been exhausted and no other options are available.

- Patient education and counseling regarding this condition is also a neglected entity and should be tackled judiciously.

# 11

# Management of Abdominal Aortic Aneurysms

*Jaisom Chopra*

## ■ DEFINITION

Aortic abdominal aneurysm is the dilatation of the abdominal aorta exceeding the normal diameter of the abdominal aorta by more than double. About 90% are infrarenal but they may be pararenal (at the level of the kidneys) or suprarenal (above the level of the kidneys). They may extend into one or both the iliac arteries, in the pelvis (Fig. 1).

## ■ INTRODUCTION

- Aortic abdominal aneurysm (AAA) occurs most commonly in the 65–75 years age group.
- The normal outer diameter of the aorta is 2 cm and is considered aneurysmal if it increases to >3 cm. It is considered large >5.5 cm.
- It is more common in the male smokers.

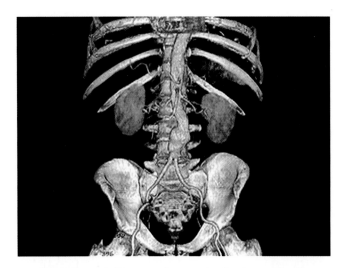

**Fig. 1** Computed tomography reconstruction image of aortic abdominal aneurysm

- They are mostly asymptomatic, although back and abdominal pain may be because of the pressure on the surrounding tissue and leg pain may be because of the disturbance of blood flow.
- The major complication of AAA is rupture leading to death within minutes. The classical triad to diagnose rupture is severe abdominal pain, shock, and pulsating abdominal mass. The mortality of rupture repair is 60–90%.
- Elective surgery is recommended when the size is >5.5 cm diameter—the risk of surgery being 1–6%.
- In open surgery, the graft replaces the diseased portion of the artery, whereas in endovascular surgery, the replacement graft is inserted through the groin artery.
- Screening of patients >65 years in the community is helpful.
- There are about 150,000 admissions to the hospitals every year from AAA and it is the tenth leading cause of death from rupture of AAA, which accounts for 16,000 deaths every year.

## ■ RISK FACTORS

- Over 90% of AAA patients are smokers or have given up smoking.
- Atherosclerosis is a secondary factor in the development of AAA and affects by weakening the wall further but is not the primary factor responsible as considered earlier.
- Age, male gender, hypertension, and chronic obstructive pulmonary disease (COPD) place the patient at higher risk.
- The influence of genetic factors is highly probable and is most notable in males. 15% of the AAA patients have a first degree relative with AAA and have a decreased type III collagen within the aortic wall, which weakens it. There is also an increase in Hp-2-1 haptoglobin phenotype, Kell positive as well as MN blood groups in patient with AAA. Alpha-1 antitrypsin deficiency could be a major factor,

whereas others favored X-linked mutation. Connective tissue disorders like Marfan's syndrome and Ehlers–Danlos syndrome are strongly associated with AAA.

- There is also a decrease in the incidence of AAA in patients with A negative blood group.
- Aortic abdominal aneurysm is degenerative in nature with polygenic inheritance pattern.
- Rare causes are cystic medial necrosis, trauma, dissection, vasculitis, and infection.

## PATHOGENESIS

- The striking changes are seen in the tunica media and the intima.
- There is lipid accumulation in the foam cells, extracellular free cholesterol crystals, calcification, thrombosis, and ulceration and rupture of the layers.
- In AAA, there is marked inflammation and imbalance between the production and degradation of structural extracellular matrix proteins.
- Disruption and degradation of medial elastin and collagen is particularly prominent feature of AAA formation. It is very likely there is an increased local production of enzymes (matrix metalloproteinases) that degrade elastin and collagen.
- There is reduction of vasa vasorum in the AAA wall—tunica media, which now gets its nutrition by diffusion making it more susceptible to damage.

## ETIOLOGY

- Degenerative (Fig. 2)
  - Abnormal matrix (collagen-elastin) degradation
  - Atherosclerosis
- Connective tissue disorders
  - Cystic medial necrosis
  - Marfan's syndrome
  - Ehlers–Danlos syndrome
- Trauma
- Dissection
- Vasculitis
  - Takayasu arteritis
- Mycotic
  - Bacterial (*Staphylococcus* species).

## CLINICAL FEATURES

- Mostly asymptomatic.
- Abdominal pain in a patient with AAA is an ominous symptom and one has to make sure this pain is aortic in origin or not (Fig. 3).
- Pain in the feet with cyanosis in a patient with AAA points toward "trash foot" due to emboli from the AAA. The thrombus breaks free due to the flow of the blood and is carried distally to the feet as emboli.
- Massive hematemesis in a patient warns of aortoduodenal fistula.
- Normal aortic pulsation is the thumb width and AAA is suspected when aortic pulse is expansile and over 2 cm.
- Extension of the pulsation to the costal margin—suspect thoracoabdominal or suprarenal aneurysm.
- Tenderness over the aneurysm is a bad sign—impending rupture.
- Prominent anterior pulsation in a thin patient—ectatic nonaneurysmal aorta (Fig. 4).
- It is not easy to palpate an infrarenal aorta as it bifurcates at the umbilicus.

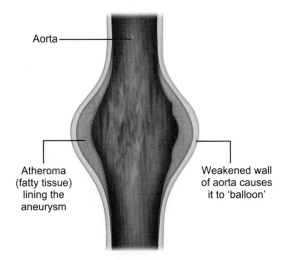

Aorta

Atheroma (fatty tissue) lining the aneurysm

Weakened wall of aorta causes it to 'balloon'

**Fig. 2** Details of aortic aneurysm

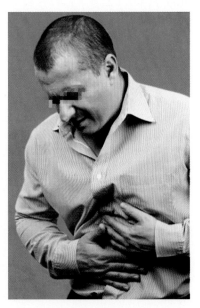

**Fig. 3** Abdominal pain from rupture of AAA

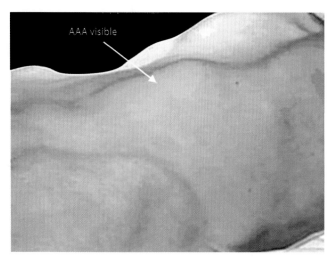

**Fig. 4** Aneurysm visible on inspection

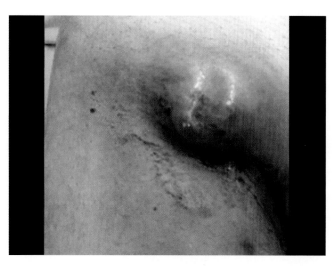

**Fig. 6** Femoral artery aneurysm in right groin

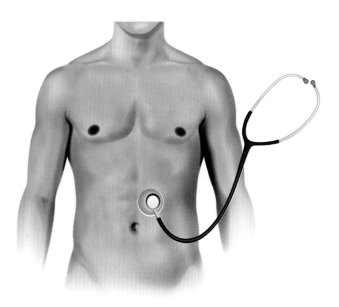

**Fig. 5** Auscultating for bruit

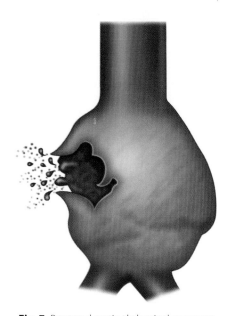

**Fig. 7** Ruptured aortic abdominal aneurysm

- Asymptomatic abdominal bruit is common in elderly and due to narrowing of the aorta, renal or mesenteric artery stenosis (Fig. 5).
- Physical examination alone is unreliable especially in obese—in one study, proven AAA patients were examined by experienced clinicians and were unable to diagnose in 50% of the patients.

## Concomitant Aneurysmal Disease

Patient with AAA must be examined for femoral artery and popliteal artery aneurysms as there is a 14% chance (Fig. 6). Conversely, if a patient has a femoral artery aneurysm, he will have an 80% chance of having AAA, whereas if he has a popliteal artery aneurysm, he has a 60% chance.

## Clinical Features of a Ruptured AAA

- The classical triad—acute hypotension, abdominal or back pain, and a palpable abdominal mass—is not present in all cases (Fig. 7).
- It may present as exacerbation of chronic back pain or abdominal, back pain radiating to the groin.
- Differential diagnosis—diverticulitis, renal colic, irritable bowel syndrome, inflammatory bowel disease, appendicitis, and ovarian torsion.

- Bedside ultrasonography is a must and accurately confirms the diagnosis of ruptured AAA.
- If patient is suspected of having a ruptured AAA, he should be transported to the OT complex at once as symptomatic AAA is an acute surgical emergency and needs operative intervention.

## ■ DIAGNOSIS

Once the diagnosis is suspected, the regimen given in Flow chart 1 should be followed.

Plain X-ray of the abdomen and the lumbosacral region should be done in anteroposterior (AP) and lateral projections to see the lumbosacral (LS) spine and the outline of a calcified outer aortic wall.

## Ultrasound (Fig. 8)

This noninvasive, patient friendly and inexpensive test provides useful and reliable information regarding the size and diameter of AAA. It correlates closely with the operative findings. Errors are attributed to inexperience, lack of interpretive skills, or excessive bowel gas (Fig. 9).

## CT Scan (Fig. 10)

This is always advised if intervention is planned and has an accuracy of 91%.

It is more accurate than ultrasound in determining:
- Aortic abdominal aneurysm wall integrity
- Location and amount of calcification within the vessel wall

**Flow chart 1** Investigating suspected aortic abdominal aneurysm

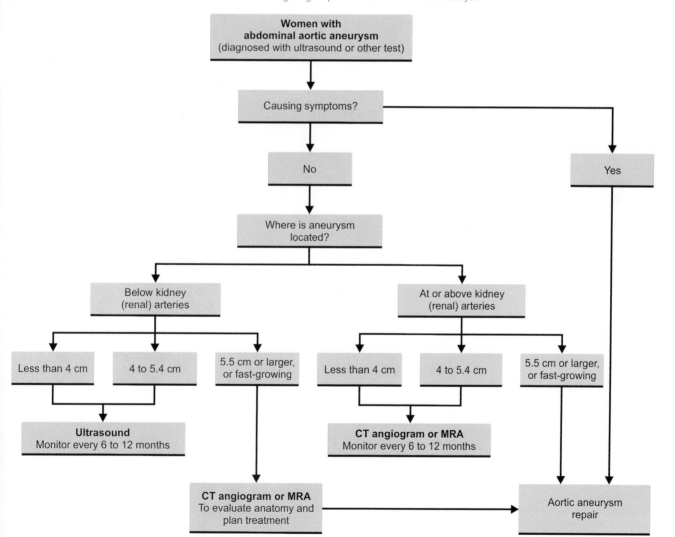

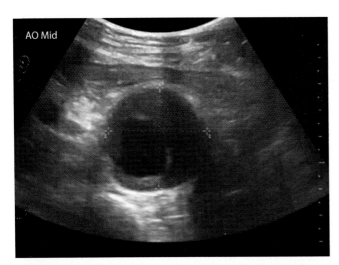

**Fig. 8** Ultrasound showing aortic abdominal aneurysm with thrombus

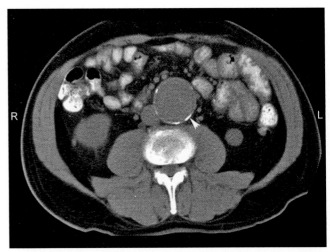

**Fig. 10** CT scan showing aortic abdominal aneurysm

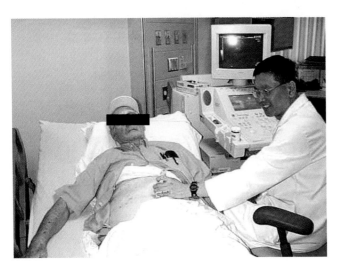

**Fig. 9** Bedside Doppler test for aortic abdominal aneurysm

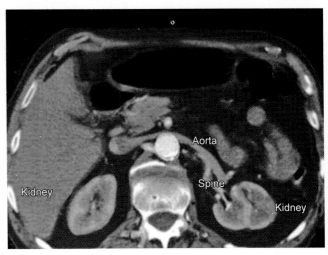

**Fig. 11** Ruptured aortic abdominal aneurysm on CT scan showing blood in the abdominal cavity

- Venous anomalies
- Retroperitoneal blood (Fig. 11)
- Aortic dissection
- Infection or inflammation of the wall
- Proximal and distal extent of the aneurysm.

CT may also demonstrate other pathologies, we are unaware of, and help to plan the procedure.

*Limitations of CT include:*
- The iodinated contrast is nephrotoxic
- Radiation exposure
- Increased cost.

Spiral or helical CT is superior to conventional CT and provides better images. It provides a roadmap for AAA repair or endoleaks.

## Magnetic Resonance Angiography

- Uses non-nephrotoxic gadolinium with breath hold technique.
- The images are based on T1 relaxation rather than the blood flow, which is good because slow blood flow does not adversely affect the image.
- It has a specificity of 94% and a specificity of 98%.
- To see if endografts are in place in patients with chronic renal failure (CRF) (creatinine >1.5 mg%).

*Limitations of MRA include:*
- Inability to scan patients with pacemakers or defibrillators
- People with claustrophobia
- Metallic objects like vascular stents can obscure images
- Inability to image calcified plaque.

## Catheter-based Angiography (Fig. 12)

- Angiography with digital subtraction is very useful.
- Intravascular ultrasound (IVUS) is especially helpful in assessing the neck of the aneurysm as CT oversizes the neck of the aneurysm.
- Both angiography and IVUS help identifying the cephalad extent of the aneurysm, the number and location of the renal vessels, state of the iliac arteries, and state of the occlusive disease in the lower limb arteries.

*Complications of angiography include:*
- Bleeding or arterial occlusion at the puncture site
- Atheroembolism
- Impairment of the renal function because of the iodine-induced contrast nephrotoxicity.

## ■ MANAGEMENT

- Ruptured AAA is a very serious complication with a very high mortality.
- According to Laplace's law, the increase in aortic wall pressure occurs with linear increase in aortic wall size. Thus, a twofold increase in size (2–4 cm) increases the pressure fourfold (pressure/cm$^2$) on the aortic wall.
- The elastic aortic wall tissue loses its integrity with age.
- Acquired risk factors like smoking and hypertension or genetic factors hasten the process and add to the risk of AAA expansion.
- Expansion over 6 mm/annum increase suggests an unstable AAA and calls for early intervention if it is 5 cm in diameter.
- An asymptomatic AAA 5 cm in diameter carries a 10% risk of rupture over 2–3 years. Greater AP diameter, COPD, and diastolic hypertension independent increase the risk of rupture.

- Therefore, a 5 cm AAA in patient with COPD or diastolic hypertension is a matter of worry as it has a mortality of over 30% per annum.
- The mortality from ruptured AAA is very high. About 60% die before reaching the hospital and only 50% of those who are operated survive. Thus, a ruptured AAA carries a mortality of over 80%.

## Surgical Therapy (Fig. 13)

Elective surgery by open technique or endovascular graft dramatically reduces the chances of mortality due to rupture AAA. The overall mortality after elective surgical repair was 5.6%, but surprisingly in women it was 10.7% compared with 6.8% in men.

The risk factors responsible for a poor surgical outcome and increase in hospital mortality by over eightfold are:
- Female gender
- Age over 65 years
- Ruptured AAA
- Lack of experience in aortic surgery.

## Conventional Surgical Treatment of Intact AAA (Fig. 14)

Increased surgical mortality is seen in:
- Operations over 5 hours increase cardiopulmonary complications
- Hypothermia
- Excessive blood loss
- Coagulopathy
- Need for supraceliac aortic cross-clamping.

Surgical approaches—transperitoneal or retroperitoneal—are dependent on surgeon's preference and aortic pathology. The transperitoneal approach is preferred when the right renal artery is to be dealt with or the aneurysmal disease extends onto

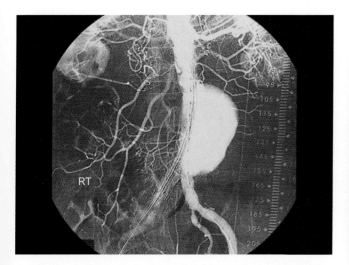

**Fig. 12** Angiography showing aortic abdominal aneurysm with diseased iliac artery

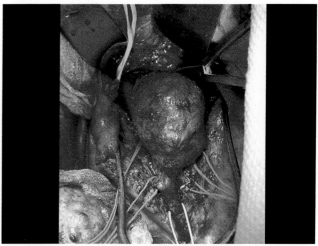

**Fig. 13** Aortic abdominal aneurysm during surgery

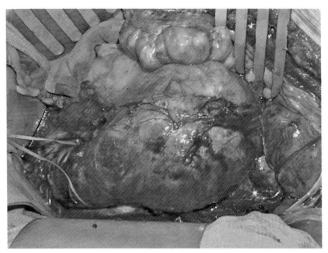

**Fig. 14** Surgical treatment of intact aortic abdominal aneurysm

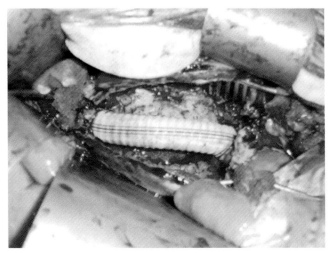

**Fig. 15** Graft in place during surgery

the right iliac artery. The retroperitoneal approach is preferred in obese or those with multiple laparotomies for various reasons. The retroperitoneal approach has no specific advantage over the transperitoneal approach as it does not reduce the mortality or the cardiopulmonary morbidity, although there is early return of postoperative bowel mobility.

In the past thrombotic complications due to the aortic clamping and renal failure were disastrous. Now prior to clamping, anticoagulant is given IV and adequate diuresis is maintained using mannitol or loop diuretics. Both are undertaken before clamping the aorta.

Now the aneurysm is incised and the clot is removed before sewing the polytetrafluoroethylene (PTFE) aortic graft in place (Fig. 15). With the graft in place, it is covered with aneurysm sac to prevent intestines coming in contact with the graft thus avoiding life-threatening graft enteric erosion (Fig. 16).

Postoperatively all patients with aortic grafts must receive antibiotics before any invasive procedure like dental procedure.

### Conventional Surgical Treatment of Ruptured AAA (Flow chart 2)

The purpose is to save life and 50% die in the first 1 month of emergency surgery due to complications. Attention during surgery must be pain to:
- Controlling hemorrhage
- Restoring aortic blood flow
- Avoiding reconstruction of less-diseased vessels like asymptomatic renal artery stenosis or minimal iliac artery aneurysmal disease.

A supraceliac aortic clamp is initially applied to control the bleeding and then shifted to below the renals once the infrarenal neck has been isolated and occluded. Adequate blood replacement and the maintenance of normothermia

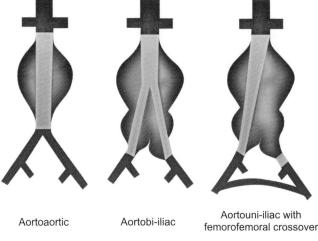

Aortoaortic          Aortobi-iliac          Aortouni-iliac with femorofemoral crossover

**Fig. 16** Various options during surgical repair for aortic abdominal aneurysm

are critical to the management and successful outcome. Following a successful reconstruction, one must look for bowel ischemia and the flow to the lower extremities.

One should consider delayed abdominal closure as massive fluid resuscitation and retroperitoneal hematoma may cause the usual abdominal closure to result in compartment syndrome with decrease blood perfusion to the splanchnic and renal circulations. Delayed abdominal closure using an open IV bag or vacuum pack dressing improves survival in some patients with rupture AAA.

### Endovascular Surgical Treatment of Intact AAA

Two endovascular grafts were approved by Food and Drug Administration (FDA) in 1999 for the treatment of infrarenal AAA and two more have been approved in 2004 (Fig. 17).

**Flow chart 2** Management of ruptured aortic abdominal aneurysm

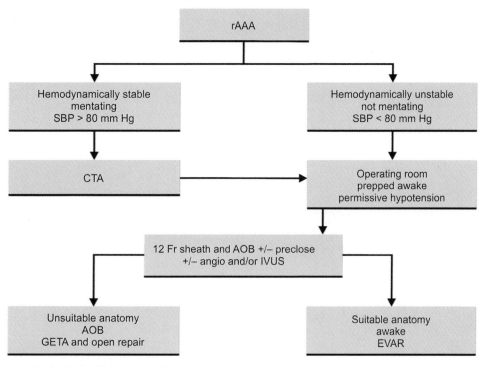

*Abbreviations:* rAAA, ruptured abdominal aortic aneurysm; SBP, systolic blood pressure; CTA, computerized tomography angiogram; AOB, aortic occlusion balloon; GETA, general endotracheal anesthesia; EVAR; endovascular aortic repair

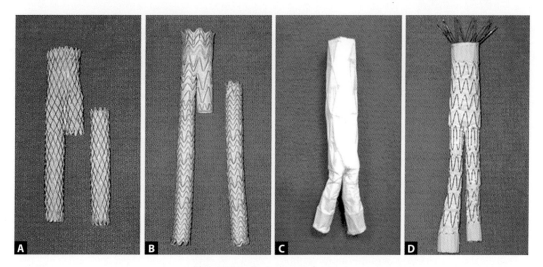

**Figs 17A to D** Endovascular stents

These are basically covered stent grafts and deployed as an aortic prosthesis with an ipsilateral iliac artery limb followed by docking of a contralateral iliac artery graft limb. These grafts have hooks mounted on Z-stents at the proximal and distal ends of the grafts. When the grafts are in place, they are dilated and the hooks become embedded into the aortic and the iliac walls. These grafts have been abandoned because of the high incidence of endovascular leaks and new grafts are being evaluated to take care of the endoleaks. Once again open infrarenal AAA repair is being done. The failure was attributed to the graft not fitting snugly into the artery as the graft was tailored after looking at the angiogram and the CT scan. Now IVUS is used to evaluate the graft designing. Failure also occurs because of the retrograde flow from the

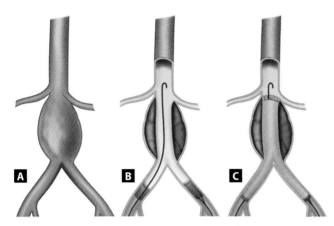

**Figs 18A to C** Procedure of endovascular stenting in aortic abdominal aneurysm

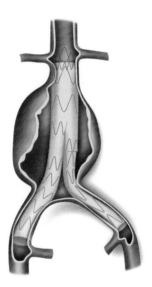

**Fig. 19** Diagrammatic representation of graft in place

lumbar and inferior mesenteric arteries into the gap between the aneurysmal wall and the graft (Figs 18A to C and 19).

## ■ PROGNOSIS AND FOLLOW-UP

Currently, open surgical repair is done with the replacement of the aneurysmal sac with prosthetic graft. The procedure has a mortality of less than 2.5%. Endovascular repair has been shown to have lower early postoperative morbidity compared with open surgery. With efficient postoperative care following conventional surgery for infrarenal AAA both morbidity and mortality are on the decline. Most mortality following open surgery is from myocardial infarction (MI). There are effective guidelines to assess preoperatively the cardiac risk from AAA surgery. The risk factors predicting the postoperative cardiac event are given further.

- Advanced age
- Male gender
- Diabetes needing medication
- Previous MI
- Congestive heart failure.

Elective intact AAA surgery has lower morbidity and mortality then emergency ruptured AAA repair. Even after elective intact repair, the prognosis worsens if the patient has:
- Coronary artery disease
- COPD
- Renal insufficiency
- Disease involving the renal and visceral vessels.

Over the years, the mortality and morbidity rates have declined with superior pre- and postoperative care in elective intact AAA repair but the mortality still remains over 50% in emergency ruptured AAA repair.

Early complications following elective intact AAA repair are:
- Cardiac event (15%)
- Pulmonary insufficiency (8%)
- Renal insufficiency (6%)
- Bleeding (4%)
- Embolization (3%)
- Wound infection (2%).

Late postoperative complications are:
- Graft infection (1%)
- Aortoenteric fistula (1%)—happens 3–5 years after aortic surgery.

Recent studies have suggested early safety and efficacy of endovascular grafting over open AAA surgery. Another study has recommended endovascular repair in ruptured AAA. There were 25 patients in the study of whom five needed conversion to open surgery and only two deaths were reported with mortality of 10% compared with 50% with open surgery.

The most common complication of endovascular repair is endoleak, which is defined as persistent blood flow into the aneurysmal sac even after placement of endovascular graft. Leaks may be:
- Graft related—failure of the endovascular graft seal at either end of the graft or from the fabric of the graft itself.
- Graft unrelated—filling of the aneurysmal sac by back bleeding from branch arteries.

Plain abdominal X-ray is used to follow-up graft migration, predictive to type 1 endoleak. In a large study of endovascular AAA repair, the following was the outcome:

Early endoleak rate was 15%—and of these:
- 35% sealed spontaneously
- 18% sealed after second intervention
- 3% had to be converted to open repair
- 7% died within 30 days of unrelated causes
- 12% had persistent leak at late follow-up
- 27% were lost to follow-up
- 18% had no postoperative leak and developed a leak on late follow-up—leaks may develop at a much later date after the graft placement.

## Classification of Endoleaks

- Leak at the attachment site
  - Proximal end of the graft
  - Distal end of the graft
  - Iliac occluder
- Branch leak
  - Simple or to-and-fro (from only one patent branch)
  - Complex or flow-through (from two or more patent branches)
- Graft defect
  - Junctional leak or modular disconnect
  - Fabric disruption (mid graft hole):
    - Minor (<2 mm, e.g. suture hole)
    - Major (>2 mm)
- Graft wall (fabric) porosity (<30 days after graft placement).

## ■ CONCLUSION

- There is increased detection of AAA along with increased awareness.
- Physical examination alone is often unreliable especially in obese.
- Diagnosis of AAA by ultrasound is reliable and cost-effective and is considered part of the screening for high risk cases.
- CT scan is investigation of choice when intervention is being considered.
- The current treatment of choice is open surgery and graft replacement—the mortality is less than 2.5%.
- Endovascular treatment in selected cases of AAA is safe.
- Widespread use of endovascular grafting as the primary therapy is hampered by the high incidence of endoleaks and awaits the maturation of device technology.

## PRACTICAL POINTS

- The classic triad of hypotension, back or abdominal pain, and palpable abdominal mass may not be seen in all ruptured AAAs.
- There is a 14% incidence of femoral and popliteal artery aneurysms in male patients with AAA. However, there is 80% incidence of AAA in patients with femoral artery aneurysm and a 60% incidence of patients with popliteal artery aneurysms having AAA.
- Aortic abdominal aneurysm over 5.5 cm in diameter is life-threatening and should be operated as a routine case in low-risk patients.
- 3–5 cm AAA rupture with unpredictable frequency. Diastolic hypertension and COPD are independent risk factors for rupture of small AAA.
- Aneurysmal expansion more than 6 mm per year suggests an unstable AAA and calls for early intervention just as it approaches 5 cm diameter.
- Ultrasounds are good for screening but CT scan is a must if intervention is planned.
- Elective AAA repair carries a mortality of 3–6% with women fearing worse than men. Emergency repair of ruptured AAA carries a mortality of 50%. The overall mortality of ruptured AAA including that cannot make it to the hospital is 80%.

# 12

# Thoracic Aortic Aneurysm

*VS Bedi, Anand Chandrasekar, Ajay Yadav, Ambarish Satwik, Kamran Ali Khan*

## ■ INTRODUCTION

A thoracic aortic aneurysm (TAA) is defined as a permanent abnormal dilatation of the thoracic aorta. Although the aortic diameter increases slightly with age, the normal diameter of the midascending aorta should always be less than 4 cm, and that of the descending aorta no more than 3 cm.[1] Multidetector computed tomographic (MD-CT) angiography is routinely performed for the diagnosis and evaluation of thoracic aortic aneurysms (TAAs), having essentially replaced diagnostic angiography.

The thoracic aorta consists of the aortic root, ascending aorta, aortic arch, and descending thoracic aorta (Fig. 1). The ascending aorta extends from the root to the origin of the right brachiocephalic artery; the arch, from the right brachio-cephalic artery to the attachment of the ligamentum arteriosum; and the descending aorta, from the ligamentum arteriosum to the aortic hiatus in the diaphragm. The aortic root is defined as that part of the ascending aorta that contains the valve, annulus, and sinuses. The arch may be subdivided into proximal (right brachiocephalic artery to left subclavian artery) and distal (left subclavian artery to attachment of the ligamentum arteriosum) segments. The distal arch, also referred to as the isthmus, may be narrower than the proximal descending aorta.

## ■ MEAN AORTIC DIAMETERS IN MALE AND FEMALE

Current screening and detection of asymptomatic aortic aneurysms is based largely on uniform cut-point diameters. Average diameters of the thoracic and abdominal aorta by computed tomography are larger in men when compared with women, vary significantly with age and body surface area, and are associated with modifiable cardiovascular disease risk factors, including diastolic blood pressure and cigarette smoking as shown in Table 1.[2]

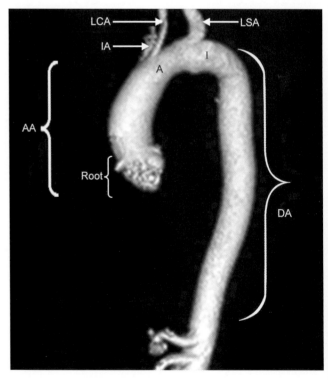

**Fig. 1** Three-dimensional volume-rendered (VR) image shows the anatomic segments of the thoracic aorta

*Abbreviations:* A, arch; AA, ascending aorta; DA, descending aorta; I, isthmus; IA, innominate artery (brachiocephalic trunk); LCA, left common carotid artery; LSA, left subclavian artery.

These mean aortic diameters has got strong correlation ($p < 0.0001$) with age and body surface area in age-adjusted analyses, and these relations remained significant in multivariate regression analyses.[2] Positive associations of diastolic blood pressure with AA and DTA diameters in

**Table 1** Mean aortic diameter with respect to the gender[2]

|  | Men | Women |
| --- | --- | --- |
| Ascending aorta | 34.1 mm | 31.9 mm |
| Descending thoracic aorta | 25.8 mm | 23.1 mm |
| Infrarenal aorta | 19.3 mm | 16.7 mm |
| Lower abdominal aorta | 18.7 mm | 16.0 mm |

both genders and pack-years of cigarette smoking with DTA diameter in women and IRA diameter in men and women were observed.[2]

# PATHOLOGY

An aneurysm can be characterized by its location, shape, and cause. Thoracic aortic aneurysms (TAAs) can involve the aortic root, ascending aorta, arch, descending aorta, abdominal aorta (TAAA) or a combination of these locations. The shape of an aneurysm is described as being fusiform or saccular which helps to identify a true aneurysm. The majority of aneurysms are degenerative; other causes include traumatic, mycotic and pseudoaneurysms. A true aneurysm involves all three layers of the arterial blood vessel wall. The more common fusiform-shaped aneurysm bulges or balloons out on all sides of the aorta. A saccular-shaped aneurysm bulges or balloons out only on one side. A pseudoaneurysm, or false aneurysm, is an enlargement of only the outer layer of the blood vessel wall. A false aneurysm may be the result of prior surgery or trauma. Once formed, an aneurysm will gradually increase in size and there will be a progressive weakening of the aneurysm wall.

Diseases affecting the ascending aorta, such as thoracic aortic aneurysms and dissections, are primarily associated with medial necrosis on pathologic examination. Medial necrosis is characterized by fragmentation and loss of elastic fibers, loss of smooth muscle cells, and interstitial collections of collagenous tissue and basophilic ground substance as shown in Figure 2.

# INCIDENCE AND PREVALENCE

Aortic aneurysms are found in about 3.4% of autopsies performed for other reasons.[3] Males are affected 9.4 times as often as females. Sixty percent of thoracic aortic aneurysms involve the aortic root and/or ascending aorta, 40% involve the descending aorta, 10% involve the arch, and 10% involve the thoracoabdominal aorta (with some involving >1 segment). The etiology, natural history, and treatment of thoracic aneurysms differ for each of these segments.[4] The incidence and prevalence of TAAAs have been increasing over the last several decades. The incidence of thoracic aortic disease rose by 52% in men and 28% in women to reach 16.3 and 9.1 per 100,000 per year, respectively. Olsson and

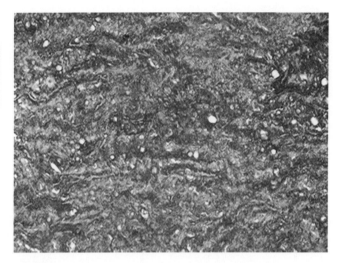

**Fig. 2** This mucin stain of the wall of the aorta demonstrates cystic medial necrosis. Pink elastic fibers, instead of running in parallel arrays, are disrupted by pools of blue mucinous ground substance

colleagues concluded that the prevalence and incidence of thoracic aortic disease were higher than previously reported and increasing.[5] The increasing prevalence of TAAAs has been attributed to a number of factors, including improved imaging techniques, an aging population, and increased patient and physician awareness.[6]

# ETIOLOGY

TAAAs are primarily a disease of the elderly. The average age of patients with TAAAs is 65 years, with a male-female ratio of 1.7:1.[7] The TAA and TAAAs clearly have a genetic component in that more than 20% of patients will have a first-degree relative affected by aneurysm disease.[8] Medial necrosis occurs as part of the normal aging of the aorta but is accelerated by other conditions, including hypertension and genetic alterations that predispose persons to these aortic diseases. The etiologies of many of the genetic syndromes, such as Marfan syndrome, that predispose persons to thoracic aortic aneurysms and dissections are understood.[9]

Many risk factors are common in patients with AAAs, including hypertension, smoking, and atherosclerosis in other arteries, are also common in patients with TAAAs (Table 2).[10]

## Risk Factors for Rupture

Because most patients with TAAAs are asymptomatic, treatment is aimed at preventing rupture (Table 3). Natural history studies of TAAAs are rarer than those of isolated infrarenal AAAs, probably related to their much less frequent occurrence. Aneurysm diameter is the most important risk factor for rupture. The expansion rate of thoracic aortic

**Table 2** Etiology of thoracoabdominal aortic aneurysms and the relative percentage contributing to disease

| Risk factors associated with TAA and TAAA |
| --- |
| Degenerative (associated with atherosclerosis)[11]—80% |
| Dissections[12]—20% |
| Connective tissue disorders such as Marfan's syndrome, EDS... |
| Infection[13]—*Salmonella* (57%), staphylococci (14%), and *Mycobacterium* (11%) |
| Takayasu's arteritis |
| Giant cell arteritis |
| Trauma |
| Miscellaneous—ankylosing spondylitis, rheumatoid arthritis |

**Table 3** Risk factors associated with rupture of thoracoabdominal aortic aneurysm[17]

| Risk factor | Relative risk |
| --- | --- |
| Age | 2.6 |
| Pain | 2.3 |
| Chronic obstructive pulmonary disease | 3.6 |
| Descending aortic diameter | 1.9 |
| Abdominal aortic diameter | 1.5 |

aneurysms may be an important and clinically relevant index of the risk of rupture.[14] Dapunt and coworkers documented that TAAAs >8 cm have an 80% risk for rupture within 1 year of diagnosis.[15] However, the size at which TAAAs rupture is unpredictable. Similar to AAAs, it appears that aneurysm

growth rates play a role. The average expansion rate of a TAAA is approximately 0.10 to 0.42 cm/year.[16]

## Others

- Smoking
- Uncontrolled systemic hypertension
- Dissection (type A > type B)
- Annual expansion rate > 1 cm/year[18]
- Chronic kidney disease[19]
- Mural thrombus
- Saccular aneurysm
- Mycotic aneurysm.

## Pathogenesis

The development of a TAAA is a multifactorial event that involves a complex interaction of genetic factors, cellular imbalance, and altered hemodynamic factors.[20] Recent studies have suggested that genetic variation in extracellular matrix (ECM) actin and myosin may contribute to the development of TAAAs.[21] TAAA formation is a complicated, dynamic process involving both extracellular and cellular processes, similar to other aneurysms. A large body of evidence suggests that ECM degradation by matrix metalloproteinases (MMPs) exceeds matrix production and repair during average function as shown in Figure 3. It is important to emphasize that there are significant differences in the composition of the aortic wall as one progress from the ascending aorta to the iliac bifurcation.

The ascending aorta has a greater concentration of elastin and is therefore more compliant than the descending aorta. This alteration in elastin concentration leads to a progressive

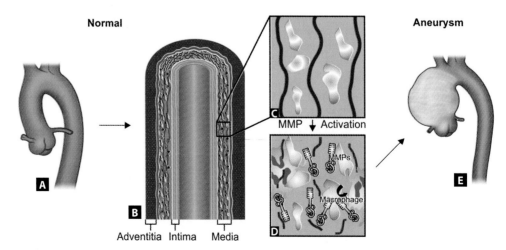

**Figs 3A to E** Medial elastin breakdown contributes to thoracic aortic aneurysm disease. (A) Normal structure of the thoracic aorta; (B) Cross-section of aorta showing adventitial, medial and intimal layers; (C) Normal medial architecture showing elastin layers interspersed with vascular smooth muscle cells; (D) Infiltration of the media by inflammatory cells such as macrophages may result in release of specific activated protease systems such as the matrix metalloproteinases (MMPs) which degrade medial elastin and weaken the aortic wall; (E) Aortic wall weakening may cause aneurysm formation

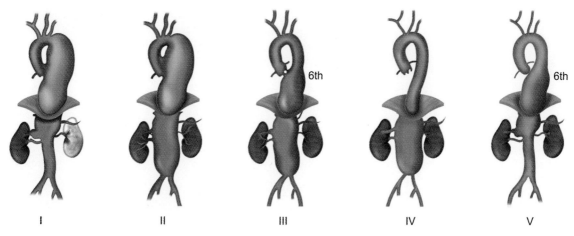

**Fig. 4** The classification of thoracoabdominal aortic aneurysms as proposed by Crawford and modified by Safi

decrease in the elastin-collagen ratio as the aorta progresses from the ascending aorta to the abdominal aorta.[22] Recent studies had documented the overexpression and increased activity of various ECM proteinases, specifically the MMPs, in human TAAAs.[23] These proteolytic enzymes, which have been more extensively studied in AAAs, are clearly critical as well during the formation of TAAAs also.

## ANATOMICAL CLASSIFICATION

Classification of thoracoabdominal aortic aneurysms (Fig. 4) has important diagnostic and therapeutic implications.[24] Type I, accounting for 25% of thoracoabdominal aortic aneurysms, involves most of the thoracic aorta with the distal portion extending to the upper abdominal aorta; type II (in nearly 30%) are those involving most of the descending thoracic aorta and most or all of the abdominal aorta; type III (less than one-quarter) involves the distal descending thoracic aorta extending to most of the abdominal aorta; and type IV (less than one-quarter) is limited to most or all of the abdominal aorta (including the visceral arteries).[25]

## CLINICAL FEATURES AND SYNCHRONOUS ANEURYSMAL RISK

Data on the natural history of descending and thoracoabdominal aneurysms are limited to a few studies. They demonstrated that, independent from the different mechanisms of injury and degeneration affecting the structural integrity of the aortic wall, the biologic fate of all aneurysms is progressive enlargement and rupture. Laminated thrombus and calcification do not prevent this process.

Synchronous aneurysms typically involving the ascending aorta or arch have been observed in ≈10% of patients being evaluated for TA/TAA repair, and a familial history of aneurysmal disease has been identified in 8.4–21% of patients presenting for evaluation of TAAA.[26] Prior operation

for aortic aneurysm disease is seen in one-third of patients being evaluated for TA/TAA repair, the most common of which is a previous infrarenal aneurysm repair.[27]

The natural history is markedly influenced by size, location, symptoms, and etiology of thoracic aneurysms.[28] They may develop symptoms related to mechanical compression of adjacent structures, but more frequently they are asymptomatic until rupture occurs.

The most common initial symptom in patients with TAAAs is vague pain, which occurs in the chest, back, flank, or abdomen. The differential diagnosis in a patient with a symptomatic TAAA includes angina, aortic dissection, and spine problems. The chronic pain associated with TAAAs may easily be dismissed in patients with TAAAs before the diagnosis of a TAAA has been made. Typical of most aneurysms when enlarging, pain may increase in severity dramatically. Symptoms may also occur in patients with TAAAs from compression of the thoracic aorta by structures in the thoracic cavity. Hoarseness of voice in patients with TAAAs indicates compression of the left recurrent laryngeal nerve. Other features like tracheal deviation, persistent cough, or other respiratory symptoms may also be present.[29] Dysphagia is an uncommon complaint reported by patients with TAAAs that is due to compression of the aneurysm by the esophagus.[30] Sudden and catastrophic hemoptysis or hematemesis may occur as a result of erosion of the TAAA into the bronchial and pulmonary space or the esophagus (aortoesophageal fistula), respectively. Patients with TAAAs may rarely have neurologic deficits, including paraplegia. This is much more common in those with aortic dissection. Embolization to the visceral, renal, and lower extremity arteries has also been reported.[31] Most patients with symptoms have TAAAs that have attained a diameter greater than 5 cm.

Patients with TAAAs generally might not have obvious physical findings in the chest area unless tracheal deviation is present.[32] Patients with an abdominal component of their TAAA may have a pulsatile abdominal mass similar to pure AAAs.

## ■ DIAGNOSTIC EVALUATION

### Imaging

A chest radiograph or plain films of the abdomen in patients with TAAA may suggest an enlarged thoracic aorta (Fig. 5). Indirect findings suggestive of TAAA on chest radiography include a widened mediastinum, enlargement of the aortic knob, and tracheal deviation.

The main imaging method used for assessment of TAA/TAAA is a dynamic fine cut contrast enhanced CT angiography which provides the following information:

- Accurate assessment of aneurysm size and extent.
- A baseline study with which future images may be compared (either follow-up in case of small aneurysms or postoperative follow-up especially post-thoracic endovascular aneurysm repair (TEVAR)).
- Determination of anatomic suitability for endovascular repair.
- If open surgery is required, the anatomic extent of resection and at least inference regarding the risk of subsequent spinal cord ischemia.

Axial images are most useful images for assessment of aortic diameters at various levels, osteas of visceral vessels and the multiplanar reconstructions are used for assessment of aortic length (Figs 6A to C).

A general assessment of other organs in the chest, abdomen, and pelvis is also obtained with CT, which allows the detection of other pathologies that might affect patient management and surgical planning.[33] CTA further documents the presence of intraluminal thrombus, surrounding inflammatory changes, dissection and retroperitoneal

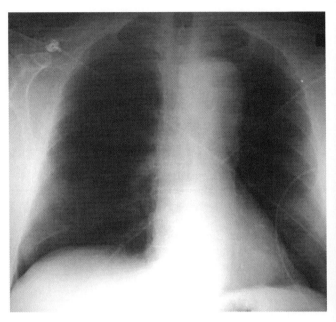

**Fig. 5** A case of thoracic aortic aneurysm showing prominent aortic knuckle

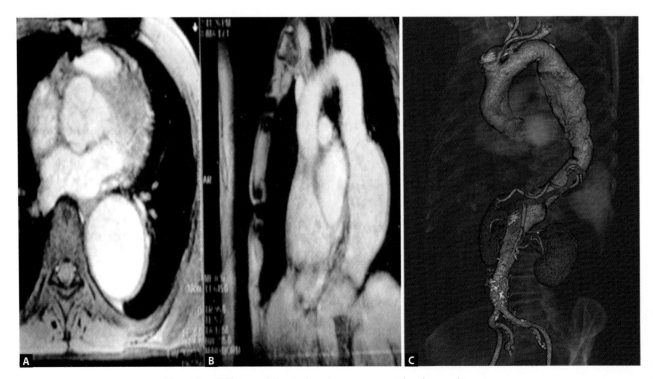

**Figs 6A to C** Thoracoabdominal aortic aneurysm: axial and coronal images

collections suggestive of a ruptured aneurysm. The advantages of CT scanning over magnetic resonance imaging (MRI) include its being less expensive, quicker to perform and thus least chance for claustrophobia-inducing, useful in patients with previous implanted ferromagnetic devices and widely available. Because of the nephrotoxicity of iodinated contrast agents, in the elective surgery and endovascular therapy setting CTA is best delayed for at least 24 hours after CT angiography. The administration of *N*-acetylcysteine and intravenous hydration are current strategies used to limit contrast-induced nephropathy.[34] If contrast-induced nephropathy does occur, elective repairs should be delayed until renal function returns to baseline.

Magnetic resonance angiography (MRA) can be considered when evaluating patients with TAAAs, especially those with renal insufficiency as it avoids the use of iodinated contrast. Although MRI is believed to provide better contrast resolution, its spatial resolution is poorer than that of CT scanning. The concerns are the requirement of gadolinium especially in patients with renal insufficiency has made the use of MRA less attractive for aortic aneurysms. MRA is also technically limited in that thrombus and calcium are not prominently displayed. In addition, the increased time required to acquire the images, the associated claustrophobia, the increased cost, and interference from metallic implants make MRA of limited use in the treatment of aortic aneurysms in general.

Angiography is presently has a very limited role especially for special situations, such as attempting to map the spinal cord circulation, evaluation of branch anatomy in a patient with a TAAA, occlusive disease in the cerebrovascular, visceral, renal, or iliac beds when one wants to limit the use of iodinated contrast material in those with chronic renal failure.

## ■ MANAGEMENT

### Medical Therapy

The goals of medical therapy have traditionally been to reduce shear stress on the aneurysmal segment of the aorta by reducing blood pressure and contractility (dP/dt). Although there is no level A or B evidence to prove that cardiovascular risk factor reduction influences outcome in aortic aneurysm to a great degree. More recently, numerous reports have been published of plausible therapies that aim to affect the underlying pathophysiological changes in aortic aneurysms, thus modifying the disease process as opposed to only trying to delay its complications.

*Role of beta blockers:* β-blockers may be beneficial for reducing the rate of aortic dilatation. This is thought to be due to the effect of β-blockers in reducing left ventricular dP/dt and reducing shear stress. In addition, β-blockers reduce dP/dt in the aorta and might be beneficial via this mechanism and the resultant effect on shear stress in the aorta.[35]

*Role of statins:* Statin treatment is one of the cornerstone therapies in cardiovascular diseases. Statins reduce the progression of atherosclerosis and improve clinical outcomes. In addition, they also reduce oxidative stress by blocking the effects of reactive oxygen species on aneurysms. This effect is independent of their lipid-lowering properties. Aneurysm expansion rate has also been shown to be reduced in AAA patients on statins in observational studies.[36]

*Role of ACE inhibitors/ARB:* Multiple regression analysis revealed that medical treatment with angiotensin II type 1 receptor blockers suppressed expression of reactive oxygen species in TAAA.[37] Losartan, an angiotensin I receptor blocker (ARB), seems to exert its beneficial effect through blocking transforming growth factor-β, thereby reducing matrix degradation in a Marfan's syndrome mouse model.[38]

### Selection of Treatment

The decision when to operate on a patient with a TAAA involves assessment of the likelihood of aortic rupture versus the operative risk and also the life-expectancy of the individual patient. Broadly, the patient's physiologic reserve and vascular anatomy, play a significant role in determining whether a patient is best suited for open repair or an endovascular approach.

Till now the maximum diameter of the aneurysmal sac is the single most important factor for intervention. But unlike AAA the size criteria for TAA and TAAA is not well studied. This issue is further complicated by the fact that degenerative TAAAs are often not uniform in size and involve aortic segments of varying diameters and also in morphology. In addition, it is important to recognize the impact of body size on aortic size and also the presence or absence of connective tissue disorders. Adjustment for body surface area or height needs to be incorporated into decision making about the threshold for repair and risk for rupture.[39]

### Preoperative Evaluation[27]

Patients treated for degenerative aneurysms average 70 years in age, and a history of hypertension is nearly universal.[27] Cigarette smoking and/or significant chronic obstructive pulmonary disease (COPD) are encountered frequently. Pulmonary function studies have been routinely performed before open operation, and 25% of patients will have significant COPD, as manifested by an $FEV_1$ of <50%.[27] Patients can also be placed on an exercise program to improve lung capacity and lose weight if obesity accompanies their lung disease.

Because most of these patients undergoing TAAA repair are elderly, impaired myocardial function and coronary artery disease are common in patients undergoing aneurysm repair.[40] Echocardiography, most often transesophageal echocardiography (TEE), is helpful in demonstrating left ventricular function and concomitant valvular abnormalities.

TEE is also useful in evaluating the ascending and descending thoracic aorta, especially in the presence of aortic dissections. Role of routine coronary evaluation in asymptomatic patients is still debatable. The procedure-related complications in patients undergoing coronary artery revascularization are frequent and often lead to delays in the intended vascular surgery. In patients with stable coronary artery disease, coronary artery revascularization before elective major vascular surgery does not improve long-term survival or reduce short-term postoperative outcomes such as death, myocardial infarction (MI), or length of hospital stay.[41] Thus, current recommendations are that coronary artery bypass grafting (CABG) or percutaneous coronary intervention (PCI) be reserved for selected patients with unstable cardiac symptoms or advanced coronary disease for which a survival benefit with coronary revascularization is clear.

Associated visceral and renovascular occlusive disease has been reported in 30% of patients.[42] A full 15% of patients with TAAAs will have some degree of chronic renal insufficiency, as defined by a creatinine level of 1.8 mg/dL (159 μmol/L) or greater.[43] The coexistence of renovascular disease and some degree of renal insufficiency is especially commonplace in patients with TAA and has important implications for accurate assessment of perioperative risk and long-term preservation of renal function. Because the majority of patients with TAA present with involvement of the entire visceral aortic segment, occlusive lesions of the mesenteric and renal arteries or total ostial occlusion of 1 or more of these vessels frequently accompanies aneurysmal dilation of this region of the aorta. In many series, the presence of an abnormal preoperative serum creatinine level is at least a univariate correlate of perioperative mortality.[44] Thus, assessment of renal function and associated renovascular disease is an important component of patient evaluation and choice of therapy.

## Open Surgery and Its Results

### Preoperative Planning

Computed tomography (CT) is the most widely used tool for preoperative planning because it provides information to classify the aneurysm according to location, extent, and diameter. Assessment of aneurysm morphology is essential prerequisite for selection of sequential clamp sites when distal aortic perfusion is used. Preserving spinal cord circulation during DTAA and TAAA repair is of eminent importance. The watershed area in spinal cord is more prone to ischemic injury during thoracic aortic operations, and its circulation is often dependent on the largest extrinsic radiculomedullary artery, known as the artery of Adamkiewicz. The artery of Adamkiewicz itself arises in the T8-L2 region in some 72% of patients.[45] Sometimes, the spinal cord blood supply comes from lumbar vessels and even the branches of internal iliac arteries. Both were major contributors to the spinal cord

circulation in 16% and 8% of cases, respectively.[46] Open surgery for DTAA and TAAA, especially type II, poses a major risk for the patient. Because the most frequent complications include myocardial infarction, pulmonary insufficiency, renal failure, and stroke, evaluation of these organ systems is essential for preoperative risk assessment and reduction of risk.

### End Organ Protection

Advances in intraoperative monitoring and anesthetic techniques and the ability to replace volume and blood rapidly have improved the outcome of patients requiring thoracic and thoracoabdominal aortic surgery. Monitoring and vascular access lines include radial arterial pressure line, a pulmonary artery (or Swan-Ganz) catheter, and large bore intravenous lines.

### Extracorporeal Circulation

Left atrium to left femoral A (atriofemoral) bypass is commonly been performed during the open repair of TAA/TAAA mainly to maintain the distal perfusion during aortic cross clamping. Also the left ventricular unloading will be facilitated (Fig. 7).

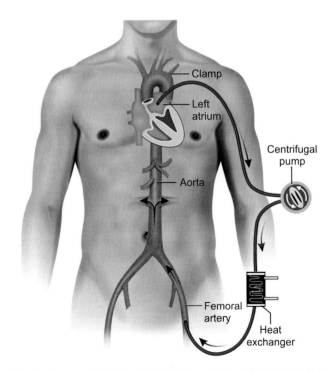

**Fig. 7** Diagram of left heart (LA-FA) bypass. The left atrium and the left femoral artery are cannulated, and a centrifugal pump is used with heparin-coated tubing. A heat exchanger may be added into the circuit for cooling and rewarming *(http://web.squ.edu.om/med-Lib/MED_CD/E_CDs/anesthesia/site/content/v04/040098r00.HTM)*

Since anticoagulant-impregnated tubing is used, only a modest dose of heparin is required; an in-line heat exchanger can provide moderate systemic hypothermia and rewarming during later stages of the reconstruction. Bleeding complications with this technique are greatly reduced when compared with full cardiopulmonary bypass. In patients in whom the aneurysm involves the origin of the left subclavian artery, the optimal approach is to avoid aortic clamping and the risk of cerebral embolization by utilizing femoral cardiopulmonary bypass and profound hypothermic circulatory arrest.[32] Other least commonly used methods of extracorporeal bypass are Gott shunt and external axillo-femoral bypass.

## Spinal Cord Protection

Paraplegia is the most dreaded and severe complication of surgery on the descending thoracic aorta (TAA) and thoracoabdominal aorta (TAAA). During open repair a variety of adjunctive measures can be performed to reduce spinal cord ischemia. They can be broadly classified as measures that seek to preserve cord blood supply (e.g. CSF drainage, intercostal artery reimplantation) and using neuroprotective adjuncts such as variations of hypothermia and endorphin receptor blockage.[47]

*Evoked potential monitoring:* The functional integrity of the spinal cord can be monitored by means of intraoperative recording of myogenic-evoked responses after transcranial electrical stimulation (transcranial motor evoked potential) and somatosensory-evoked potential (SEP) monitoring.[48] In SSEP monitoring, the dorsal tibial nerve is stimulated and the signal is conducted through the dorsal columns of the spinal cord and is recorded from the scalp. MEPs can be stimulated by electrical or magnetic transcranial stimuli and are typically recorded at the level of the anterior tibial muscle and compared with recordings at the thenar muscles, which are independent of the spinal cord blood supply (Fig. 8).[49] MEP is very sensitive and reliable in detecting earlier onset of spinal cord ischemia during the repair. Changes in spinal cord function as measured by SSEPs or MEPs influence the operative strategy.

*Cerebrospinal fluid drainage:* Paraparesis and paraplegia complicate surgical repair of thoracic and thoracoabdominal aneurysms in 6–40% of patients.[50] The rationale of using adopting CSF drainage is that aortic cross-clamping both decreases arterial spinal cord pressure and increases CSF pressure.[51] This produces spinal cord ischemia (similar to the compartment syndrome elsewhere). CSF drainage, both during and after surgery, decreases CSF pressure and

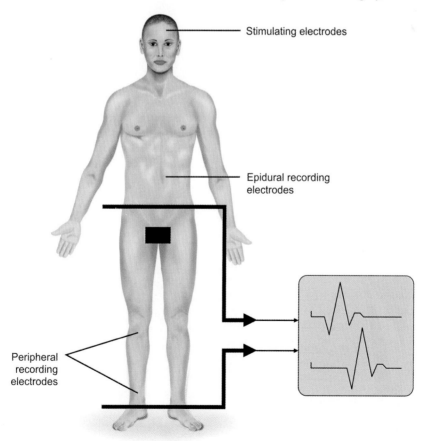

**Fig. 8** Schematic representation of MEP monitoring

increases the relative spinal cord perfusion pressure. CSF pressure was typically maintained at less than 10 mm Hg and maintained for 72 hours. Major complications like subdural hematoma, meningitis can also occur related to the CSF drainage.

*Other measures:* Intrathecal papaverine injection, intraoperative administration of naloxone, use of steroid or barbiturate agents are also used to a variable extent.

### Renal and Visceral Organ Protection

In TAA/TAAA repair with a distal cross-clamp above the celiac artery, continuous visceral and renal perfusion is possible when using a distal aortic perfusion method. If this method is combined with moderate systemic hypothermia, the kidneys and intestines should have minimal ischemic insults. Mean arterial pressure in the renal artery should be approximately 70–80 mm Hg.

## Surgical Technique

The choice of specific surgical technique is dependent on the aneurysm anatomy, including arch involvement and/or distal extent of the lesion. Variations on surgical techniques include organ-specific protective adjuncts and/or some form of extracorporeal circulatory support. In circumstances in which proximal cross-clamp application is neither possible nor desirable, total cardiopulmonary bypass with deep hypothermic circulatory arrest can be utilized. However, because of the bleeding and pulmonary complications that often accompany this technique, most surgeons believe that it should be utilized when no other technical option exists for repair of TAAA.[52]

The patient is positioned in a right lateral decubitus position with the upper body and torso perpendicular to the table, while keeping the pelvis flattened (the left hip 60° from the edge of the table) to allow to both groins (Fig. 9).

In general, a posterolateral thoracotomy via the sixth intercostal space provides excellent access to the entire descending thoracic aorta, although adequate access to the proximal descending aorta requires an approach via the fifth intercostal space. Sometimes resection of the sixth rib will be required to facilitate the exposure. Adequate preparation of the proximal clamp position is crucial. This includes the identification of vagus and recurrent laryngeal nerves; transection of the ligamentum arteriosum; dissection of aorta from the esophagus to avoid later prosthetic-esophageal fistula formation. The abdominal aorta is exposed (in TAAA repair) via retroperitoneal approach after division of the diaphragm. The abdominal aorta, origins of celiac A, superior mesenteric artery (SMA) and left renal artery are exposed.

Only limited heparinization (0.5 mg/kg) with an activated clotting time of approximately 200 seconds is required. Normothermia is maintained during the procedure to maintain the cardiac contraction. Once partial cardiopulmonary bypass

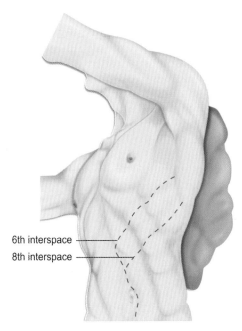

6th interspace
8th interspace

**Fig. 9** Position of patient in open repair

is instituted (as shown in Fig. 7), the aorta cross-clamped proximally with two clamps. Mean arterial pressure in the distal aorta should be maintained above 70 mm Hg. Once proximal anastomosis is completed the distal aorta is clamped and aneurysmal sac is opened and thrombus evacuated. Intercostals branches in the proximal aorta are controlled with suture ligatures. Typically the patent intercostals at the T8-L1 level are reimplanted into the side of the graft and the clamps shifted distally. Distal anastomoses will be completed in DTAA whereas in TAAA visceral revascularization has to be performed.

The distal aorta (i.e. abdominal aorta) is prepared depending on the extent of the abdominal involvement. If the aneurysm extends to the celiac artery and visceral arteries but not beyond (as in type I), the abdominal aorta can be partially divided tangentially and the distal anastomoses performed without separate reimplantation of the visceral vessels. If the abdominal component of the aneurysm is more extensive as in type 2, 3 and 4, the visceral and right renal arteries may be reimplanted using the graft inclusion method as one large 'island' with the left renal artery reimplanted as a separate button.

The distal neck of the aneurysm is defined and the graft sewn to it in an end-to-end fashion. After sequential flushing of air and debris from the graft and aorta, the aortic clamps are released and the patient weaned from cardiopulmonary bypass. The divided diaphragm is reapproximated and the thoracic and abdominal incisions closed.

### Postoperative Management

Because of the extent of operation and consequent physiologic disturbances, there are considerations unique to patients undergoing DTA and TAAA repair. Intraoperatively and in the early postoperative period, the patient requires close monitoring, adequate analgesia, aggressive volume resuscitation, ventilator support and correction of any electrolyte disturbances. The patient is transfused with packed red blood cells as necessary. The use of cardiopulmonary bypass in the operation often leads to a coagulopathy that persists into the postoperative period. Thus, the patient's coagulation status is frequently evaluated and corrected with transfusions of blood components, such as platelets and fresh frozen plasma. Mean arterial pressures have to be maintained >100 mm Hg.

# ■ COMPLICATIONS

## Mortality

For patients undergoing repair of thoracoabdominal aortic aneurysm, the overall operative 30-day mortality rate was 5–12%.[53] The presence of increasing numbers of comorbid conditions can naturally be expected to increase overall operative risk. Individual series have demonstrated increased operative risks in patients with antecedent coronary artery disease, significant COPD, and, in particular, preoperative renal insufficiency.[54] Conrad MF and colleagues had found that the 30-day mortality is commonly associated with preoperative serum creatinine level of 1.8 mg/dL or more ($p = 0.005$), intraoperative hypotension ($p = 0.01$), intraoperative transfusion requirement ($p = 0.0008$), postoperative SCI ($p = 0.02$), and postoperative renal failure ($p < 0.0001$).[26]

## Cardiac

The aortic cross-clamp time, level of cross-clamp placement, declamping and its hemodynamic changes are directly related to postoperative complications. In general, aortic cross-clamping increases the after load which increases the myocardial oxygen demand. Declamping is associated sudden decrease in the peripheral vascular resistance along with electrolyte imbalance causes tachycardia and hence causing perioperative cardiac events. Postoperative cardiac complications, reported in 12–25% of patients. These include myocardial infarction, arrhythmias, congestive heart failure and unstable angina.[55]

## Pulmonary

The overall incidence of pulmonary complications ranges between 32% and 49%.[55] COPD, smoking status and associated other comorbidities is associated with requirement of prolonged ventilator support. Intraoperative factors associated with pulmonary complications are related to collapse of left lung, operative trauma, transection of diaphragmatic fibers or left phrenic nerve paralysis and also inflammatory mediators associated with reperfusion injury.

## Spinal Cord Injury

A particularly troubling complication of extensive replacement of the thoracic and abdominal aorta is paraplegia, which is related to intraoperative or postoperative spinal cord ischemia. Repair of type I TAAA is associated with a paraplegia or paraparesis rate of 15% and for type III is 7–20%.[25] Replacement of the entire abdominal aorta (type IV) has a paraplegia risk of 2–4%.[25] Rupture of the thoracoabdominal aortic aneurysm is associated with a paraplegia risk of over 25%.[25] If the patient required replacement of the entire descending thoracic aorta and all of the abdominal aorta (type II), the paraplegia or paraparesis rate can range up to 30%.[57] Risk factors for postoperative paraplegia include more extensive repair (type II), duration of aortic cross-clamp, presence of collaterals, spinal cord cooling, CSF drainage, persistent hypotension and use of neuroprotectives. Despite the use of various strategies for the prevention of spinal cord ischemia, paraplegia and paraparesis continue to occur after thoracoabdominal aortic aneurysm (TAAA) repair. Coseli JS and colleagues found that incidence of paraplegia in the immediate post operative period was 13% without CSF drainage and 2.6% in patients with CSF drainage ($p = 0.03$). They had concluded that CSF drainage reduces the relative risk of paraplegia by 80%.[56] Because of multiple mechanisms and processes involved in ischemic neuronal death like intracellular calcium overload, nitric oxide, eicosanoids, apoptosis, inflammation, and reactive oxygen species, the usage of current pharmacological measures alone is unlikely to improve on the clinical outcome.[60]

## Renal

Postoperative renal failure is one of the significant problems contributing to adverse outcomes as it increases the risk for early mortality by 10-fold.[58] The preoperative risk factors for developing renal failure in the postoperative period includes smoking, old age, serum creatinine >1.8 mg%, diabetes, systemic hypertension, presence of renal artery stenosis. The intraoperative factors include warm ischemia time, distal aortic perfusion (mean arterial BP >70 mm Hg), use of renal protective measures (like cold crystalloid perfusion or normothermic blood perfusion), reperfusion injury. For patients undergoing descending thoracic aortic aneurysm repair, the risk of renal insufficiency or failure is approximately 5%.[59] In patients undergoing extensive thoracoabdominal aneurysm repair, renal failure occurs in 13%.[25]

## Graft-related Complications

Aortoesophageal and aortobronchial fistulae are known to occur following open repair. In literature, many case reports or limited series are described, and therefore the exact incidence of these complications cannot be assessed.

These complications are mostly associated graft infection presenting with massive hematemesis or hemoptysis. The close anatomic relationship between the descending thoracic aorta and esophagus explains the potential risk for fistulae, especially if anastomotic sutures injure or even include the esophagus. Complete separation of esophagus from the proximal neck and closing the aneurysmal sac around the prosthetic graft virtually eliminates this type of complication. Endovascular treatment is considered as a lifesaving procedure and to be used as a bridge to final treatment, which if necessary, consists of esophageal resection and replacement of the aorta with a homograft or extra-anatomic aortic bypass from the ascending to the descending aorta.

## Survival

Lifelong follow-up is generally recommended although not as frequent as in post-endovascular repair where repeated imaging is required. Patients who have associated connective tissue disorders are more prone for aneurysmal dilatation of the remaining native aorta. Late survival following open repair of TAA and TAAA varies with case series as there are multiple factors other than just the operative technique are involved. Schepens et al. in his series had concluded that avoidance of postoperative problems such as dialysis and neurologic deficits and performing elective surgery on relative young patients with unimpaired ventricular function will increase the likelihood of late survival. TAAA repair appears to be a durable operation, with a reasonable 5-year patient survival rate and a low-risk of postoperative paraplegia or additional aortic events (Table 4).

## ■ ENDOVASCULAR AND ITS RESULTS

Dake and coworkers introduced the concept of stent-graft exclusion for the thoracic aorta in December 1994.[64] They had used custom designed self-expanding stainless steel stents

**Table 4** Long-term survival following open repair of TAAA

| Author | Year | Disease | No of surgeries | Follow-up year | Survival |
|---|---|---|---|---|---|
| Cambria et al.[43] | 1997 | TAAA | 157 | 1 | 86 ± 2.9% |
| | | | | 5 | 62 ± 5.8% |
| Schepens et al.[61] | 2007 | TAAA | 500 (95% CI) | 1 | 83% |
| | | | | 5 | 63% |
| | | | | 10 | 34% |
| | | | | 15 | 16% |
| | | | | 20 | 6% |
| Estrera et al.[62] | 2005 | DTAA | 355 | 5 | 64% |
| | | | | 10 | 35% |
| Dardik et al.[63] | 2002 | TAAA | 257 | 5 | 53% |

covered with woven dacron grafts. TEVAR for descending thoracic aortic aneurysms (DTAAs) became a mainstream technology with the release of commercial endografts starting with the TAG device (WL Gore and Associates, Flagstaff, AZ) in early 2005. Most of the clinical information about TEVAR originates from industry-sponsored nonrandomized comparisons to open repair of DTAA, as well as single-center experiences or registry data that combine different pathologies and indications. Nonetheless, TEVAR has emerged as an attractive option for the treatment of DTAA and has shown very good early and midterm results.

## Preoperative Planning

### Indications

The size criteria which applies for the open repair, is well applicable for TEVAR. In general, the commonly followed size criteria include a size of 6 cm or larger, a saccular configuration, annual expansion rate >1 cm/year and symptomatic aneurysms, including rupture. The size recommendations are somewhat variable as no randomized trials exist to guide the decision-making process. Apart from the size criteria, relevant anatomy is required for TEVAR. This includes good proximal and distal landing zones, no access vessel issues.... especially in patients with multiple comorbidities. TEVAR has gained its popularity as it avoids aortic cross clamping which is associated with complications. A number of case-series studies and reviews have shown reduced early morbidity and mortality rates in a range of thoracic aortic diseases for TEVAR in comparison to open surgical repair. However, there is a lack of robust clinical data to suggest any improvement in long-term overall survival.[65]

## Suitable Anatomy for TEVAR

Achieving safe and successful endovascular access for introduction and deployment of the stent-graft device is a crucially important and often challenging step during TEVAR. The currently available thoracic endografts have a large profile. Consequently, arterial access injury has been, and continues to be an all-too-common occurrence, with external iliac artery (EIA) rupture ranking high as a cause of procedure-related mortality to this day. Assessment of iliac artery for diameter (minimum 8 mm is required), tortuosity, extent of calcification, presence of stenosis and angulations at the aortic junction. In general, women tend to have more access vessel issues due to small iliac and femoral arterial segments.

Adequate fixation of a stent-graft to both proximal and distal landing zones is essential for successful performance of TEVAR. To standardize comparisons, Ishimaru's group classified the thoracic aorta into five landing zones (Fig. 10) in the proximal landing zone.

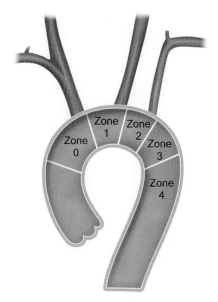

**Fig. 10** Showing the landing zones in TEVAR. An endografting procedure at Zone 3 is an ideal situation and requires no surgical complementary step for both aneurysms

*Source:* (Int J Mol Sci. 2010; 11(11):4687-96). http://www.ncbi.nlm.nih.gov/pmc/articles/PMC3000108/

Sometimes aneurysms may impinge on one or more visceral arterial branch (as in TAAA) that must be occluded for adequate sealing. In these situations, the safety of such branch sacrifice must be balanced against further observation of the aneurysm or open repair. The alternative would be surgical bypass or "debranching" to maintain perfusion while extending the sealing zone or snorkel technique or using a branched aortic devices. TEVAR should be contraindicated when the anatomy of the aneurysm prevents safe and effective performance of stent-graft exclusion of the DTAA.

## Contraindications

The majority of patients, however, do not have perfect anatomy for TEVAR and the risk-benefit assessment becomes more complex. Severe tortuosity of the aneurysm or the access vessels can also increase morbidity. Severe aortoiliac occlusive disease, rapid taper of the aorta, aortic size

outside the range of available devices and circumferential thrombus at the attachment sites are contraindications for any endovascular repairs. Endovascular repairs should also be avoided in patients with life-threatening allergic reaction to intravenous contrast material, patients with significant chronic renal insufficiency (because of precipitation of end-stage renal failure), and those who are not suitable for frequent follow-up.

## Approved Devices for TEVAR

There are three commercially manufactured, FDA-approved devices currently available. These include the TAG (WL Gore and Associates, Flagstaff, AZ), Zenith TX2 (Cook Medical, Bloomington, IN), and Talent Thoracic (Medtronic, Santa Rosa, CA) (Table 5).[66]

## TEVAR for TAA

### Operative Planning

Preoperative planning begins with imaging studies. The primary modality for such planning is computed tomographic angiography (CTA), which has mostly supplanted the additional use of catheter angiography in preoperative planning and is capable of providing most of the preoperative anatomic information. The 64- slice computed tomography (CT) scanner is the latest technology and provides fine definition and very fast scan times. It also offers three-dimensional volume rendering, as well as maximum intensity projections and sagittal and coronal reconstructions, which aid in the analysis of angles and relationships to adjacent vessels.

The preoperative CTA should include the chest, abdomen, and pelvis with and without contrast enhancement (from aortic arch to mid thigh) to fully evaluate the access vessels, as well as the extent of calcification and angulations throughout. Tortuosity is best delineated by a three-dimensional reconstruction. The arteries of importance in maintaining the spinal cord perfusion are:

- Left subclavian A (via left vertebral A and anterior spinal artery).
- Posterior intercostals arteries especially the artery of Adamkiewicz.

**Table 5** FDA-approved devices for TEVAR

| Name of the device | Composition | Access sheath size | Available sizes | Specific characters |
|---|---|---|---|---|
| TAG device | External nitinol self-expanding stent with an internal ePTFE graft | 20–24 F | 26–40 mm | The device is supplied without a sheath. The graft opens from the center outwards toward both ends |
| Zenith TX 2 device | External self-expanding stainless steel barbed Z-stent with a Dacron graft | 20–22 F | 28–42 mm | The device is supplied preloaded within a delivery device to be deployed through a sheath |
| Talent thoracic endograft | Self-expanding nitinol stents arrayed along the length of a woven polyester graft | 22–25 F | 22–46 mm | The device is supplied preloaded within a delivery device |

- Lumbar arteries.
- Internal iliac arteries.

Hence, assessment of all these vessels in CTA is important for planning purpose, especially when left subclavian artery needs to be covered for adequate sealing.

## Spinal Cord Protection

Similar to open repair, TEVAR is also associated with spinal cord ischemia as the artery of Ademkiewicz will be covered by the stent graft.

Risk factors for developing spinal cord injury following TEVAR:
- Extensive coverage of the thoracic aorta
- Previous AAA repair
- Diseased internal iliac arteries
- Left subclavian artery (LSA) covers without revascularization.[67]

## Strategy for Spinal Cord Protection

- LSA revascularization
- CSF drainage (maintaining CSF pressure <10 mm Hg)
- Maintaining the MAP >100 mm Hg
- Use of neuroprotectives like naloxone.

## Indications for Left Subclavian A Revascularization

- Dominant left VA
- Patent left internal mammary bypass to a coronary artery
- An aberrant right SA
- An anomalous origin of the left VA from the arch
- Patent AV access in left upper limb.

# Operative Technique

## Anesthetic Management

Main advantage of TEVAR over open surgery is it can be done under regional anesthesia with arterial line for hemodynamic monitoring. The right radial is preferred if left brachial puncture is anticipated CSF drain, if required, is to be placed. The use of heparin during the procedure is associated with spinal hematoma.

## Access

Based on the preoperative planning, one side common femoral artery is chosen and exposed for the insertion of the device and other side is for diagnostic angiogram. The side, which has fewer issues, is preferred. Otherwise right side is the most favored site. When a conduit is needed, the common iliac artery exposed by retroperitoneal approach and brought into the groin to allow straight access to the iliac artery. A 10-mm Dacron graft is commonly used as a conduit.

At the end of the procedure, the conduit may be converted to an iliofemoral bypass graft.

## Imaging

Angiography of the aortic arch and descending thoracic aorta are the primary procedural guidance tools in accurate placement of the thoracic aortic stent graft. Therefore, the proper performance of angiography is critical. The imaging equipment used must be able to perform multiple digitally subtracted angiographic examinations with steep tube angulation (mainly to visualize the origin of the important branches and also to image the aortic arch) without tube cooling requirements. High-quality live fluoroscopy and roadmapping capabilities are critical to accurate and safe deployment of devices.

Diagnostic angiography of the aortic arch relies on high contrast rate and volume, due to the large size of and high flow in the arch. Inadequate contrast bolus for angiography will cause misleading imaging with inadequate demonstration of branch vessel origins. Arch angiography should, therefore, be performed with a flush catheter with a pressure injector, with contrast flow rates compatible with the patient's arch aortic diameter.

A final, critical element of quality imaging for the procedure is minimization of patient motion. This can be achieved best through the use of suitable anesthesia. In case of regional anesthesia, patient has to be instructed for breath holding during the angiography.

## Operative Procedure

Once the common femoral artery is exposed and the opposite femoral artery is accessed with 6 F sheath, a graduated pigtail catheter is taken across the aneurysmal sac to be kept in the proximal neck. A flush aortogram is done to assess the proximal landing zone. Left brachial puncture is required if the proximal landing zone is close to the LSA.

The advantage of keeping a stiff guidewire across the origin if LSA is:
- It can serve as a marker during deployment of the device.
- In case of inadvertent coverage of LSA, a stent can be inserted via the guide wire (Chimney technique).

Once the landing zone is confirmed, the main device of suitable size (20% over sizing with respect to the diameter of the neck) is positioned under fluro guidance. For imaging the arch of the aorta, left anterior oblique is required though the angulation varies with each case. Usually for distal aorta, a lateral view is used to view the origins of celiac and SMA. Once the device is position, careful and staged deployment of the device is performed as per the instructions which vary with the device. Typically an aortic neck of 2–3 cm is required for adequate sealing. During deployment, systemic BP and heart rate is lowered to decrease the windsock effect (that may result in placement of the endograft more distally than desired). At this step a check angiography is done to see for type 1A endoleak and also coverage of major aortic branch if any. When more than one device is required, the overlapping between the devices should be minimum 5 cm for adequate sealing.

Once the device is deployed, the delivery system is carefully removed under fluroguidance. Most important is to maintain the guidewire across while removing the device as inadvertent injury to the iliac bifurcation can happen. In case of iliac injury, a balloon to be inserted under the fluoro guidance and to be inflated to control the bleeding. Insertion of a covered stent at the site of rupture has to be done to cover the site of rupture.

Finally a completion angiogram is done to see for endoleaks and to confirm the patency of nearby important branches. Type 1 (A and B) and type 3 endoleaks has to be addressed on table. Type 2 endoleak is very common (from the posterior intercostals arteries) and to be left for follow-up.

Procedural 'technical' success is achieved when the endograft is deployed accurately and the aneurysm is excluded from the circulation (i.e. absence of type I or III endoleak) (Fig. 11). Evaluation of clinical success requires follow-up examinations of the patient demonstrating complete thrombosis and shrinkage of the aneurysm sac and in the absence of complications.

## Steps for Thoracic Endovascular Aortic Repair with Debranching of Left Carotid Artery

1. Vertical incision along sternomastoid on both sides.
2. Exposure of both common carotid arteries.
3. Creation of a retropharyngeal space from right to left by blunt dissection to enable passage of ringed PTFE graft.
4. Systemic heparin given.
5. Small arteriotomy vertically over right CCA after clamping and aortic punch used to make a 6 mm hole.
6. 6 mm ringed PTFE graft anastomosed using CV-7 PTFE suturing after tunneling the other end to left.

7. Thereafter, clamps released with deairing protocol.
8. Graft anastomosed similarly to left side.
9. Left carotid ligated proximally with 2 "O" silk to prevent endoleak of the restoring flow from graft.
10. Closure in layers.
11. Groin exposure of common femoral artery (CFA) through vertical incision.
12. Arteries looped and 6 "F" sheath inserted into the CFA.
13. Pigtail/JR catheter advanced up to ascending aorta using Terumo guidewire which is subsequently replaced with a super stiff Amplatz/Lunderquist wire.
14. Opposite femoral punctured and a pigtail placed in ascending aorta. Left brachial artery also punctured and 5 F sheath inserted.
15. The thoracic endograft is then taken up from the groin over the superstiff wire and positioned just proximally to the innominate and first deployed using check angio through the pigtail.
16. Device repositioned just distal to origin of innominate artery and deployed completely using check angio.
17. Compliant aortic balloon then used for proximal and distal end of endograft to seal the ends after removing the delivery system.
18. Check angio done with pressure injector.
19. If no endoleak, no active treatment.
20. If there is a leak from left subclavian, an amplatzer plug of appropriate size or coils can be inserted.
21. If no further intervention, the wires are removed and arteriotomy closed and wound closed.

## Patients Requiring Subclavian Artery Revascularization

Due to dominant vertebral/aneurysm/dissection extending up to abdominal aorta.
1. Standard subclavian artery exposure through supraclavicular approach.
2. Jump graft from left common carotid to left subclavian in a similar fashion tunneling the graft behind internal jugular vein.

## Steps for Total Debranching of Arch Vessels with TEVAR

1. Sternal split/sternotomy.
2. Ascending aorta side biting clamp after heparinization.
3. Bilateral incisions similar to carotid-carotid bypass.
4. A 12/6 mm on 14/7 mm bifurcation graft anastomosed to proximal ascending aorta using CV-4 PTFE sutures (Fig. 12)
5. Graft tunneled to both carotids in a subcutaneous plane.
6. Anastomosis to both carotids. End-to-side using CV-7 PTFE suturing.
7. Closure after placing a Liga clip just distal to anastomosis which will act as a marker for placing the endograft.

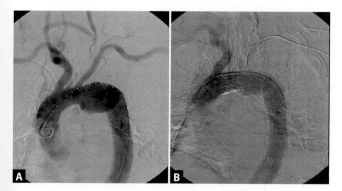

**Figs 11A and B** Operative image of TEVAR

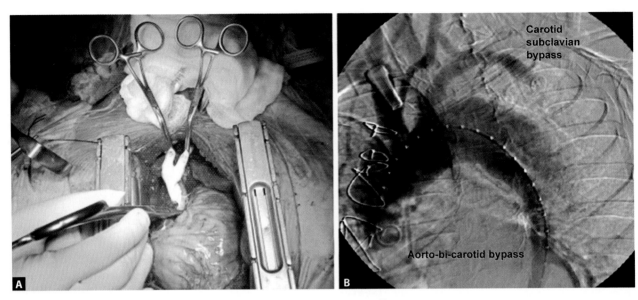

**Figs 12A and B** Aorto-bi-carotid bypass

8. Rest of the steps as per the previous part.
9. Right brachial puncture and on completion of TEVAR, as amplatzer plug of appropriate size to be placed at the origin of innominate artery.

## Steps for Visceral Debranching Including Renal Arteries

1. Midline incision over abdomen xiphipubic.
2. Common hepatic artery identified in Calot's triangle and gastroduodenal branch also identified and looped.
3. Through a standard approach to aorta through the ligament of Treitz, the superior mesenteric artery is felt just above the left renal vein.
4. The artery is dissected through thick tissue and looped.
5. The left renal artery is similarly identified and looped just below the renal vein.
6. Through the medial visceral rotation of right colon, the right renal artery is located posteriorly going behind the IVC and looped.
7. Both external iliac arteries are looped just after bifurcation.
8. A ringed 8 mm PTFE graft is used for SMA to prevent kinking and the same is anastomosed distally into left EIA after heparinization using CV-6 PTFE sutures.
9. The SMA is then transected just distal to its origin and end-to-end anastomosis done giving a little laxity to the graft for movement.
10. A 6 mm graft can be piggy backward from 8 mm graft or separately anastomosed to left EIA and anastomosed end-to-end with left renal artery after perfusing the Kidney with chilled saline and transection of the Artery from Aorta (Fig. 13).

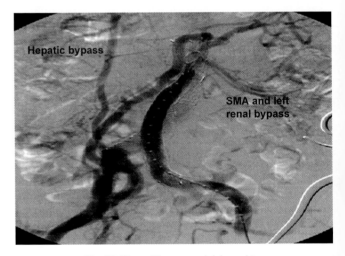

**Fig. 13** Visceral bypass and debranching

11. The common hepatic artery, which is prone to spasm is handled very delicately and if space available proximal to gastroduodenal artery, end-to-side anastomosis done from a bifurcation graft (12/6 mm) taken from right EIA. The anastomosis is done end to side. It can be converted to end to end in case of a kink.
12. The right renal artery similarly anastomosed using the second arm of bifurcation graft after perfusing the kidney with chilled saline.
13. Right colon repositioned leaving the grafts posteriorly and posterior peritoneum closed on left.
14. Tube drains placed in Calot's triangle and pelvis.
15. Closure in layers.
16. EVAR is carried out at the same sitting or it is staged separately after a couple of days.

## Perioperative Complications

When compared to open repair, the 30-day mortality is low for TEVAR. Etezadi V and colleagues had found that in their series of 133 TEVAR the 30-day mortality rates in emergency and elective TEVAR procedures were 23.9% and 4.5% ($p = 0.005$).[68] However, TEVAR is not without complications. Complications related to the usage of contrast media includes type 1 hypersensitivity reaction, contrast induced nephropathy and flash pulmonary edema (in patients who are on dialysis).

Complications related to access vessel issues are failure to manipulate the device successfully. Causes may be use of large sheaths in an already diseased vessels, tortuous iliac arteries, female. Other complications related to access vessel issues includes access site thrombosis, atheroembolization, iliac artery injury all these can add on to morbidity and mortality.

Neurological complications are mainly stroke and spinal cord ischemia. Deployment of the proximal end of the endograft in zone 2 is strongly associated with perioperative stroke, probably secondary to manipulation of the arch with catheters, wires, balloons, and stent-grafts at the origin of the cerebral vessels, i.e. either atheroembolization or in situ thrombosis. Ullery BW and colleagues noted that in a series of 424 TEVARs, the incidence of spinal cord ischemia was 2.8%.[69] Czerny M and colleagues had concluded that, extensive coverage of intercostal arteries alone by a thoracic stent-graft is not associated with symptomatic SCI. However, simultaneous closure of at least 2 vascular territories supplying the spinal cord is highly relevant, especially in combination with prolonged intraoperative hypotension (PPV 0.75, 95% CI 0.38 to 0.75, $p < 0.0001$).[70] They emphasize the need to preserve the left subclavian artery during TEVAR.

## Endoleaks

Type 1 and 3 endoleaks are usually managed and their incidence is very low. Type 2 endoleaks are the most common as there is a tendency to observe these leaks. They are typically seen in CT angiogram during the venous phase as the collaterals get filled up. Majority of the type 2 endoleaks stops spontaneously in 6 months duration. Persistent type 2 endoleaks (> 6 months duration) with associated increase in the sac size warrants reintervention.

Other delayed complications include retrograde type A dissection, aneurysmal dilatation of the proximal and distal aorta leading to type 1 endoleak, stent migration and fracture leading to type 3 endoleak, endotension, device failure, infection, aortoesophageal fistula and aortobronchial fistula all these leads to secondary interventions.

## ◼ CONCLUSION

The complications of elective thoracic aneurysm repair using an open surgical technique are higher than most elective surgical procedures, given anatomical constraints and operative complexity. TEVAR was initially developed to treat patients who were considered to not be open surgical candidates but is not considered suitable alternative to open surgery in most cases.

## ◼ REFERENCES

1. Aronberg DJ, Glazer HS, Madsen K, Sagel SS. Normal thoracic aortic diameters by computed tomography. J Comput Assist Tomogr. 1984;8:247-50.
2. Rogers IS, Massaro JM, Truong QA, Mahabadi AA, Kriegel MF, Fox CS, et al. Distribution, determinants, and normal reference values of thoracic and abdominal aortic diameters by computed tomography (from the Framingham Heart Study). Am J Cardiol. 2013;111(10):1510-6. doi: 10.1016/j.amjcard.2013.01.306. Epub 2013 Mar 13.
3. Young R, Ostertag H. Incidence, etiology and risk of rupture of aortic aneurysm. An autopsy study. Dtsch Med Wochenschr. 1987;112(33):1253-6.
4. Isselbacher EM. Thoracic and abdominal aortic aneurysms. Circulation. 2005;111:816-28. doi: 10.1161/01.CIR.0000154569.08857.7A.
5. Olsson C, Thelin S, Stahle E, et al. Thoracic aortic aneurysm and dissection: increasing prevalence and improved outcomes reported in a nationwide population-based study of more than 14,000 cases from 1987 to 2002. Circulation. 2006;114:2611-18.
6. LaRoy LL, Cormier PJ, Matalon TA, et al. Imaging of abdominal aortic aneurysms. AJR Am J Roentgenol. 1989;152:785-92.
7. Bickerstaff LK, Pairolero PC, Hollier LH, et al. Thoracic aortic aneurysms: a population-based study. Surgery. 1982;92:1103-8.
8. Coady MA, Davies RR, Roberts M, et al. Familial patterns of thoracic aortic aneurysms. Arch Surg. 1999;134:361-7.
9. Hasham SN, Guo DC, Milewicz DM. Genetic basis of thoracic aortic aneurysms and dissections. Curr Opin Cardiol. 2002;17(6): 677-83.
10. Moreno-Cabral CE, Miller DC, Mitchell RS, et al. Degenerative and atherosclerotic aneurysms of the thoracic aorta. Determinants of early and late surgical outcome. J Thorac Cardiovasc Surg. 1984;88: 1020-32.
11. Panneton JM, Hollier LH. Nondissecting thoracoabdominal aortic aneurysms: Part I. Ann Vasc Surg. 1995;9:503-14.
12. Cambria RP, Davison JK, Zannetti S, et al. Thoracoabdominal aneurysm repair: perspectives over a decade with the clamp-and-sew technique. Ann Surg. 1997;226:294-303.
13. Hsu RB, Lin FY. Infected aneurysm of the thoracic aorta. J Vasc Surg. 2008;47(2):270-6. doi: 10.1016/j.jvs.2007.10.017.
14. Shimada I, Rooney SJ, Pagano D, Farneti PA, Davies P, Guest PJ, Bonser RS. Prediction of thoracic aortic aneurysm expansion: validation of formulae describing growth. Ann Thorac Surg. 1999;67(6):1968-70; discussion 1979-80.
15. Dapunt OE, Galla JD, Sadeghi AM, et al. The natural history of thoracic aortic aneurysms. J Thorac Cardiovasc Surg. 1994;107: 1323-32.
16. Davies RR, Goldstein LJ, Coady MA, et al. Yearly rupture or dissection rates for thoracic aortic aneurysms: simple prediction based on size. Ann Thorac Surg. 2002;73:17-27.
17. Juvonen T, Ergin MA, Galla JD, et al. Risk factors for rupture of chronic type B dissections. J Thorac Cardiovasc Surg. 1999;117: 776-7.
18. Coady MA, Rizzo JA, Hammond GL, et al. What is the appropriate size criterion for resection of thoracic aortic aneurysms? J Thorac Cardiovasc Surg. 1997;113:476-91.

19. Cambria RA, Gloviczki P, Stanson AW, et al. Outcome and expansion rate of 57 thoracoabdominal aortic aneurysms managed nonoperatively. Am J Surg. 1995;170:213-7.

20. Barbour JR, Spinale FG, Ikonomidis JS. Proteinase systems and thoracic aortic aneurysm progression. J Surg Res. 2007;139: 292-307.

21. Guo DC, Pannu H, Tran-Fadulu V, et al. Mutations in smooth muscle alpha-actin (ACTA2) lead to thoracic aortic aneurysms and dissections. Nat Genet. 2007;39:1488-93.

22. Andreotti L, Bussotti A, Cammelli D, et al. Aortic connective tissue in ageing—a biochemical study. Angiology. 1985;36:872-9.

23. Ikonomidis JS, Barbour JR, Amani Z, et al. Effects of deletion of the matrix metalloproteinase 9 gene on development of murine thoracic aortic aneurysms. Circulation. 2005;112 (9 Suppl):I242-8.

24. Crawford ES, Snyder DM, Cho GC, Roehm JO. Progress in treatment of thoracoabdominal and abdominal aortic aneurysms involving celiac, superior mesenteric, and renal arteries. Ann Surg. 1978;188:404.

25. Fann JI. Descending thoracic and thoracoabdominal aortic aneurysms. Coronary Artery Disease. 2002;13:93-102.

26. Conrad MF, Crawford RS, Davison JK, Cambria RP. Thoracoabdominal aneurysm repair: a 20-year perspective. Ann Thorac Surg. 2007;83:S856-S61.

27. Conrad MF, Cambria RP. Contemporary management of descending thoracic and thoracoabdominal aortic aneurysms: endovascular versus open. Circulation. 2008;117:841-52 doi: 10.1161/CIRCULATIONAHA.107.690958.

28. Coselli JS, de Figueiredo LF. Natural history of descending and thoracoabdominal aortic aneurysms. J Card Surg. 1997;12(2 Suppl): 285-9; discussion 289-91.

29. McNamara JJ, Pressler VM. Natural history of arteriosclerotic thoracic aortic aneurysms. Ann Thorac Surg. 1978;26:468-73.

30. Furukawa H, Tsuchiya K, Osawa H, et al. Saccular descending thoracic aortic aneurysm with dysphagia. Jpn J Thorac Cardiovasc Surg. 1999; 47:277-80.

31. Arnold SE, Biller J. Spontaneous cerebral embolism from descending thoracic aortic aneurysm—a case report. Angiology. 1991;42:69-72.

32. Fann JI. Descending thoracic and thoracoabdominal aortic aneurysms. Coronary Artery Disease. 2002;13:93-102.

33. Loutsidis A, Koukis I, Argiriou M, Bellenis I. Incidental finding of lung cancer in a patient with thoracic aortic aneurysm—simultaneous management. A case report. Eur J Cancer Care (Engl). 2007;16:387-9.

34. Schweiger MJ, Chambers CE, Davidson CJ, et al. Prevention of contrast induced nephropathy: recommendations for the high risk patient undergoing cardiovascular procedures. Catheter Cardiovasc Interv. 2007;69:135-140.

35. Danyi P, Elefteriades JA, Jovin IS. Medical therapy of thoracic aortic aneurysms. Circulation. 2011;124:1469-76 doi: 10.1161/CIRCULATIONAHA.110.006486

36. Sukhija R, Aronow WS, Sandhu R, Kakar P, Babu S. Mortality and size of abdominal aortic aneurysm at long-term follow-up of patients not treated surgically and treated with and without statins. Am J Cardiol. 2006;97:279-80.

37. Ejiri J, Inoue N, Tsukube T, et al. Oxidative stress in the pathogenesis of thoracic aortic aneurysm: protective role of statin and angiotensin II type 1 receptor blocker. Cardiovasc Res. 2003;59:988-96.

38. Habashi JP, Judge DP, Holm TM, Cohn RD, Loeys BL, Cooper TK, et al. Losartan, an AT1 antagonist, prevents aortic aneurysm in a mouse model of Marfan syndrome. Science. 2006;312:117-21.

39. Davies RR, Gallo A, Coady MA, et al. Novel measurement of relative aortic size predicts rupture of thoracic aortic aneurysms. Ann Thorac Surg. 2006;81:169-77.

40. Hertzer NR, Young JR, Kramer JR, et al. Routine coronary angiography prior to elective aortic reconstruction: results of selective myocardial revascularization in patients with peripheral vascular disease. Arch Surg. 1979;114:1336-44.

41. McFalls EO, Ward HB, Moritz TE, et al. Coronary-artery revascularization before elective major vascular surgery. N Engl J Med. 2004;351:2795-2804.

42. Coselli JS. Thoracoabdominal aortic aneurysms: experience with 372 patients. J Card Surg. 1994;9:638-47.

43. Cambria RP, Davison JK, Zannetti S, L'Italien G, Atamian S. Thoracoabdominal aneurysm repair: perspectives over a decade with the clamp-and-sew technique. Ann Surg. 1997;226:294-303.

44. Cox GS, O'Hara PJ, Hertzer NR, Piedmonte MR, Krajewski LP, Beven EG. Thoracoabdominal aneurysm repair: a representative experience. J Vasc Surg. 1992;15:780-7.

45. Nijenhuis RJ, Jacobs MJ, Schurink GW, et al. Magnetic resonance angiography and neuromonitoring to assess spinal cord blood supply in thoracic and thoracoabdominal aortic aneurysm surgery. J Vasc Surg. 2007;45:71-7.

46. Jacobs MJ, de Mol BA, Elenbaas T, et al. Spinal cord blood supply in patients with thoracoabdominal aortic aneurysms. J Vasc Surg. 2002;35:30-7.

47. Cambria RP, Giglia JS. Prevention of spinal cord ischaemic complications after thoracoabdominal aortic surgery. Eur J Vasc Endovasc Surg. 1998;15:96-109.

48. van Dongen EP, Schepens MA, Morshuis WJ, ter Beek HT, Aarts LP, de Boer A, Boezeman EH. Thoracic and thoracoabdominal aortic aneurysm repair: use of evoked potential monitoring in 118 patients. J Vasc Surg. 2001;34(6):1035-40.

49. Jacobs MJ, de Mol BA, Elenbaas T, et al. Spinal cord blood supply in patients with thoracoabdominal aortic aneurysms. J Vasc Surg. 2002;35:30-7.

50. Murray MJ, Bower TC, Oliver WCJ, Werner E, Gloviczki P. Effects of cerebrospinal fluid drainage in patients undergoing thoracic and thoracoabdominal aortic surgery. J Cardiothorac Vasc Anesth. 1993;7:266-72.

51. Saether OD, Juul R, Aadahl P, et al. Cerebral haemodynamics during thoracic- and thoracoabdominal aortic aneurysm repair. Eur J Vasc Endovasc Surg. 1996;12:81-5.

52. Safi HJ, Miller CC III, Subramaniam MH, Campbell MP, Iliopoulos DC, O'Donnell JJ, et al. Thoracic and thoracoabdominal aortic aneurysm repair using cardiopulmonary bypass, profound hypothermia, and circulatory arrest via left side of the chest incision. J Vasc Surg. 1998;28:591-8.

53. Crawford ES, Crawford JL, Safi HJ, Coselli JS, Hess KR, Brooks B, et al. Thoracoabdominal aortic aneurysms: preoperative and intraoperative factors determining immediate and long-term results of operations in 605 patients. J Vasc Surg. 1986;3:389.

54. LeMaire SA, Miller CC III, Conklin LD, Schmittling ZC, Coselli JS. Estimating group mortality and paraplegia rates after thoracoabdominal aortic aneurysm repair. Ann Thorac Surg. 2003;75:508-13.

55. Coselli JS, Bozinovski J, LeMaire SA. Open surgical repair of 2286 thoracoabdominal aortic aneurysms. Ann Thorac Surg. 2007;83: S862-S4.

56. Coseli JS, LeMaire SA, Koksoy C, Schmittling ZC, Curling PE. Cerebrospinal fluid drainage reduces paraplegia after thoraco-abdominal aortic aneurysm repair: Results of a randomized clinical trial. J V Surg. 2002;35(4):631-9.

57. Safi HJ, Winnerkvist A, Miller CC III, Iliopoulos DC, Reardon MJ, Espada R, et al. Effect of extended cross-clamp time during thoracoabdominal aortic aneurysm repair. Ann Thorac Surg 1998;1204-9.

58. Kashyap VS, Cambria RP, Davison JK, L'Italien GJ. Renal failure after thoracoabdominal aortic surgery. J Vasc Surg. 1997;26:949-55.

59. Livesay JJ, Cooley DA, Ventemiglia RA, Montero CG, Warian RK, Brown DM, et al. Surgical experience in descending thoracic aneurysmectomy with and without adjuncts to avoid ischemia. Ann Thorac Surg. 1985;39:37-46.

60. De Haan P. Pharmacologic adjuncts to protect the spinal cord during transient ischemia. Sem Vasc Surg. 2000;13:264-71.

61. Schepens MA, Kelder JC, Morshuis WJ, Heijmen RH, van Dongen EP, ter Beek HT. Long-term follow-up after thoracoabdominal aortic aneurysm repair. Ann Thorac Surg. 2007;83(2):S851-5; discussion S890-2.

62. Estrera AL, Miller 3rd CC, Chen EP, et al. Descending thoracic aortic aneurysm repair: 12-year experience using distal aortic perfusion and cerebrospinal fluid drainage. Ann Thorac Surg. 2005;80:1290-6.

63. Dardik A, Krosnick T, Perler BA, et al. Durability of thoraco-abdominal aortic aneurysm repair in patients with connective tissue disorders. J Vasc Surg. 2002;36:696-703.

64. Dake MD, Miller DC, Semba CP, et al. Transluminal placement of endovascular stent-grafts for the treatment of descending thoracic aortic aneurysms. N Engl J Med. 1994;331:1729-34.

65. Cao CQ, Bannon PG, Shee R, Yan TD. Thoracic endovascular aortic repair—indications and evidence. Ann Thorac Cardiovasc Surg. 2011;17(1):1-6.

66. FiFindeiss LK, Cody ME. Endovascular repair of thoracic aortic aneurysms. Semin Intervent Radiol. 2011;28(1):107-17.

67. Buth J, Harris PL, Hobo R, et al. Neurologic complications associated with endovascular repair of thoracic aortic pathology: Incidence and risk factors. a study from the European Collaborators on Stent/Graft Techniques for Aortic Aneurysm Repair (EUROSTAR) registry. J Vasc Surg. 2007;46:1103-10.

68. Etezadi V, Schiro B, Peña CS, Kovacs M, Benenati JF, Katzen BT. Endovascular treatment of descending thoracic aortic disease: single-center, 15-year experience. J Vasc Interv Radiol. 2012;23(4):468-75. doi: 10.1016/j.jvir.2011.12.005. Epub 2012 Feb 1.

69. Ullery BW, Cheung AT, Fairman RM, Jackson BM, Woo EY, Bavaria J, et al. Risk factors, outcomes, and clinical manifestations of spinal cord ischemia following thoracic endovascular aortic repair. J Vasc Surg. 2011;54(3):677-84. doi: 10.1016/j.jvs.2011.03.259. Epub 2011 May 14.

70. Czerny M, Eggebrecht H, Sodeck G, Verzini F, Cao P, Maritati G, et al. Mechanisms of symptomatic spinal cord ischemia after TEVAR: insights from the European Registry of Endovascular Aortic Repair Complications (EuREC). J Endovasc Ther. 2012; 19(1):37-43. doi: 10.1583/11-3578.1.

## PRACTICAL POINTS

- Average diameter of the thoracic and abdominal aorta as determined by CT scan are larger in men when compared with women and vary significantly with age and body surface area.

- Majority of aneurysms are degenerative while others may be traumatic, mycotic, and pseudoaneurysms.

- The expansion rate of thoracic aortic aneurysm may be an important and clinically relevant index of the risk of rupture.

- TAAA formation is a complicated, dynamic process involving both extracellular and cellular processes. ECM degradation by matrix metalloproteinase (MMP) contributes to thoracic aortic aneurysm disease.

- The most common initial symptom in patients with TAAA is vague pain which occurs in the chest, back, flank or abdomen. Most patients with symptoms have TAAA is that have attained a diameter of greater than 5 cm. Other symptoms may be due to compression of the thoracic structures.

- The main imaging method used for the assessment of TAA/TAAA is a dynamic fine cut contrast enhanced CT angiography and provides information about anatomy, surgical/endovascular planning and acts as baseline for follow-up scans. Magnetic resonance angiography can be considered in patients with renal insufficiency. Angiography at present has little role.

- Medical therapy aims to reduce shear stress on the aneurysmal segment of the aorta by reducing blood pressure and contractility (dP/dt).

- Decision of open/endovascular repair is broadly based on patient's physiological reserve and vascular anatomy.

- Surgical repair is indicated if TAAA is 6 cm or larger, has a saccular configuration, an annual expansion rate >1 cm/year and symptomatic aneurysm, including rupture.

- TEVAR in patients with or without involvement of the abdominal aorta has gained acceptance as a reasonable alternative to open surgery. While no randomized trial data is available to compare the two strategies, observational data suggests equivalent or better patient outcomes with TEVAR.

- When TAAA involves major aortic branches, the options are use of branched aortic stent grafts, chimney technique and hybrid approach.

- Follow-up: Recommended follow-up schedules typically include a CT scan of the chest with and without contrast enhancement, preferably with delayed imaging to detect slow endoleaks at 1, 6 and 12 months during the first year. Yearly follow-up is then recommended for life.

# 13

# Approach to the Management of Mesenteric Vascular Disease

*Jaisom Chopra*

## ■ INTRODUCTION

Mesenteric ischemia may be acute or chronic.
Acute mesenteric ischemia could be due to:

- Embolic arterial occlusion
- Thrombotic arterial occlusion
- Nonocclusive mesenteric arterial insufficiency
- Mesenteric venous occlusion.

Chronic mesenteric occlusion is due to the progressive atherosclerotic narrowing of the arteries. Because of multiple causes of mesenteric ischemia, the diagnosis goes unnoticed and has a high morbidity and mortality (Fig. 1).

## ■ CLINICAL ANATOMY

The gastrointestinal tract is supplied by the celiac trunk, the superior mesenteric artery (SMA) and the inferior mesenteric artery (IMA).

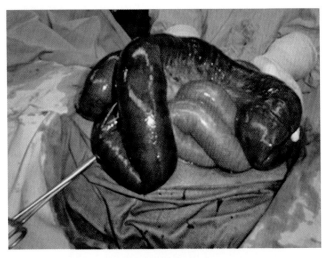

**Fig. 1** Mesenteric ischemia showing dead gut

## Celiac Trunk (Fig. 2)

- Arises anteriorly from the aorta at the level of T12 vertebra and branches into the common hepatic, splenic, and the left gastric arteries.
- The left gastric supplies the lesser curvature of the stomach and anastomosis with the right gastric, a branch of the hepatic artery.
- The common hepatic artery gives of the hepatic artery and the gastroduodenal artery, which supplies the distal stomach and the duodenum.
- The greater curvature of the stomach is supplied by the gastroepiploic artery, a branch of the gastroduodenal artery.

## Superior Mesenteric Artery (Fig. 3)

- This is located 2 cm below the celiac trunk at the level of L1 vertebra and has a 20–30° caudal angle to the aorta.
- It supplies the pancreas, duodenum, jejunum, ileum, and the right half of colon.
- The branches of SMA are inferior pancreaticoduodenal artery, the jejunal and ileal arteries, the ileocolic artery, the right colic artery, and the middle colic artery.

## Inferior Mesenteric Artery (Fig. 4)

- Arises from the aorta at the level of L3 vertebra 5 cm below the SMA.
- It supplies the distal transverse, left colon, sigmoid colon, and the rectum as the left colic artery, sigmoid artery, and the superior rectal artery.
- The SMA and IMA collateralize via the artery of Drummond and the meandering mesenteric artery.

The venous system follows the arterial system with the vasa recta forming the venous arcade that drains the small bowel and proximal colon via the ileocolic, middle colic, and right colic veins that join to form the superior mesenteric vein, which in

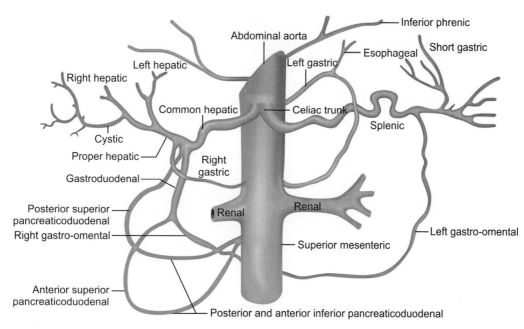

**Fig. 2** Anatomy of the celiac axis

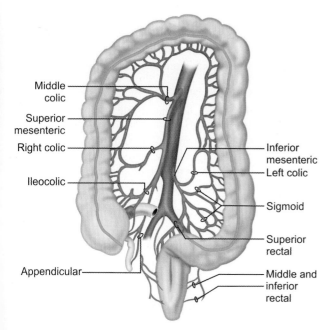

**Fig. 3** Anatomy of superior mesenteric artery

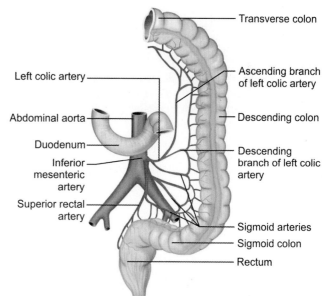

**Fig. 4** Anatomy of inferior mesenteric artery

turn joins the splenic veins to form the portal vein to the liver (Fig. 5).

There are three areas vulnerable to ischemia during low flow states because of their more remote position between the arteries.

These are the hepatic flexure between the ileocolic and middle colic arteries of the SMA, the splenic flexure between the middle colic and the left colic arteries, and the distal sigmoid and the rectum.

## ■ CLINICAL FEATURES AND DIAGNOSIS (TABLE 1)

### Acute Mesenteric Ischemia

This could be due to:
- Embolism
- Acute thrombosis on pre-existing atherosclerotic disease or
- Low flow state caused by systemic illness.

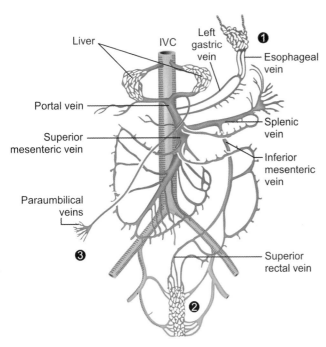

**Fig. 5** Mesenteric venous system

**Table 1** Clinical features differentiating the reason for gut ischemia

|  | Acute embolic occlusion | Acute thrombotic occlusion | Nonocclusive mesenteric ischemia |
|---|---|---|---|
| Clinical features | Sudden abdominal pain | Gradual progressive postprandial pain | Several days of vague abdominal pain and distension |
| Gender (M:F) | 2:1 | 1:2 | 1.5:1 |
| Diagnostic study | Operative diagnosis | Angiography | Angiography |
| Pathology | Embolic occlusion of SMA | Atherosclerosis | Low cardiac output; vasospasm from medications |
| Treatment | Embolectomy | Bypass or endarterectomy | Improve cardiac output, vasodilators, and IV fluids |

Even with aggressive treatment, the mortality is 40–50%, so early diagnosis is mandatory. Because it is an exceptionally difficult diagnosis to make, a high degree of suspicion is needed.

## Acute Embolic Mesenteric Artery Occlusion

The mesenteric arteries become occluded by embolus. SMA receives 3–4% of all arterial emboli. The common sources of emboli are:
• Atrial fibrillation with left atrial thrombus
• Mitral thrombosis with left atrial thrombus

• Transmural myocardial infarction with mural thrombus
• Proximal aortic atheroma
• Left atrial myxoma
• Paradoxical emboli from venous circulation.

### Clinical Features

• There is sudden onset of acute abdominal pain out of proportion to the examination, which initially is cramp like but later becomes constant.
• The patient has one or more of the above cardiac risk factors but has no history of previous intestinal angina or weight loss.
• Rapid evacuation of the bowel sometimes occurs.
• There is leukocytosis, hemoconcentration, and metabolic acidosis. Elevated serum amylase, alkaline phosphatase, and creatinine phosphokinase indicates bowel infarction.
• Early physical examination is generally inconclusive but later the patient has abdominal distension, signs of peritoneal irritation, and gastrointestinal bleeding.

### Investigations

• Blood tests
  – Hematology—leukocytosis, hemoconcentration, and metabolic acidosis
  – Biochemistry—elevated serum amylase, alkaline phosphatase, and creatinine phosphokinase indicate bowel infarction.
• Abdominal X-ray
  – There are no early findings to suggest bowel infarction or ischemia.
  – Free air within the abdomen would reveal perforation.
  – Other causes like obstruction may be ruled out by multiple fluid levels or distended bowel loops.
  – Renal or biliary calculi or chronic calcified pancreatitis could be excluded by plain abdominal X-ray.
  – Late findings are "thumbprinting" signifying intramural edema or hemorrhage.
  – Portal vein gas signifies bowel infarction.
• Ultrasound abdomen: Has not been as helpful as expected in acute abdomen due to bowel infarction of ischemia because of:
  – Poor quality image in obese
  – Poor visualization with bowel gas
  – Tortuosity of vessels
  – Technical inexperience.
• Angiography
  – It is still the gold standard with delayed venous phase films
  – Lateral angiography should be done to visualize the arterial origin
  – Selective cannulation is generally done in celiac artery, SMA and IMA
  – The rate of injection of dye must match the rate of flow in each vessel which is 10 mL/s in celiac trunk, 8 mL/s in SMA, and 3 mL/s in IMA

- Digital subtraction angiography (DSA) is hampered by bowel gas and should not be done
- "Meniscus" sign in SMA (4–6 cm from origin) is conclusive for embolus
- Emboli usually lodge distal to the origin of the middle colic artery or first jejuna branch of SMA and so proximal jejuna branches fill rapidly, whereas distal jejuna and ileal branches fill slowly.

## Acute Thrombotic Mesenteric Artery Occlusion

### Clinical Features

- It commonly occurs in females between 60 and 70 years.
- These patients have weight loss, altered bowel habit, and chronic abdominal pain.
- There is generally pre-existing atherosclerosis of SMA.
- Other causes are fibromuscular dysplasia, hypercoagulable states, inflammatory arteritis, and aortic dissection.

### Diagnosis

- The gold standard once again is angiography.
- Atherosclerosis affects the first few centimeters of the SMA. There is mostly a sharp cut off in the first 3 cm of the SMA and extensive collateral circulation is seen from the celiac artery or the IMA.

## Acute Mesenteric Venous Thrombosis (Table 2)

### Clinical Features

- The presentation ranges from asymptomatic to portal venous occlusion with associated liver failure and extensive bowel necrosis.
- This accounts for 10% of the mesenteric occlusions.
- The causes of mesenteric vein occlusion are:
  - Hypercoagulable states
  - Abdominal malignancies

- Abdominal operations
- Oral contraceptives use
- Inflammatory bowel disease.

When the mesenteric vein occludes the fluid accumulates within the wall of the intestine. Thrombosis may extend to the vasa recta and the intramural venous collaterals. This results in increased capillary pressure resulting in edema and finally arterial compromise.

Acute mesenteric venous occlusion may give rise to bowel infarction and peritonitis.

In subacute mesenteric venous occlusion, persistent abdominal pain for days to weeks without bowel infarction or variceal hemorrhage.

In chronic venous occlusion, there are complications of portal or splanchnic venous thrombosis leading to variceal bleeding. There is no pain due to the extensive collateral formation.

### Diagnosis

- Routine blood tests and physical examination is not helpful
- Abdominal X-ray may be difficult to interpret
  - Look for "thumbprinting", which is blunt semi-opaque indentation of bowel lumen indicative of bowel mucosal edema.
  - Bowel infarction may show as gas within the intestinal wall or the portal vein or free peritoneal air.
  - Thus, barium contrast is not indicated.
- Abdominal ultrasound can show portal vein thrombosis, intestinal edema, and ascitis.
- CT abdomen is the investigation of choice
  - Acute thrombosis will show as lucency in mesenteric vein.
  - It shows enlargement of the superior mesenteric vein (SMV) with a sharply defined vein wall and a rim of increased density.
  - Persistent enlargement of the bowel wall with pneumatosis intestinalis and portal vein gas are late findings.
  - Extensive collaterals in the mesentery and retroperitoneum shows the venous thrombosis is weeks old.

**Table 2** Causes of mesenteric venous thrombosis

| Post-thrombotic state | Hematologic disease | Inflammatory disease | Postoperative state | Others |
|---|---|---|---|---|
| Antithrombin III deficiency | Polycythemia vera | Pancreatitis | Abdominal operation | Cirrhosis |
| Protein C deficiency | Paroxysmal nocturnal hemoglobinuria | Peritonitis | Splenectomy | Portal hypertension |
| Protein S deficiency | Essential thrombocythemia | Ulcerative colitis | Sclerotherapy | Abdominal trauma |
| Factor V Leiden | | Crohn's disease | | Decompression sickness |
| Antiphospholipid antibodies | | Diverticulitis | | |
| Hyperhomocysteinemia | | | | |
| Oral contraceptives pregnancy Neoplasms | | | | |

- Angiography
  - Distal arterial spasm with stretching of the arterioles over the wall edema.
  - There is prolonged capillary phase of the study.
  - There is generally no venous phase due to the blockage.

## Nonocclusive Mesenteric Ischemia (Table 3)

### Clinical Features

- This is the most common cause of acute mesenteric ischemia.
- Elderly males and females are equally affected.
- It occurs in low cardiac output states or those with sustained mesenteric vasoconstriction.
- This disease is as a direct result of the effects of systemic process on mesenteric circulation.
- A combination of low flow state and vasoconstriction must be severe enough to overwhelm the compensatory mechanism found in normal intestinal state.
- In hypovolemia due to shock, bowel ischemia may be aggravated by drugs needed to promote cardiac output like vasopressors and digitalis, which cause vasoconstriction.
- Prolonged vasoconstriction damages the intestinal wall unless the vasoconstriction can be decreased and the splanchnic perfusion improved.
- The splenic flexure of the colon is the most vulnerable area due to the watershed blood supply.

### Diagnosis

- Gradual onset of lower abdominal pain is the norm and there are minimal physical signs.
- Unfortunately, the diagnosis is delayed due to the attention paid to the critically ill patient.
- Routine bloods and X-rays are not helpful.
- A high level of suspicion is needed for the diagnosis.
- Angiography is the gold standard. A normal proximal SMA with tapering of the distal branches finally becoming opacified and absent suggests severe vasospasm.

## Chronic Mesenteric Ischemia

### Clinical Features

- It is rare and there is insufficient blood to the small bowel resulting in ischemia.

**Table 3** Causes of nonocclusive mesenteric ischemia

| Low cardiac output states | Mesenteric vasoconstriction |
|---|---|
| Congestive heart failure (CHF) | Medications—digitalis, vasopressors |
| Cardiac arrhythmia | Hypovolemia |
| Postcardiac surgery | Septic shock |
| Cardiomyopathy | Hemoconcentration |
|  | Postabdominal surgery |

- The most common cause is atherosclerosis but may be caused by trauma or fibromuscular disease.
- All three—celiac axis, SMA, and IMA—have ostial disease and occlusions in the proximal few centimeters of the arteries.
- Two or three of these splanchnic vessels may have severe stenosis responsible for bowel ischemia.
- At rest, generally, there is enough blood flow and the patient is asymptomatic; however, with increased demand after a meal, there is not enough blood to cope with the increased demand and these results in intestinal angina.

### Diagnosis

- More common in females in 50s and 60s and have atherosclerotic disease at other sites also like peripheral artery disease, coronary artery disease, and cerebrovascular disease.
- The most common complaint is abdominal pain after eating. It is colicky epigastric pain coming on 15–20 minutes after eating and lasting 2–3 hours.
- These patients have marked weight loss.
- Physical examination shows weight loss and generalized atherosclerosis.
- Plain abdominal X-ray, CT scan, and endoscopy are all unreliable.
- Ultrasound is needs a very skilled operator, well prepared patient with reduced bowel gas. Velocities of over 275 cm/s in the celiac axis, over 200 cm/s in the SMA point toward a 70% stenosis in the respective arteries. This is 90% sensitive and specific as compared with angiography.
- Magnetic resonance angiography (MRA) is turning out to be the investigation of choice. Angiography shows extent of the disease and collateral flow.

## Chronic Mesenteric Venous Thrombosis

### Clinical Features

- These patients, unlike acute mesenteric venous thrombosis are generally asymptomatic.
- CT for some other cause may reveal non-visualization of SMA and extensive venous collaterals.
- There is no need for angiography.
- If portal and splenic veins are involved then portal hypertension with esophageal varices and splenomegaly are present.
- Pancreatitis and pancreatic neoplasm should be excluded.

## ■ MANAGEMENT

### Acute Mesenteric Ischemia

- This is generally embolic and proven by angiogram.
- The treatment of choice is embolectomy.

- Following adequate reperfusion time the bowel viability is assessed using Doppler ultrasound, IV fluorescein with woods lamp illumination, and clinical assessment.
- If doubt remains, a second look surgery should be planned in 12–24 h.
- SMA embolectomy is successful in majority. However, because of the poor general condition of the patient and the delayed diagnosis the mortality is high (over 70%).
- Thrombolysis is an option.
- The late complication of thrombolysis is development of stricture after about 2 months of a successful thrombolysis.
- It is only indicated when we are sure of occlusion and there are no signs of peritoneal irritation as yet.
- Bowel necrosis has a mortality of over 90%.
- Lysis and angioplasty are associated with unacceptably high rates of hemorrhage.
- Surgical exploration is not mandatory in cases of acute mesenteric vein occlusion if there is no peritonitis.
- It is only indicated if peritonitis develops.
- Necrotic bowel must be resected even without perforation.
- If the thrombus is fresh then thrombectomy may be done only in the superior mesenteric vein.
- Arterial spasm that may accompany venous thrombosis treated with papaverine and anticoagulation.
- Intra-arterial thrombolysis is associated with increased survival and decreased recurrence rates.
- Acute abdomen needs broad-spectrum antibiotic cover.
- In the absence of bowel infarction, mesenteric vein occlusion is managed medically.
- Systemic anticoagulation is started immediately after giving bolus, the infusion is adjusted by regular activated partial thromboplastin time (aPTT) tests which are maintained at two times control levels.
- This anticoagulation is started even with intestinal bleeding if the benefit from preventing bowel necrosis is greater than the risk from bleeding.
- Warfarin is started when the risk of bowel necrosis no longer exists.
- Despite variceal bleeding, the benefits of long-term anticoagulation should not be underestimated.
- The duration of anticoagulation depends on the cause of mesenteric occlusion. If there is no ongoing thrombotic cause, anticoagulation may be stopped within 6 months to 1 year.
- During systemic anticoagulation, it is important to continue with IV fluid resuscitation and bowel decompression with an NG tube.
- Chronic mesenteric thrombosis is treated with the idea of preventing esophageal variceal bleeding.
- Long-term anticoagulation is given to patients with prothrombotic state.

In nonocclusive mesenteric states, the cause is treated.
- Inotropic support to increase cardiac output, aggressive diuresis for CHF, and fluid resuscitation for hypovolemia should be the goal.

- Avoid digitalis and alpha-agonists.
- Pulmonary artery catheter is needed for fluid resuscitation.
- Bowel decompression with rest is a must.
- While addressing all these underlying problems, it is important to institute vasodilatation of the mesenteric vessels.
- Selective catheter directed drugs are the treatment of choice. A continuous infusion of papaverine 30–60 mg/h is started and only terminated when angiography shows vasodilatation. Epidural infusion of papaverine and systemic glucagon has also been advocated but no studies prove their efficacy.
- The mortality in this condition remains very high at 60%.

## Chronic Mesenteric Ischemia

- Surgical revascularization is recommended but the overall operative mortality remains high at 7.5%.
- The surgical possibilities remain visceral endarterectomy, antegrade supraceliac aorta to visceral bypass or a retrograde infrarenal aorta to visceral bypass.
- Preoperatively total parenteral nutrition may be beneficial.
- In the antegrade technique, the chances of paraplegia are there because of the aortic cross clamping at this level.
- Retrograde SMA bypass is most commonly performed because of the easier approach but care must be taken the graft does not kink.
- Antegrade procedure is advocated when infrarenal aorta is markedly atherosclerotic.
- Endarterectomy has the lowest rate of recurrence followed by antegrade technique and then retrograde procedure.
- Endovascular stenting is emerging the procedure of choice.

## ■ SPECIAL ISSUES

## Median Arcuate Ligament Syndrome

- The median arcuate ligament of the diaphragm causes compression of the celiac trunk in middle-aged females.
- There is abdomen pain with weight loss.
- There is generally a bruit in the upper abdomen.
- Lateral angiographic films reveal celiac compression by the ligament on deep expiration.
- Surgical division of the ligament is the treatment of choice.

## Mesenteric Aneurysms

### Splenic Artery Aneurysm (Fig. 6)

- It is the most common of the visceral artery aneurysms and is due to degeneration of the media of the arterial wall.
- It is more common in females of childbearing age.
- Fibromuscular dysplasia occurs in 15%.
- 10% patients with splenic artery aneurysm have portal hypertension, whereas 5% have renal artery disease.

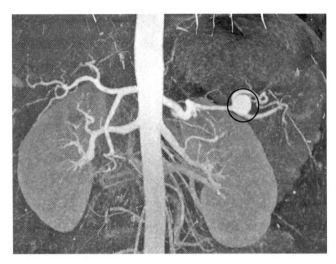

**Fig. 6** Splenic artery aneurysm

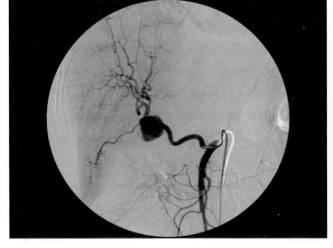

**Fig. 7** Hepatic artery aneurysm

- Generally patients are asymptomatic or have vague upper abdominal pain.
- Plain abdominal X-ray may show signet ring calcification.
- Angiography shows aneurysm which is saccular and occurs at bifurcation usually at the distal one-third of splenic artery.
- In nonpregnant females, the rupture rate is 2% and mortality 25%.
- In pregnant, the rupture rates are high and the maternal and fetal mortality is 70% and 75%, respectively.
- The treatment is excision of the aneurysm or ligation and splenectomy if aneurysm is very distally placed.
- A pseudoaneurysm in pancreatitis patient is treated by distal pancreatectomy and splenectomy along with resection of aneurysm.
- Catheter embolization is only recommended is very sick patients.

## Hepatic Artery Aneurysm (Fig. 7)

- These account for 20% of all visceral aneurysms.
- The cause is atherosclerosis, trauma, infection, and degeneration of the media in the arterial wall.
- Most are extrahepatic with common hepatic accounting for the majority.

Intrahepatic aneurysms are mostly due to trauma.
- It occurs in men over 60 years.
- They may be asymptomatic or have pain in the right upper abdomen radiating to the shoulder and in large aneurysms there may be jaundice from compression of the common bile duct.

- The diagnosis is by angiography and 20% rupture with a mortality of 35%.
- Repair is advocated regardless of the size. Intrahepatic aneurysms are treated by catheter directed embolization and extrahepatic aneurysms are excised or excluded. Common hepatic aneurysms are excluded with proximal and distal ligation. The main hepatic artery aneurysms are excised and interposition venous graft put to restore the blood flow.

## Celiac Trunk Aneurysms (Fig. 8)

- They occur because of atherosclerosis, trauma, infection, and medial degeneration.
- They affect middle-aged males and females equally.
- The patient has significant abdominal pain diagnosed by angiography.
- Because of the high incidence of rupture, they should be repaired and blood flow restored even though they are asymptomatic.

## SMA Aneurysms (Fig. 9)

- It has equal incidence in males and females.
- Infection from nonhemolytic *Streptococcus* from left sided endocarditis causes most though trauma, atherosclerosis, medial degeneration, and illicit drug abuse can also be responsible.
- They present with epigastric pain.
- Plain X-ray abdomen may show calcification.
- Angiogram gives the diagnosis.

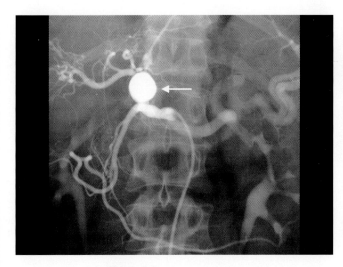

**Fig. 8** Celiac artery aneurysm

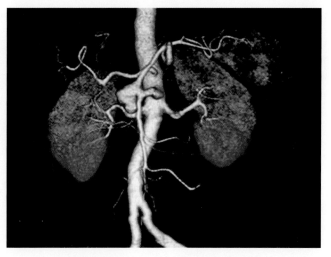

**Fig. 9** Superior mesenteric artery aneurysm

- Although rupture rate is low, thrombosis rates are high and therefore most should be treated.
- Excision of the aneurysm and arterial reconstruction to restore the flow are recommended.
- The operative mortality is 15% and that of rupture is 50%.

## ■ CONCLUSION

- Mesenteric vascular disease represents a vast number of conditions that have a high mortality, if left untreated.
- Doctors must have a high degree of suspicion to treat these conditions.

- Only early diagnosis and aggressive treatment can reduce the high mortality rates
- Angiography is the gold standard to the diagnosis of acute mesenteric ischemia due to embolism, thrombosis, and nonobstructed mesenteric occlusion.
- CT scan has a 90% sensitivity in diagnosing mesenteric venous thrombosis.
- Mesenteric venous thrombosis can be managed by medications alone if there is no bowel infarction. Anticoagulation is started immediately in the operating theater.
- Visceral aneurysms are repaired in most cases.

## PRACTICAL POINTS

- There are three areas in the colon that are prone to ischemia—(i) Hepatic flexure between ileocolic and middle colic branches of the SMA; (ii) The splenic flexure between the middle colic and the left colic arteries; (iii) The distal sigmoid and rectum.
- Urgent surgery if mesenteric embolism and acute thrombosis are suspected, without angiogram.
- There is abrupt change from ischemic to normal bowel in arterial thromboembolism.
- IMA is commonly involved in arterial thromboembolism and rarely in venous thrombosis.
- Thrombolysis is useful in arterial thromboembolism but rarely in venous thrombosis.
- Infection from nonhemolytic *Streptococcus* from left sided endocarditis accounts for most SMA aneurysms.
- The splenic artery is the most common visceral artery to become aneurysmal.
- Three conditions are associated with splenic artery aneurysm—(i) fibrodysplasia; (ii) portal hypertension with splenomegaly; and (iii) multiparity.

# 14

# Approach to the Patient with Upper Extremity Arterial Disease

*Jaisom Chopra*

## ■ INTRODUCTION

- Upper extremity arterial disease (UEAD) accounts for only 5% of all arterial cases.
- It is uncommon because of the extensive collateral network and the low incidence of atherosclerosis in the upper extremity.
- Unlike lower extremity where arterial disease is caused exclusively by atherosclerosis, UEAD is caused by multiple causes that make diagnosis difficult.
- The clinical features of these multiple etiologies may be similar, making the diagnosis difficult.

## ■ PROBLEMS

- Upper extremity arterial disease may be a part of the systemic disease or it may be local disease.
- The disease pattern depends on the etiology.
- Upper extremity arterial disease is divided into large vessel (above the wrist) and small vessel (below the wrist) arterial disease.
- Large vessel arterial disease has four causes:
  - Embolic
  - Aneurysmal
  - Vasculopathy (vasculitis and atherosclerosis)
  - Entrapment
- Atherosclerosis involves the inflow arteries—brachiocephalic and subclavian.

*Differential diagnosis of large vessel obstructive disease of the upper limb:*

- Atherosclerosis
- Aneurysmal—thoracic outlet syndrome (TOS) and trauma
- Embolic—from heart, arch of the aorta, and proximal great vessels

- Entrapment—TOS
- Vasculitis—giant cell (Takayasu's) and radiation.

There are many conditions causing small vessel arterial disease, which are difficult to differentiate from history and examination alone and need additional diagnostic studies. These studies are noninvasive or invasive and define the etiology and treatment planning.

*Differential diagnosis of small vessel arterial disease of the upper limb:*

- Blood dyscrasias—cryoglobulins, myeloproliferative disease, and multiple myeloma
- Buerger's disease
- Embolic—sites include
  - Atheromatous plaque (heart, innominate, subclavian)
  - Aneurysms (innominate, subclavian, axillary, brachial, and ulnar)
- Henoch-Schönlein purpura
- Hypercoagulable states—antiphospholipid syndrome, deficiency of antithrombin III, protein C and S, lupus anticoagulant, and heparin-induced thrombocytopenia
- Vasculitis—scleroderma, CREST (calcinosis, Raynaud phenomenon, esophageal dysmotility, sclerodactyly, and telangiectasia), rheumatoid arthritis, systemic lupus erythematosus, and polymyositis.
- Miscellaneous—frostbite.

## ■ ANATOMY AND PHYSIOLOGY OF UPPER EXTREMITY CIRCULATION

This is important to understand the manifestations of disease in the upper limbs.

### Physiologic Vasospasm

This is a mechanism for thermoregulation. The cutaneous circulation of the hands is regulated by the sympathetic nervous system via the alpha-adrenergic receptors. Emotional states, cold exposure, and respiratory reflexes cause arteriolar constriction. The presence of many arteriovenous (AV) shunts helps rapid regulation of blood flow to the hands in response to body temperature and strong emotional states. Normal vasospasm never causes cessation of blood flow whereas in Raynaud's phenomenon blood flow ceases.

## Anatomy of Upper Extremity Arterial Circulation (Fig. 1)

The inflow arteries of the upper limb are the brachiocephalic and the subclavian, whereas the intrinsic arteries are the axillary, brachial, radial, ulnar, palmar, and digital arteries. On the radial and ulnar arteries crossing the wrist, they become the superficial and the deep palmar arches. These arches vary in caliber, origin, and anatomy.

The deep palmar arch from the radial gives rise to four palmar metacarpal arteries. These anastomose with the common palmar digital arteries arising from the superficial palmar arch and immediately divide into the proper digital arteries. The digital arteries lie on the medial and the lateral sides of the fingers and anastomose at the tip of the finger (Fig. 2).

The parallel arterial system—radial and ulnar—and the digital arteries on the medial and lateral aspect of the digits allow normal upper limb perfusion despite significant arterial occlusion. Normal pressures are maintained even if one of the parallel arteries is totally occluded (Fig. 3).

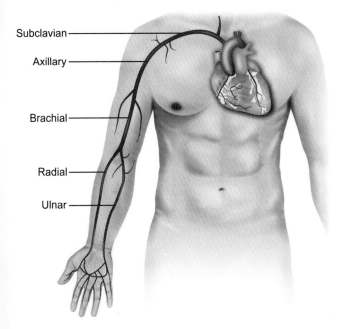

**Fig. 1** Arterial supply of the upper limb

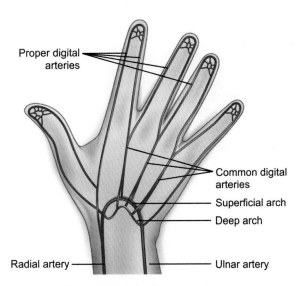

**Fig. 2** Arterial circulation of the hand

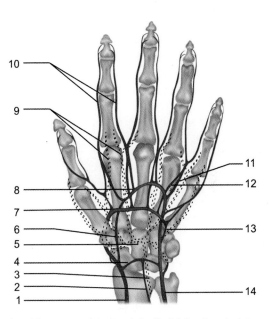

**Fig. 3** Arterial anatomy of the hand. 1 = Radial; 2 = Anterior interosseus; 3 = Posterior interosseus; 4 = Palmar carpal branch; 5 = Dorsal carpal branch forming the dorsal carpal rete; 6 = Superficial palmar branch of the radial artery; 7 = Deep palmar arch; 8 = Superficial palmar arch; 9 = Dorsal metacarpal arteries; 10 = Proper palmar digital arteries; 11 = Common palmar digital arteries; 12 = Palmar metacarpal; 13 = Deep palmar branch of the ulnar artery; 14 = Ulnar artery

Adapted from Atlas of Normal and Variant Angiographic Anatomy. Kadir, Saadoon. W.B Saunders Company, 1991

## Anomalous Circulation

This can lead to the wrong diagnosis. Thus, one must be aware of the common and multiple variants of the upper limb circulation.

## Variant Percent of Population

### Arch of Aorta and Great Vessels

- Common origin of right brachiocephalic and left common carotid arteries—22%
- Left vertebral artery origin directly from the aorta—4-6%.

### Brachial Artery

- Radial artery origin from the brachial or axillary—15-20%
- Ulnar artery origin from the brachial or axillary—1-3%
- Accessory (duplicate) brachial artery and rejoins original
- Brachial artery in the elbow—0.1-0.2%.

### Radial Artery

- Origin from brachial or axillary artery—15-20%
- Aplasia, hypoplasia, and duplication—<1%.

### Ulnar Artery

- High origin (axillary/brachial)—1-3%
- Low origin (5-7 cm below the elbow joint)—1%
- Persistent median artery—<0.1%
- Persistent interosseous branch—<0.1%.

### Palmar Arch Variants

Incomplete deep and superficial palmar arches—0.5-1.5%.

## Collateral Pathway in Upper Extremity

These are multiple tributaries present that serve as collaterals in obstructive disease. These delay the outcome of ischemic symptoms and so if patients with UEAD become symptomatic, it is always more advanced than expected. In subclavian artery stenosis, the vertebra serves as a collateral pathway (subclavian steal). In brachial artery occlusion, collaterals from the distal arm to the forearm beyond the occlusion are seen. In radial or ulnar occlusions, collaterals from mid arm are seen to the distal forearm beyond the occlusion. There may be retrograde filling from the palmar arch.

## ■ HISTORY AND PHYSICAL EXAMINATION

## History

- Detailed description of symptoms and associated illnesses.
- Occupational and exposure history—vinyl chloride exposure with Raynaud's.

- Traumatic history—hypothenar hammer syndrome or vibratory tool history with Raynaud's.
- Drug history—migraine and other vasospastic medications.
- Tobacco use.
- Upper extremity ischemia is often associated with collagen and hematologic disorders and so the history must exclude rashes, myalgia, arthralgia, fever, weight loss, fatigue, dysphagia, xerostomia, and xerophthalmia.
- Large artery involvement of the upper limb presents as claudication in arm and hand with finger pain.
- Small vessel disease gives rise to only hand and finger pain along with cyanosis, ulcers, and gangrene.
- In all UEAD, there is always some element of Raynaud's phenomenon.
- Unilateral versus bilateral limb involvement—unilateral is evaluated for proximal embolic source, whereas bilateral is generally systemic cause.
- Intermittent versus constant symptoms—nonobstructive disease shows intermittent symptoms with normal asymptomatic periods in between. Obstructive arterial disease shows constant Raynaud's symptoms.
- Acuteness of symptoms does not suggest acute disease process as most acute symptoms are caused by progression of chronic obstruction, which manifests when the collateral circulation is compromised.
- Vasculitis is responsible for digital ulcerations in 50-75% cases. The common causes of vasculitis are Buerger's disease, atherosclerosis-related complications like embolism, progressive sclerosis scleroderma (PSS)/CREST.

## Physical Examination

### General Examination

- Cardiovascular examination to exclude embolic source—atrial fibrillation, atrial myxoma, valvular disease, left ventricular (LV) thrombus, paradoxical embolic due to atrial septal defect (ASD) or patent foramen ovale (PFO). These may need an echocardiogram.
- Rashes suggest underlying collagen disease.
- Petechiae may suggest hematological malignancy.
- Signs of endocarditis—Osler's nodes—must be noted.

### Upper Extremity Examination

- Pulsatile mass in the supraclavicular region suggests a subclavian artery aneurysm.
- Palpation of the supraclavicular region may reveal a cervical rib or tenderness over scalene muscle suggesting thoracic outlet syndrome (TOS).
- Bruit over subclavian suggests stenosis, whereas a continuous murmur suggests AV fistula.

- Aneurysms of the brachial and axillary arteries occur because of trauma, iatrogenic cardiac catheterization, and fibromuscular dysplasia but are rare.
- Radial artery aneurysms are rare and due to trauma or iatrogenic.
- Ulnar artery aneurysms are seen in mechanics and carpenters with hypothenar hammer syndrome.

*Allen's test and TOS maneuvers (Adson's abduction external rotation and costoclavicular maneuvers):* In all these maneuvers, the radial pulse is felt digitally or with the help of a Doppler at rest and after a provocative maneuver. The positive test is the reduction in the pulse amplitude.

*Adson's test:* The patient sitting upright is asked to take a deep breath and look upward and turn the face to the affected side. There is reduction in the pulse tracing.

*Hyperabduction maneuver:* The patient is made to hyperabduct the upper extremity. The pulse disappears due to compression of the artery in the event of compression syndrome and reappearance with normal position.

*Costoclavicular maneuver:* Both shoulders are thrust backward and downward maximally—the radial pulse is lost.

*EAST maneuver (external rotation—abduction stress test):* It is the most reliable. The patient adopts the "stick-up posture"—arms extended and externally rotated behind the head. The patient repeatedly makes fists for 3 minutes and the pulse is felt at the end of this period.

*Branham's sign:* This is done when an AV fistula is suspected. Pressure on the artery proximal to the fistula will cause it to disappear with loss of bruit as well as a fall in pulse.

About 15% patients will have positive test despite being asymptomatic. A negative test does not rule out TOS.

Majority patients with TOS have neurological signs rather than vascular compromise.

## ■ DIAGNOSTIC TESTING

## Segmental Limb Pressures and Doppler Pulse Contours

This is the first noninvasive test that should be performed with cuffs around the brachial, upper elbow, and the wrist, recording the Doppler pressures and recording waveforms at these levels. The difference of the pressure levels at two adjacent sites of the same limb or at the same level of the contralateral limb should be <7 mm Hg. A difference of over 15 mm Hg means hemodynamically significant stenosis. A brachial/brachial, forearm/forearm or a wrist/wrist index should be 0.85–1. If it is <0.85, it is significant for a stenosis. Normally, pulse contours in the upper extremity are biphasic or triphasic.

*Interpretation:* A pressure difference of >15 mm Hg between the two upper limbs or an index <0.8 shows significant disease while monophasic wave from also shows disease.

## Finger Pressure and Pulse Contours (Figs 4A to C)

The pressure in all 10 fingers is measured using a cuff 1.2 times the diameter of the finger around the proximal phalanx. Brachial to finger index on the same side is 1. In obstructive lesions, a brachial–finger pressure index <0.7 or an absolute finger pressure <70 mm Hg is significant, whereas a finger–wrist pressure gradient >30 mm Hg or a finger–finger pressure gradient >15 mm Hg is abnormal. Normal pressures at the proximal phalanx do not rule out distal disease and can be tested by digital waveform on photoplethysmography. Normal contours are specific for the absence of disease.

### Interpretation (Flow chart 1)

- If arm pressure is abnormal (disease in axillary or brachial) with sparing of the palmar/digital arteries, the pressure in all fingers is symmetrically reduced and the wrist finger ratio is normal.
- If the arm pressure is abnormal with further drops in the pressures beyond the brachial or elbow with abnormal wrist finger ratio then there is arterial disease in all vessels of the limb.
- If arm pressures are normal and all digital pressures are equally reduced the critical lesion must involve the palmar arch or the distal radial and ulnar arteries.
- Abnormal pressures on only one side of the hand show critical lesion in a segment of the palmar arch.
- Reduction of pressure in a single digit indicates occlusion of the digital artery in that finger.
- Patients with primary Raynaud's have normal digital pressures and waveforms.
- Patients with palmar and digital obstructive disease without inflow disease have abnormal finger pressures and waveforms. This could be seen in secondary Raynaud's and is in both hands while it is unilateral in peripheral embolization.

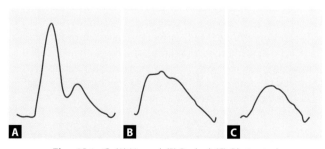

**Figs 4A to C** (A) Normal; (B) Peaked; (C) Obstructed

**Flow chart 1** Diagnostic approach to the patient with upper extremity ischemia

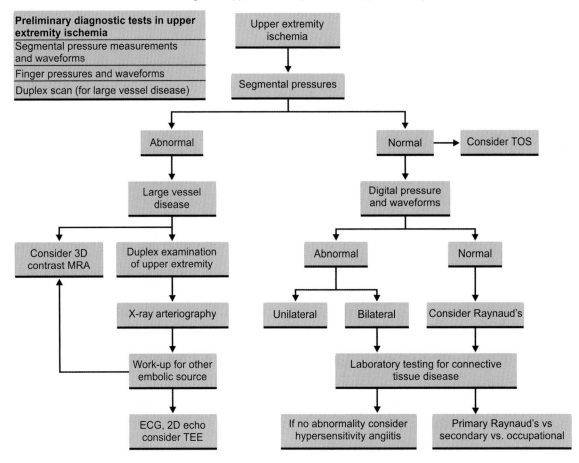

## Duplex Scans

Color Doppler scans are very accurate in locating anatomic and physiological information on stenosis up to the digital vessels (sensitivity and specificity for occlusion >90%). Subclavian artery has a blind spot behind the clavicle but segmental pressures provide useful information. The anatomy and physiology are tracked down to the digital vessels from the subclavian. For digital vessels, a high frequency transducer gives excellent information.

### Allen Test with Doppler Probe

The effect of compression of the radial or ulnar artery on the palmar arch signals is assessed. Normally, there is no interruption of flow. If both are compressed simultaneously there is no flow in the palmar arch, which resumes on release. Nonresumption of flow shows occlusion in that artery. Incomplete palmar arch is a variant having normal digital pressures and waveforms.

## Radiography and Contrast Angiography

Every patient with suspected TOS should undergo X-ray cervical spine AP view to rule out cervical rib. Angiography

is recommended for embolic occlusion. Bilateral angiograms are recommended as it differentiates Raynaud's disease, which is bilateral from embolic occlusive disease, which is unilateral.

## Magnetic Resonance Angiography

It is a good alternative to conventional angiography. Recent advances provide excellent resolution of the palmar arch and the digital arteries. In magnetic resonance angiography (MRA), aorta can be seen along with plaques.

## Laboratory Tests for Primary Raynaud's Disease (Nonobstructive Disease)

Complete blood count (CBC), erythrocyte sedimentation rate (ESR), biochemistry, antinuclear antibody (ANA), and rheumatoid factor.

## Laboratory Tests for Secondary Raynaud's Disease and Obstructive Disease

Hypercoagulability studies, ANA, and anti-dsDNA, rheumatoid factor, homocysteine levels, serum protein electrophoresis, cryoglobulins, complement levels, hepatitis screen, and anti-centromere antibodies.

## Ancillary Studies

Two-dimensional echo and ECG are a must to see cardiac status in proximal emboli.

## Capillary Microscopy

This provides prognostic information in a patient with cold sensitivity. Abnormal results suggest eventual development of connective tissue disease. In this, an ophthalmoscope is used at maximum magnification. Abnormal findings are dilated capillary loops and avascular areas. Giant capillaries are seen in PSS and CREST variants. Presence of abnormal capillaries in Raynaud's syndrome predicts connective tissue disorder in future.

## Cold Immersion Testing

It measures the time to recovery after exposure to cold (Porter method). A sensitive thermometer is attached to the finger and the hand immersed in iced water for 10 s. Normally temperature returns to normal in 10 minutes but in Raynaud's, it takes >20 minutes. The sensitivity is over 85% and the specificity over 75%.

## ■ IMPLICATIONS OF TESTING FOR UPPER EXTREMITY DISEASE

*Primary Raynaud's syndrome:* If segmental pressures, digital pressures, waveform studies duplex imaging, and laboratory tests are all normal in a patient with bilateral cold sensitivity and no other physical manifestations then a diagnosis of primary Raynaud's syndrome is made. 3% of these patients develop collagen vascular disease in the next 5 years.

*Secondary Raynaud's syndrome* has laboratory abnormalities (positive ANA and abnormal electrophoretic pattern but do not have rheumatologic illness) along with abnormal noninvasive vascular examination (isolated digital artery pressure disease or peaked digital artery pressure contour), the incidence of collagen vascular disease being diagnosed in the subsequent 4 years is 35%.

## ■ CONCLUSION

- Upper extremity arterial disease is less common than lower extremity arterial disease and involves large and small vessels.
- Large vessel disease has limited causes—embolic, aneurysms, vasculopathy (vasculitis and atherosclerosis), and entrapment.
- Small vessel disease has many causes but presents with vasospastic or obstructive symptoms.
- Segmental limb pressures and pulse waveforms as well as digital pressures and waveforms are excellent initial studies after a complete history and physical examination to arrive at a tentative diagnosis. Subsequent studies depend on the finding of these studies.
- Primary Raynaud's syndrome patients need no further testing other than additional laboratory tests to rule out collagen vascular disease.

## PRACTICAL POINTS

- Raynaud's syndrome is a nonspecific symptom that may occur on its own (primary disease) or along with obstructive lesion of the hand. It does not help in the etiological diagnosis.
- Unilateral Raynaud's should be investigated for embolic source.
- Continuous symptoms due to Raynaud's exclude primary disease, as it is always intermittent with normal asymptomatic intervals.
- About 50–75% of digital ulcerations are caused by vasculitis, Buerger's, and atherosclerosis-related complications (embolism).
- Only one finger may be symptomatic but investigations show involvement of multiple vessels.
- Since digital waveforms are obtained in distal phalanx, the presence of normal pressures in proximal phalanx does not prove disease as seen by abnormal pulse contours.
- Abnormal capillaries as seen on capillary microscopy in a Raynaud's patient predict connective tissue disorder later.
- 3% patients with Raynaud's disease and abnormal laboratory and noninvasive testing develop collagen vascular disease in the following 5 years.

# 15

# Large Arteries of Upper Limb: Innominate, Subclavian and Axillary

*Jaisom Chopra*

## ■ INTRODUCTION

- The lower limb is much more commonly involved than the upper limb.
- Subclavian artery is the most common to be involved in the upper limb and that too at its origin.
- Left side is three to four times as commonly involved as the right side.
- If there is significant stenosis of the subclavian artery origin then subclavian steal syndrome (SSS) may result leading to vertebrobasilar insufficiency, upper limb claudication, and myocardial infarction due to hypoperfusion of the internal mammary artery (IMA) in patients with IMA bypass.
- Axillary artery is rarely involved by atherosclerosis but stenosis or aneurysm occurs in patients using axillary crutches.

The *common causes* of large vessel disease in the upper extremity are:
- Atherosclerosis
- Aneurysmal
  - Thoracic outlet syndrome (TOS)
  - Traumatic
  - Kawasaki's disease
- Embolic—from heart, arch of aorta, proximal great vessels
- Entrapment—TOS
- Vasculitis
  - Takayasu's disease
  - Radiation.

Takayasu disease is considered in young with upper extremity involvement.

Atherosclerosis is considered in older people.

Thoracic outlet syndrome is considered in patients with acute or chronic upper extremity symptoms.

## ■ CLINICAL FEATURES

### Innominate Disease

- Rarely involved by atherosclerosis or vasculitis.
- Seen in 5–17% cases undergoing arch of aorta angiography and mostly is an unsuspected incidental finding.
- Mostly asymptomatic but minority have right upper limb claudication, microembolization, or cerebrovascular ischemic symptoms due to vertebrobasilar involvement.

### Subclavian Artery Disease

- Mostly asymptomatic and therefore an incidental finding when investigating for carotid or vertebral disease.
- Arm claudication is very rare due to excellent collateral circulation and may happen in long occlusions and tight stenosis.
- *Subclavian steal syndrome* occurs in tight stenosis of the subclavian artery proximal to the origin of the vertebral of the same side. This leads to reversal of flow in vertebral artery as seen on angiography and is diagnostic (Fig. 1).
- The patient presents with dizziness, unsteadiness, vertigo, or visual changes on exercising that limb. The blood is circulated into the ipsilateral vertebral from contralateral posterior circulation. That is why, patients with coronary artery bypass using left IMA (LIMA) may develop angina on exertion of upper extremity because of coronary subclavian steal where blood flow is reversed in LIMA leading to myocardial ischemia.

### Giant Cell Arteritis (Takayasu's)

- Almost always involves subclavian arteries.
- Type I involves aortic arch vessels only and type II involves abdominal aorta besides the aortic arch.

- The patients are asymptomatic and the only finding is bruit over subclavian artery, absent radial pulse, and pressure difference in both the upper limbs.
- If Takayasu is suspected always take the blood pressure in all four limbs.

## Thoracic Outlet Syndrome

- It is defined as compression of the neurovascular bundle at the upper thoracic outlet.
- Anatomically the scalene triangle is a narrow space bounded by the first rib or cervical rib, scalenus muscle, and costoclavicular ligament (Fig. 2).
- 95% patients have neurological symptoms compared with only 5% having arterial involvement.
- Arterial compression may present with upper limb claudication, ulcers on the finger tips, gangrene, or Raynaud's phenomenon. This is due to proximal arterial thrombosis leading to distal embolization.
- In suspected cases, record the blood pressure in both upper limbs and feel radial pulse. Listen to bruit over the subclavian.
- Noninvasive tests include, duplex studies, plethysmography, pressure studies in positions that cause symptoms of TOS.
- Angiography is gold standard.
- Treatment is surgical decompression of the neurovascular bundle by division of the abnormal structures like cervical rib or first rib and scalene muscles. The same is the treatment of poststenotic dilatation and subclavian artery aneurysms.

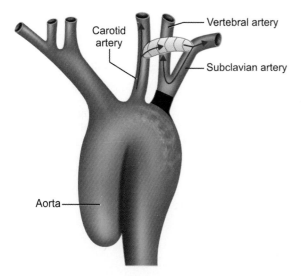

**Fig. 1** Subclavian artery stenosis leading to steal syndrome

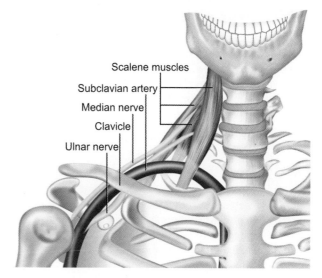

**Fig. 2** Anatomy of thoracic outlet

## Aneurysms of the Subclavian and Axillary Arteries

### Subclavian Artery Aneurysms

- This can result from atherosclerosis, trauma, TOS, and collagen diseases.
- It is an unusual site for aneurysms so look for aneurysms elsewhere.
- They present with neck pain, embolization distally and pressure symptoms due to the compression of adjacent structures like nerve and vein. Rarely recurrent laryngeal nerve compression gives rise to hoarseness, tracheal compression leads to dyspnea and TIAs due to retrograde embolization in vertebral and carotid arteries.
- Pulsatile mass above the clavicle is usually due to tortuous artery and rarely due to aneurysm. Aneurysms in the distal subclavian are due to TOS (almost always cervical rib).

### Kommerell's Diverticulum and Aneurysm of the Aberrant Right Subclavian Artery

- Aberrant right subclavian artery arises from left side of aortic arch distal to the origin of the left subclavian and crosses the midline between the spinal column and the esophagus in 0.4–2% of the population.
- In 60%, its origin from the aortic arch is saccular (Kommerell's diverticulum).
- It is mostly asymptomatic and discovered per chance on CXR or endoscopy.
- It may cause dysphagia for solids intermittently—dysphagia lusoria. There is a high risk for rupture.

### *Axillary Artery Aneurysms*

Mostly traumatic in people using crutches (crutch aneurysm), blunt, or penetrating trauma as in vehicle accidents, fracture humerus, or anterior shoulder dissection. They present as upper limb ischemia with absent radial and brachial pulse because they are mostly thrombosed. It should also be suspected in brachial plexus injury having a pulsatile mass in the axilla. Angiogram is diagnostic.

## ■ DIAGNOSIS

Subclavian artery or innominate involvement may go unnoticed and is suspected with a weak or absent radial pulse, a distinct blood pressure difference between the two arms (>15 mm Hg) and presence of a bruit over the subclavian or carotid arteries. Presence of distal embolization should make one suspect proximal innominate or subclavian artery disease.

Reduced blood pressure bilaterally should alert one of bilateral subclavian artery involvement secondary to TOS.

To diagnose the condition, there are maneuvers that unfortunately are not very reliable because they may be positive in normal people. However, they may be of some value with specific signs and symptoms. In each of the maneuvers, the radial pulse is felt or Doppler used at rest and after the provocative test. A positive test is reduction in pulse amplitude with the maneuver.

- *Adson's test:* Patient sitting upright is asked to take a deep breath and turn the face upward and toward the affected side (Fig. 3).
- *Hyperabduction maneuver:* The patient hyperabducts the affected extremity (180°). This causes disappearance of pulse due to the arterial compression and reappearance in normal position (Fig. 4).

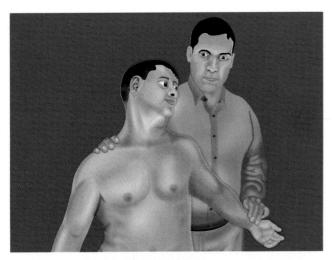

**Fig. 3** Adson's test

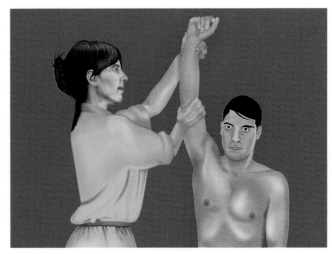

**Fig. 4** Abduction test

- *Costoclavicular maneuver:* Patient thrusts both shoulders backward and downwards maximally.
- *EAST maneuver (external rotation—abduction stress test):* It is the most reliable with arms extended, externally rotated and behind the head—"stick-up posture"—the patient makes fists repeatedly for 3 minutes and pulses are felt at the end of 3 minutes.
- *Branham's sign:* Done when an AV fistula is suspected. Pressure on the artery proximal to the fistula causes a reduction in size of the swelling and disappearance of bruit and fall in radial pulse.

About 15% of the asymptomatic patient suffering from TOS have positive tests. A negative test does not rule out TOS. All cases of suspected TOS must have cervical X-ray to rule out cervical rib.

Angiography is diagnostic but is considered when surgery is contemplated.

## Segmental Limb Pressures, Finger Pressures and Doppler Pressure Contours

Normal pressures between two levels of the same limb or same level of the contralateral limb is <7 mm Hg. A pressure difference of >10 mm Hg or an index of 0.8 indicates disease at that level. Monophasic signal indicates disease. Finger pressures must be obtained in Raynaud's disease or small vessel disease.

## Duplex Ultrasound

- This is very helpful in the large vessels, although subclavian artery under the clavicle may be difficult to study.
- Normal velocities in the subclavian artery and the innominate are 80–120 cm/s. A twofold increase in

the velocity in the stenotic zone compared with the perstenotic zone indicates a 50% stenosis. In occlusion, there is no flow in the segment of the artery.

- People with arm claudication but normal pressures should have a color Dopper 3–5 minutes after exercising.

## Magnetic Resonance Angiography

- This evaluates aortic arch vessels and upper limb arteries. Also reversal of flow may be seen in the vertebral artery in subclavian artery steal syndrome.
- Two artifacts are particularly relevant to this setting— (i) Coil dropout artifact occurs in people with high shoulders or low arch of aorta and mimic a stenosis. (ii) Venous susceptibility artifact occurs in the subclavian or innominate region if the dye in the veins is dense and obscures the arterial view. To avoid this, right arm injection is given because left arm injection is more prone to artifacts.

## Catheter-based Angiography

- It is the gold standard. Digital subtraction angiography produces high quality pictures with less contrast.
- An aortic arch angiography study (LAO 30° projection) shows origin of the vessels from the arch.
- Innominate bifurcation is best visualized right anterior oblique (RAO) 20–30° and caudally 10–20° view.
- The entire arm form the subclavian to the digital arteries must be studied.

## ■ MANAGEMENT

## Medical Management

- Asymptomatic subclavian artery stenosis should be managed medically.
- Intensive risk factor management is required to reduce risk of cardiovascular morbidity and mortality.

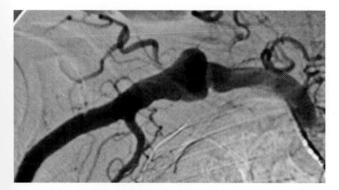

**Fig. 5** Subclavian artery aneurysm

- Antiplatelet drugs are very helpful in reducing the risk of amputation and improve the blood supply. Thus, there is need for aspirin and clopidogrel (adenosine diphosphate antagonist).
- Lipid lowering drugs must be given with a target low-density lipoprotein <100 mg/dL.

## Surgical Treatment

### Subclavian Disease

- Surgical or percutaneous revascularization is indicated for coronary or vertebral steal syndrome, severe arm claudication, or rest pain.
- In symptomatic subclavian stenosis, carotid to subclavian bypass is done if carotid is disease free on that side. The 10-year primary patency rate using polytetrafluoro-ethylene (PTFE) graft is 92%. The complication of this surgery is injury to the thoracic duct leading to a lymph fistula, injury to the sympathetic nerves, graft stenosis, and graft infection.
- Percutaneous interventions are generally preferred in these circumstances.

### Innominate Disease

Stenosis is corrected percutaneously but if this is not possible then the other options are:
- Extra-anatomic carotid to subclavian bypass is done.
- If contralateral carotid is involved percutaneous correction may suffice.

*Percutaneous treatment versus surgery of subclavian and innominate artery disease.*
Angioplasty and stenting is the preferred treatment in cases of stenosis. The advantages over surgery are:
- No surgical and anesthetic complications
- Lower morbidity
- Shorter hospital stay
- Very high success rate—nearly 100%
- Long-term follow-up showed no stenosis and patients were asymptomatic.
- The mean gradient across the lesion is reduced from 52.3 to 3.1 mm Hg.
- It is now considered the procedure of choice for stenoses of these vessels.

### Protocol for Subclavian/Innominate Artery Stenting (Flow chart 1)

- The patients are given short-acting intravenous sedation and the sheath inserted into the femoral artery.
- Aortic arch angiography study is performed (LAO 30° projection) to see the roots of the great vessels to choose catheter for selective angiography.

**Flow chart 1** A simplified approach to the patient with suspected subclavian/innominate artery stenosis

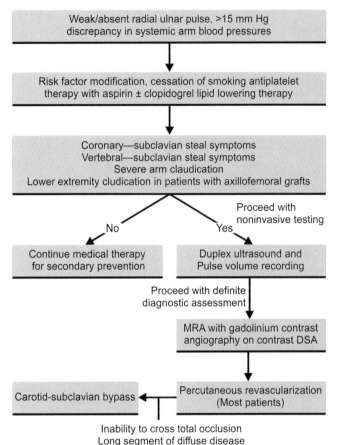

- The left subclavian artery is well visualized in this projection.
- The innominate artery is seen in the RAO (20–30°) and caudal 10–20° view.
- The carotids and the vertebrals are visualized to see extent of disease and collateral circulation. If the patient has intracranial extension of vertebral disease then correction of subclavian artery disease may not improve symptoms of vertebra-basilar ischemia.
- Unfractionated heparin 60 U/kg is given with target activated clotting time > 250 s.
- A 125 cm 5F JR4 diagnostic catheter placed inside a 90 cm 7F sheath is introduced.
- The origin of the left subclavian/innominate is negotiated with JR4 catheter and a guidewire inserted into the artery.

- The 7F sheath is advanced into the left subclavian artery over the JR4 catheter.
- The JR4 catheter is withdrawn and angiogram performed.
- An undersized balloon is used to dilate the lesion so that the stent can be passed.
- A balloon expandable stent is passed and put in place of the stenosis.
- All patients receive 325 mg aspirin and 300 mg clopidogrel prior to the procedure and discharged the following day on clopidogrel 75 mg orally 6 hourly for 4 weeks and aspirin 325 mg orally 6 hourly for life.

## Management of Subclavian and Axillary Aneurysmal Disease

- The treatment is dependent on the cause.
- In subclavian artery aneurysms, if cervical rib is the cause then thoracic outlet decompression with removal of the cervical rib is recommended (Fig. 5).
- Asymptomatic poststenotic dilatation returns to normal with this treatment alone.
- With significant dilatation of aneurysm resection or bypass is indicated with vein graft interposition.
- Always treat aneurysm whether symptomatic or asymptomatic, if double the diameter of the vessel.
- Aneurysms of the aberrant subclavian must be resected early due to the chances of rupture.
- The operative mortality is <5%.

## ■ CONCLUSION

- The most common site of upper limb arterial stenosis is origin of subclavian artery and left side is involved four times more commonly than right.
- Physical examination showing reduced pulse volume at the affected limb, reduced blood pressure on the affected site compared with the contralateral side and a bruit over the subclavian artery shows significant stenosis.
- Duplex scan and contrast magnetic resonance imaging show the subclavian artery stenosis.
- Percutaneous revascularization is the procedure of choice for symptomatic subclavian artery stenosis because of the technical success, low restenosis rate, minimal complications, elimination of general anesthesia, and low cost.
- If percutaneous revascularization is not possible because of the inability to cross the lesion, stent failure, or the extent of subclavian disease then extra-anatomic bypass is recommended and gives good results.

## PRACTICAL POINTS

- Atherosclerosis commonly affects the subclavian arteries.
- Takayasu's arteritis affects the subclavian arteries in the young.
- In suspected atherosclerosis and Takayasu's disease, always measure the BP in both upper limbs and the lower limbs.
- Evaluation of large vessel disease of upper limb is incomplete without diagnostic TOS maneuvers.
- Radiologic subclavian steal is more common than SSS.
- Clinical SSS is seen in relation to contralateral carotid, posterior circulation disease, and hypoplastic communicating arteries.
- Relationship of subclavian artery to IMA, vertebral, and other collateral arteries must be documented and understood before revascularization.
- *Percutaneous intervention points:*
    - Total occlusion of subclavian artery is easier to cross from ipsilateral brachial artery.
    - In treating right ostial subclavian artery stenosis, femoral artery access along with right brachial artery access is needed to protect origin of right common carotid artery stenosis. This is the kissing balloon technique.
    - Balloon expandable stents are indicated for ostial subclavian and innominate stenosis with stent protruding 1–2 mm into the aorta to ensure the ostium is covered with the stent.

# 16

# Vasospastic Disorders and Miscellaneous Disorders of the Extremities

*Jaisom Chopra*

## ◼ RAYNAUD'S PHENOMENON

### Introduction

- Raynaud's phenomenon (RP) is episodic vasospasm on exposure to cold.
- Classically there is blanching followed by cyanosis on exposure to cold followed by redness on rewarming. In practice, generally, there is no cyanosis but only painful pallor followed by redness.
- Initially one or two fingers get involved. Other rarer sites are the toes, nose, and ears.
- The diagnosis is made on history but investigations rule out secondary causes.
- In some cases, it may alter the quality of life in the cold months (prevalence is >5% even in warm climates).

*Risk factors include:*
- Cold weather
- Females
- Family history of the disorder
- Emotional stress
- Exposure to vibratory tools
- Chemotherapeutic agents.

### Clinical Features

The diagnosis is made by clinical history and physical examination. However, this is misleading as most of the patients do not present during the acute episode.

### Criteria for Diagnosing Primary RP
- Vasospastic attacks aggravated by cold and emotion
- Symmetric attacks involving both hands

- Normal nail-fold capillaries
- Normal erythrocyte sedimentation rate (ESR) and negative antinuclear antibody (ANA).

### How do We Differentiate Primary from Secondary RP?

History differentiates primary RP where there is intermittent vasospasm from constant symptomatic ischemia (rest pain and ulceration) due to arterial obstruction (severe secondary RP).

Features that differentiate primary from secondary RP are given in Table 1.

### Unilateral RP

Mostly secondary RP is due to embolic causes. The most common source of emboli is the upper extremity large arteries involved are:
- Atherosclerosis
- Vasculitis

**Table 1** Differences between primary and secondary Raynaud's phenomenon

| Features | Primary PR | Secondary RP |
|---|---|---|
| Age of onset (years) | 15–30 | >40 |
| Severity of symptoms | Mild | Severe |
| Tissue necrosis and gangrene | Absent | May be present |
| Risk of progression | Minimal | High |
| Autoantibodies | Absent | Present |
| Endothelial dysfunction | + | +++ |
| Circulating vasoconstrictors | + | +++ |

- Thoracic outlet syndrome (TOS)
- Buerger's disease
- Occupational- and trauma-related diseases.

## Classification

- Raynaud's phenomenon may be primary (idiopathic) or secondary.
- Secondary is due to the underlying collagen vascular diseases causing severe vasospasm.
- Only 30% primary RP suffer from severe attacks compared with 75% secondary RP.
- Tissue necrosis, advanced ischemia, and abnormal non-invasive laboratory tests exclude primary RP as the cause.

## Pathophysiology

- It is still not very clear and is multifactorial involving the endothelium, smooth muscle, neural, and circulating or paracrine mediators that regulate the cutaneous vascular tone.
- The normal neural regulation of cutaneous blood flow in response to cold is through sympathetic adrenergic vasoconstrictor fibers via the post-junctional $\alpha 2$ receptors in the vascular smooth muscle cells.
- Vasodilatation is partly through the withdrawal of the sympathetic stimulus.
- Elevation in levels of vasoconstrictors like endothelin 1, asymmetric dimethylarginine (ADMA) and thromboxane A2 has been noted in RP.
- There are also reduced fibrinolytic and increased pro-thrombotic factors.
- Genetic and hormonal factors may also be responsible as shown by females more commonly affected.

## Differential Diagnosis

The diagnosis of RP is found in only 10% and needs to be distinguished from other conditions that mimic it when exposed to cold. It must be distinguished from compressive neuropathies like carpal tunnel syndrome (CTS). Here, there is compression of the median nerve because of the localized tenosynovitis, trauma, hypothyroidism, amyloidosis, or activities related to repetitive motions of the wrist. The diagnosis of CTS is by tapping the wrist (Tinel's sign) or maintaining flexion at the wrist (Phalen's maneuver), which elicits symptoms (Figs 1A and B).

Once diagnosis of RP is made, it is important to differentiate primary from secondary RP.

- Connective tissue diseases accounts for 20% of all RP but is the cause of majority of secondary RP. They include:
  - Systemic sclerosis spectrum
  - Systemic erythematosus
  - Dermatomyositis or polymyositis
  - Rheumatoid arthritis
  - Takayasu's arthritis
  - Giant cell arthritis
  - Primary biliary cirrhosis.
- Buerger's disease (thromboangiitis obliterans) involves upper limb also with 20–50% having secondary RP with obstructive lesions to the digits.
- Mechanical injury—trauma-induced RP is seen in frostbite or crush injury or traumatic aneurysms of the ulnar and radial artery. Vascular steal syndrome following AV fistula leads to severe distal ischemia and severe RP. Hypothenar hammer syndrome occurs because of the repeated pounding of the ulnar artery leading to aneurysm and RP of the digits. Here, Allen's test is positive.
- Thoracic outlet syndrome (TOS) causes RP because of the compression of the neurovascular bundle in the neck or shoulder causing injury and distal embolization.
- Arterial disorders may give rise to embolization from involvement of the proximal large arteries due to athero-sclerosis, aneurysmal disease, and vasculitis (Takayasu's disease and giant cell arteritis).
- Toxins—heavy metal poisoning (arsenic, mercury and lead) exposes to vinyl chloride causing RP. Angiography shows multiple arterial stenosis and occlusions along with hypervascularity along areas of bony resorption.

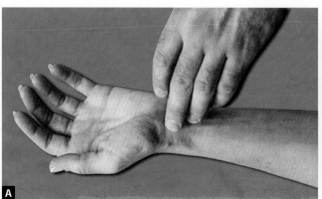 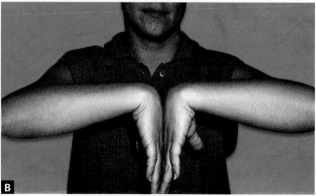

**Figs 1A and B** (A) Tinel's sign; (B) Phalen's sign

- Rheological and hematological causes—these alter the macromolecular or cellular element of the blood increasing blood viscosity may cause RP. Polycythemia, thrombocythemia, and chronic myeloid leukemia may cause RP.
- Drugs—ergot derivatives for treating Parkinson's disease and drugs or migraine headaches and amphetamines all can aggravate arterial vasospasm. β-blockers may cause RP because of the unopposed α-adrenergic vasoconstriction. Chemotherapeutic agents and interferon α/β may precipitate RP.

## Risk of Progression of RP and Prognosis

- Patients with RP and no associated symptoms and normal serology (normal ESR and normal ANA), the chances of developing rheumatologic disorder is 2% over 5 years and chances of developing increased symptoms is 6% over 10 years.
- The risk of developing rheumatologic disorder in presence of RP with positive ANA is about 50%.
- The 2-year risk of developing rheumatologic disorder in patients with RP and abnormal nail-fold examination along with positive autoantibodies is 20%.
- There are a number of specific autoantibodies that can predict the risk of ultimately developing rheumatologic disorder
  - Antismith—for SLE
  - Scl-70 (antitopoisomerase) and anticentromere antibodies—or PSS
  - Antibodies to antiribonucleoprotein (anti-RNP)—severe RP.

## Diagnosis (Flow chart 1)

Initial diagnosis is clinical. Three leading questions are:
1. Are your fingers unusually sensitive to cold?
2. Do your fingers change color when exposed to cold?
3. Do they turn white blue or both?

The diagnosis of RP is excluded, if the question no. 2 and 3 are negative. The history should include detailed review of symptoms:
- Associated illnesses
- Occupational/exposure history—vinyl chloride
- Trauma—vibratory tool and hypothenar hammer syndrome
- Drug history—drugs promoting vasospasm (β-blockers)
- Tobacco abuse.

Primary RP is differentiated from secondary RP by exclusion, physical examination, and blood testing.

By physical examination, large vessel disease is excluded due to absence of pulses.

Patients with PSS and rheumatologic diseases have abnormal capillary loops surrounded by avascular areas in capillary microscopy of nail folds (Fig. 2).

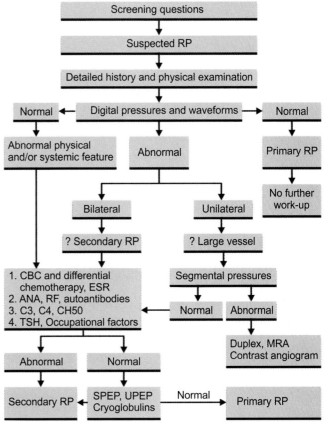

**Flow chart 1** Approach to Raynaud's phenomenon

*Abbreviations:* ANA, antinuclear antibody; RF, rheumatoid factor; C3,C4, and CH50, complement 3, 4, and hemolytic complement 50; SPEP and UPEP, serum protein and urinary protein electrophoresis; MRA, magnetic resonance angiography; TSH, thyroid stimulating hormone; CBC, complete blood count; ESR, erythrocyte sedimentation rate.

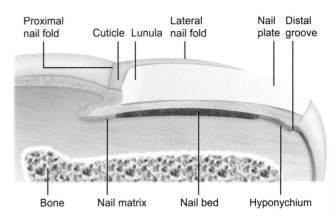

**Fig. 2** Anatomy of the nail fold where capillary microscopy is performed

Digital ulcerations are due to vasculitis (50–75%).

Segmental pressures diagnose large vessel disease and may be associated with RP.

Unilateral RP symptoms with ischemia—proximal large vessel disease like atherosclerosis TOS and Buerger's.

Digital pressures and waveform differentiate primary from secondary RP. Normal finger to ipsilateral brachial index is 1 but <0.7 suggests obstructive lesions or absolute finger pressure is <70 mm Hg.

Normal pressures at the proximal phalanx do not rule out distal disease and so waveforms by photoplethysmography is needed. Normal waveform excludes obstructive lesions.

Secondary RP have obstructive disease with abnormal pressures and waveforms. This could be bilateral as in occupational causes, trauma, and drug related.

Angiography is reserved for cases suspected for TOS and proximal embolism.

## Treatment (Flow chart 2)

It depends on the underlying cause and the severity of symptoms. The lines of treatment are:
- Conservative therapy
- Pharmacological treatment
- Surgical sympathectomy.

In secondary RP, the underlying cause must be treated along with removal of inciting stimuli.

### Conservative Therapy
- Mostly recommended in mild cases of primary RP and involves reassurance that it would never lead to amputation.

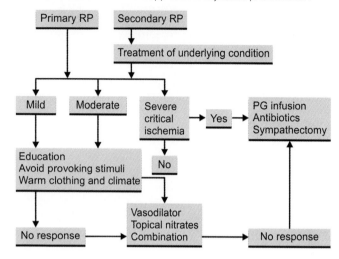

**Flow chart 2** Treatment approach in Raynaud's phenomenon

- Wear warm clothing and gloves to prevent cold exposure.
- Wash hands with warm water.
- Stop active and passive smoking
- Treating the underlying cause.

### Pharmacological Treatment

The results are modest and better in primary than secondary Raynaud's phenomenon (Table 2).

**Table 2** Pharmacologic therapies in Raynaud's phenomenon

| Agents | Mechanism of action | Dosage | Side effects |
|---|---|---|---|
| *Calcium channel blockers* | | | |
| Nifedipine SR | Vasodilator through | 30–120 mg/d | Reflex tachycardia, flushing, dizziness, hypotension, constipation, peripheral edema |
| Amlodipine | blockade of | 5–20 mg/d | |
| Felodipine | L type calcium | 2.5–10 mg/d | |
| Isradipine | channels | 2.5–5.0 mg/d | |
| Diltiazem SR | | 120–300 mg/d | |
| *Nitrates* | | | |
| Topical nitroglycerin | Nitric oxide generation and smooth muscle relaxation | 2% ointment applied locally to finger | Headache, dizziness, and hypotension |
| *Miscellaneous* | | | |
| Prazosin | An α2 agonist and vasodilator | 1–5 mg/d | Dizziness, hypotension |
| Fluoxetine | A selective serotonin reuptake inhibitor | 20–40 mg/d | Sleep disturbances, importance |
| Losartan | An angiotensin type 1 receptor antagonist | 25–100 mg/d | Hypotension |
| Cilostazol | Type III phosphodiesterase inhibitor | 50–100 mg/d | Headache, diarrhea, dizziness |
| *Prostaglandins* | | | |
| Epoprostenol | Vasodilator prostanoids that are used only in critical upper extremity ischemia associated with secondary RP | 0.5–6 ng/kg/min IV for 2–7 days | Diarrhea, flushing, headache, hypotension and rash |
| Alprostadil | | 0.1–0.4 µg/kg/min IV 6–24 h for 2–7 days | |
| Iloprost | | 0.5–2.0 ng/kg/min for 2–7 days | |

### Vasodilator Therapy

- These include calcium channel blockers, nitroglycerin, α2 agonists, angiotensin receptor antagonists, and sympathetic nervous inhibitors.
- These act by reducing the digital vascular resistance with environment cold exposure and increasing the digital systolic pressure and the skin temperature during cold.
- *Nifedipine* reduces the attacks in its frequency and severity or both primary and secondary RP by over 65%. The starting dose is 30 mg/day and increasing to 90 mg/day if there is no improvement. Side effects are hypotension, light-headedness, peripheral edema, and indigestion. Longer acting nifedipine like amlodipine are very helpful. Nitroglycerin ointment applied locally is also very helpful.
- Antiplatelets and anticoagulants are not very helpful and low molecular weight heparin (LMWH) or thrombolytic agents like tPA have not shown promising results.
- Prostaglandin E1 and prostacycline have not shown much benefit in their oral preparations. Intravenously they have shown benefit in healing necrotic tissue and in acute ischemic crisis seen in RP associated with rheumatologic disease.

## Surgical Intervention

- Cervical sympathectomy is performed in severe cases refractory to drugs treatment. The distal half of the stellate ganglion is excised via the transaxillary route or the anterior root of neck. To prevent Horner's syndrome, the upper half the ganglion is spared. The success is about 50%.
- Lumbar sympathectomy involves the removal of the 2nd and 3rd lumbar ganglia. Before sympathectomy, the ability of the peripheral vessels to dilate must be carried out through reactive hyperemic assessment of the digital pulse volume or flow. Sympathetic chemical block may also be of benefit.

## ■ COMPLEX REGIONAL PAIN SYNDROME

## Introduction

Complex regional pain syndrome (CRPS), was formerly called Sudeck's atrophy, is a regional post-traumatic neuropathic pain problem affecting one or more limbs. It was referred as causalgia, which is burning sensation following limb injury involving damage to the major peripheral nerve.

## Classification

There are two types:

*Type I*
- Pain after a painful traumatic or nontraumatic event.
- Pain may be spontaneous, hyperalgesia, or allodynia and is not consistent with distribution of a single peripheral nerve.

- There is swelling, redness in the affected area.
- No other concomitant conditions account for the pain.

*Type II*—exactly as above except pain after an identifiable trauma or nerve injury.

## Etiology

There are three main causes:
- Traumatic—burns, crush injuries, fractures, and dislocations
- Nontraumatic—myocardial infarction, deep vein thrombosis (DVT), prolonged bed rest, and neoplasms
- Idiopathic.

## Clinical Symptoms and Signs (Fig. 3)

- Burning and throbbing pain extending beyond the nerve distribution
- Allodynia and hyperalgesia in response to normal sensory stimuli
- Sudomotor and vasomotor instability causing changes in sweating patterns along with a warm and red or cold and blue limb
- Swelling may be intermittent or constant
- Atrophy of the skin and nails
- Tremor, weakness, and joint stiffness.

## Diagnosis

There are no specific tests. They are dependent on history.
- Vasomotor signs calls for vascular testing
- Electroencephalography (EEG) in case of neurological signs
- Radiological studies if bone and soft tissue are suspected
- Blood tests for infection or rheumatologic condition.

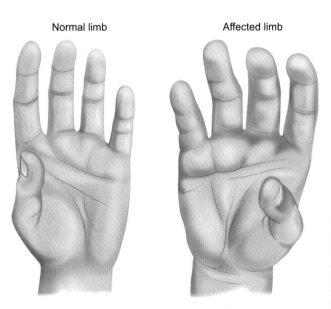

Normal limb           Affected limb

**Fig. 3** Complex regional pain syndrome

*Diagnostic testing includes:*
- Sensory evaluation.
- Sudomotor and vasomotor studies—infrared thermography to measure temperature and sweat studies on affected area.
- Radiological testing with Technetium 99m scan shows increased uptake and bone X-ray may show osteoporosis.
- Diagnostic sympathetic block—lumbar paravertebral sympathetic block for lower extremity and a stellate ganglion block for upper extremity.

## Treatment

Physiotherapy is the main treatment and medications only help physiotherapy. Medications include antidepressants like doxepin or nortriptyline (both 10–75 mg/day), opioids, and corticosteroids. Those not responding to medications and improve by sympathetic blockade need regional anesthetic blocks. Two major types of blocks are sympathetic nerve block and combined sympathetic/somatic nerve block. A daily block using local anesthetic is performed for 1–3 weeks. Cervical or lumbar blocks can be performed with the catheter placed next to the site or by daily injections. If this is not very helpful then neurolysis with neurolytic agents or radiofrequency ablation is considered.

## ■ ERYTHERMALGIA

## Introduction

Involves the extremities but can involve other parts of the body as well. There is increased temperature, burning pain, and erythema.

## Signs and Symptoms (Fig. 4)

The diagnosis of erythermalgia (EM) is historical and depends upon:
- Burning extremity pain
- Pain worsened by warming
- Pain relieved by cooling
- Redness of the affected skin
- Increased temperature of the affected skin during the attack and associated with pain and erythema.

Symptoms are intermittent and involve both lower limbs symmetrically.

Pruritus and pins and needles may precede burning pain. The duration varies from minutes to hours. Symptoms are aggravated by hot weather, dependency of lower extremities, exercise, alcohol ingestion, and excessive warmth as sleeping under quilts, wearing shoes and gloves. Relief is obtained by lowering the skin temperature or elevating the affected part. Relief with cooling is mandatory for diagnosis.

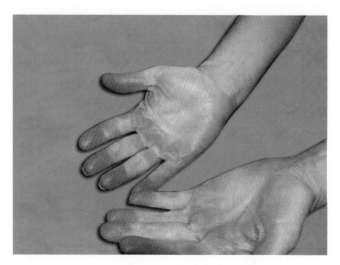

**Fig. 4** Erythermalgia

## Classification

Erythermalgia is primary or secondary.

Primary is in middle-aged men.

Secondary EM is seen in myeloproliferative disorders like polycythemia vera and essential thrombocythemia. EM may precede the diagnosis of secondary causes by several years.

## Pathophysiology

Not known but local defect in vascular and neurological function of the involved skin is proposed. Possibly arteriovenous shunts in affected skin with subsequent hypoxia and metabolic disorders are responsible.

## Differential Diagnosis

Complex regional pain syndrome and neuropathic pain.

Complex regional pain syndrome may mimic EM but EM is usually bilateral and is typically intermittent compared with CRPS, which is continuous. It may be extremely difficult to differentiate EM from neuropathic pain and differentiation may depend on skin biopsy. In EM, there are small and large fiber neuropathies.

## Treatment

This could be conservative, pharmacological, or surgical.
- Avoid precipitating factors and treat underlying cause.
- Cold water immersion is helpful but not beneficial in the long-term.
- Aspirin helps in secondary causes but not in primary EM.

- The most useful are gabapentin, diltiazem, prazosin, sertraline, amitriptyline, imipramine, fluoxetine, and paroxitine. The response is variable but substantial benefit may be obtained.
- Surgical treatment is for severe cases—neurolysis with neurolytic injections or radiofrequency ablatio.

## ACROCYANOSIS (FIG. 5)

- Bluish discoloration of the digits of hands and feet.
- It is distinguished from RP as it is persistent and not painful.
- It may extend to involve the hands and the feet. It may involve the face, elbows, and the knees.
- Cold causes vasospasm and heat, redness.
- Men and women affected equally—20-45 years.
- Vasospasm of small cutaneous arteries causing compensatory dilatation of the capillaries and post-capillary venules. Resultant decrease in blood flow and oxygen extraction causes cyanosis.

- Prognosis is good and rarely is there tissue loss.
- Treatment is to avoid cold by wearing gloves. Drugs are rarely needed.

## PERNIO (CHILBLAINS) (FIG. 6)

- This is a vasculitis disorder on exposure to extreme cold.
- There are red and blue lesions on the shin and feet on exposure to extreme cold.
- These lesions blister and ulcerate with burning sensation.
- These lesions resolve in about 10 days leaving a pigmented scar.
- Women 15-30 years are more commonly involved.
- Biopsy reveals vasculitis with intimal proliferation and perivascular infiltration of mononuclear and polymorphonuclear leukocytes along with giant cells.
- Treatment is avoiding cold and dress warmly.
- Sympathectomy and sympathetic blocking drugs are not effective.
- Nifedipine may reduce time of resolution of existing lesions and prevent new ones from developing.

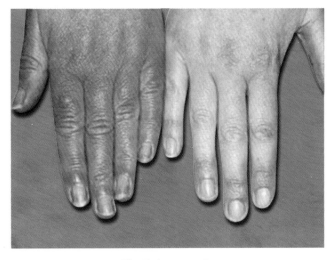

**Fig. 5** Acrocyanosis

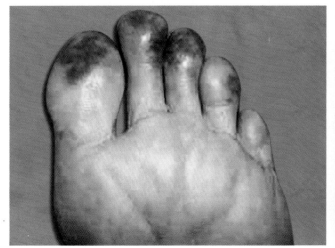

**Fig. 6** Chilblains

## PRACTICAL POINTS

- Advanced ischemia—tissue necrosis and gangrene—rules out RP.
- 2-year risk of rheumatologic disorder in patients with RP + abnormal nail fold examination + positive autoantibodies is 20%.
- Unilateral RP raises the possibility of embolic or traumatic causes (hypothenar hammer or vibrational white finger).
- Unilateral symptoms in patient with bilateral abnormal digital waveform and pressures suggest Buerger's disease.
- Upper extremity embolization takes place from proximal artery in TOS.
- Lesions of chilblains are pruritic with burning.
- Complex regional pain syndrome normally gives history of trauma or injury.
- Helpful diagnostic sympathetic block is seen in CRPS.
- Relief of pain and symptoms with cold is seen in EM and not in CRPS.

# 17

# History, Physical Examination and Diagnostic Approach to Venous Disorders

*Jaisom Chopra*

## ■ INTRODUCTION

Around 27% of the world's population, suffers from venous disorders, mainly varicose veins, whereas 1–3% suffers from chronic venous insufficiency (CVI).

Venous thromboembolism (VTE) is the third most common vascular disorder after CVA.

*Venous disorders include:*

- Varicose veins are dilated, elongated, and tortuous veins irrespective of the size. They may be:
  - Trunk veins involving the long and short saphenous veins (Fig. 1);
  - Reticular veins are subcutaneous veins arising from the trunk veins;
  - Telangiectasias are the spider veins or intradermal varicosities that are seldom symptomatic (Fig. 2).
- *Deep vein thrombosis (DVT):* Thrombus in the deep veins (Fig. 3)

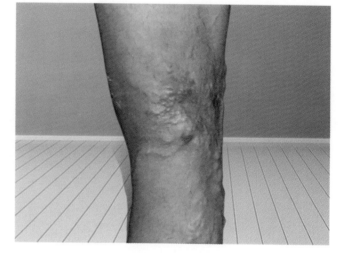

**Fig. 2** Telangiectasia

- *Superficial thrombophlebitis:* Thrombus in the superficial veins (Fig. 4). It may occur in any superficial vein in the body because of infection, trauma, hypercoagulable state including carcinoma (Trousseu's migratory thrombophlebitis, Mondor's disease, and thrombophlebitis of the superficial veins of the breast), drugs like oral contraceptives. In 10–15%, superficial thrombophlebitis may progress to DVT.
- Chronic venous insufficiency is due to venous hypertension, which occurs in chronic venous reflux as a consequence of structural abnormalities of the veins (Fig. 5). Reflux is retrograde venous flow due to incompetent valves. In 20% of the asymptomatic, over 20 years some reflux is present. Reflux is due to:
  - Perforator vein incompetence in calf, thigh, saphenofemoral, and saphenopopliteal junction

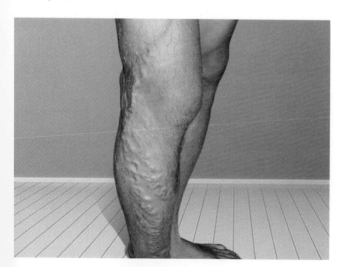

**Fig. 1** Varicose veins

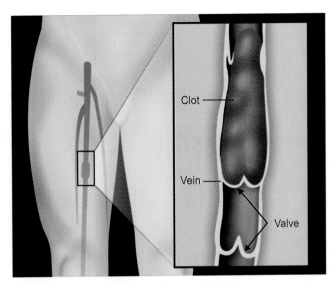

**Fig. 3** Clot in the vein

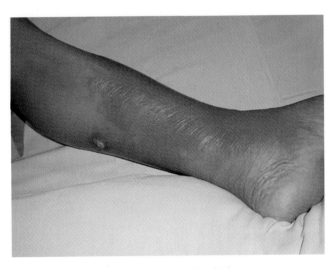

**Fig. 4** Superficial thrombophlebitis

– Incompetence of the deep vein valves due to destruction by DVT
– Ineffective calf muscle pump mechanism that makes the ejection of blood from lower limbs inadequate thus increasing the residual venous volume (VV). Venous hypertension is the result of reflux of the deep venous pressure into the low pressure superficial venous system. It presents as leg heaviness, fatigue, and ache. Chronic long-standing venous hypertension leads to cutaneous changes of CVI like edema, dilated veins, skin pigmentation, lipodermatosclerosis, and ulceration.

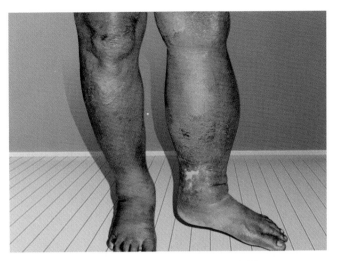

**Fig. 5** Chronic venous insufficiency in left leg

## ■ CLINICAL FEATURES

### Medical History

#### Demographics

*Age:* Incidence of VVs and CVI increase with age and so do the complications. The risk of DVT doubles with each decade of life. Venous thromboembolism in young is a consequence of thrombotic diathesis.

*Sex:* It is three to four times as common in females. There is a strong link between varicose veins and ultimately development of CVI. However, CVI seems more common in men.

*Race:* The greatest risk of VTE is in whites followed by Hispanics and then Asians. It may be due to the genetic factors that predispose to DVT like factor V Leiden.

*Obesity:* It increases the risk of VVs in females but not in males. It has a definite strong link with CVI. It is debatable, if it increases the risk of DVT, but if there is prolonged immobility due to obesity then the risk is definitely increased.

#### History of Present Illness

The most common symptoms of venous disease are pain, swelling, heaviness, and cutaneous changes. These are present in various combinations.

*Pain:* This could be due to thrombophlebitis, venous thrombosis, or CVI. Pain due to blocked veins is sudden in onset with a cord-like painful structure. Pain due to CVI is present at the end of the day and is an ache in whole of the leg.

Varicose veins are generally not painful and if they become so then it raises the doubt of phlebitis. However, patients with VVs experience tingling, pin-pricks, and burning over the vein. Extensive DVT produces a bursting pain in legs on exertion relieved by rest and leg elevation.

*Swelling:* The second most common manifestation of venous disease and is due to venous hypertension, which is the hallmark of CVI. It is the transmission of venous pressure in an unopposed manner aided by gravity due to incompetent valves in the deep system and the communicating system. Other causes of venous hypertension besides CVI are:
- Intrinsic venous thrombosis
- Extrinsic venous compression as caused by crossing of right iliac artery over left iliac vein
- Right heart failure due to venous causes.

History should include location, onset, and duration of swelling along with aggravating and relieving factors. Table 1 differentiates venous edema from other forms of edema.

History should include recent journey, prolonged immobility after recent surgery, malignant disease, and trauma.

One must enquire into the risk factors for DVT.

*Strong risk:* Knee or hip replacement, major trauma, fracture hip or knee, and spinal cord injury.

*Moderate risk:* Abdominal or thoracic surgery, arthroscopic surgery, congestive heart failure (CHF), cerebrovascular accident (CVA) with paralysis, chemotherapy, hormone replacement therapy, previous DVT, and thrombophilia.

*Low risk:* Age, bed rest over 3 days, obesity, varicose veins, laparoscopic surgery, prolonged plane or car travel, and pregnancy.

Contrary to previous beliefs prolonged travel by air or car (>8 h) is a low risk for DVT and does not cause excessive PE in the general population.

Trauma is strongly related to DVT with 50% cases of leg trauma and 40% with trauma elsewhere like chest and abdomen have evidence of DVT on duplex evaluation.

Fracture of the long bones of the lower extremity or the pelvic bones increases the risk of asymptomatic DVT.

Central venous catheters, pace makers, and infusion ports increase the incidence of DVT at the site of insertion.

## Past Medical and Surgical History

- Previous history of DVT makes the possibility of recurrent DVT likely along with CVI responsible for swelling of the leg.
- Malignancy increases the incidence of DVT and in 3–20% DVT may be the first manifestation of malignancy. Lung cancer shows highest incidence of DVT because it is the most common cancer. Gastrointestinal, genitourinary, and adenocarcinomas show increased incidence of DVT.
- Paralysis due to spinal cord injury shows highest incidence of DVT in the first 2 weeks. Incidence of PE also rises but is rare after 3 months.
- Pregnancy increases the risk of VTE in the immediate postpartum period (20 times higher). The risk is further increased by smoking, previous DVT, and inherited thrombophilias.

## Medication History

- Exposure to estrogens and oral contraceptives increases the risk. Risk of death from VTE in women on oral contraceptives is lower than the risk of death from pregnancy. The risk of DVT in postmenopausal women on HRT is two times the controls.
- People with inherited thrombophilias due to prothrombin 20210 mutation and factor V Leiden mutation carry a 120 times and 30–40 times increased risk of VTE if given oral contraceptives (Table 2).

## Family History

A first degree relative with strong family history of DVT suggests inherited disorder. Patients with antithrombin III

**Table 1** Distinction between different causes of edema

| Feature | Orthostatic | Venous | Lymphatic |
|---|---|---|---|
| Bilateral | Bilateral | Usually unequal | Usually unequal |
| Effect of elevation | Relieved totally | Relieved totally | Mild or minimal |
| Distribution | Diffuse with maximal edema in ankle and feet | Ankle and legs with feet spared | Diffuse greatest distally |
| Pain | None | Fatigue, heaviness, and bursting discomfort | Minimal pain |
| Skin changes | Shiny skin with no pigmentation or trophic changes | More on medial aspect leg with pigmentation and ulceration | Thickening of skin |

**Table 2** Inherent thrombophilias

| Syndrome | General population | Percent with DVT |
|---|---|---|
| Factor V Leiden | 3–6% | 21 |
| Prothrombin G 20210A | 1.5–3% | 6 |
| Protein C deficiency | 0.1–0.5% | 3 |
| Protein S deficiency | – | 2 |
| Antithrombin deficiency | 0.02–0.17% | 1 |

deficiency are at higher risk of VTE than other causes. History of spontaneous abortions raises the possibility of antiphospholipid antibodies.

## Physical Examination (Fig. 6)

This must include the entire vascular system. Always examine the abdomen for possible malignancy and masses.

### Inspection and Palpation

The long saphenous vein starts in front of the medial malleolus and ends at the saphenofemoral junction of the groin. Short saphenous varicosities are seen behind the lateral malleolus (Fig. 7). As the short saphenous vein is embedded in fascia, it is difficult to see its tributaries causing varicosities in the calf under venous hypertension. The Hunter's perforator incompetence is a common cause of mid-thigh varicosities, whereas Dodd's perforator is a common cause of lower thigh varicosities on the medial aspect. The Boyd perforator is on the anteriomedial aspect of calf just below the knee connecting to the short saphenous vein. It is the most common site for varicosities (Fig. 8).

### Swelling and Skin Changes

Swelling is seen in DVT, superficial thrombophlebitis, and varicosities. In veins, swelling involves the varix locally and redness is due to phlebitis locally. Lymphedema typically involves the toes (square toe sign), whereas venous edema does not. This is an important clinical clue to differentiate between the two.

- Phlegmasia cerulea dolens seen in extensive DVT with limb diffusely swollen and blue because of the concomitant arterial insufficiency.
- Stasis dermatitis is pigmentation and eczema on the medial aspect of the lower leg and is diagnostic of CVI.
- Venous ulceration is seen in long-standing stasis dermatitis and is typically seen above the medial malleolus with surrounding skin discolored due to CVI. The ulcer is shallow and never penetrates the deep fascia. The floor is covered with a moist granulating base while edge is sloping and pale blue in color.
- Always exclude DVT is all venous cases. This is done by clinical signs, which are neither specific nor sensitive for diagnosing DVT. They are:
  - *Homan's sign*—pain in the calf muscle on passive dorsiflexion.

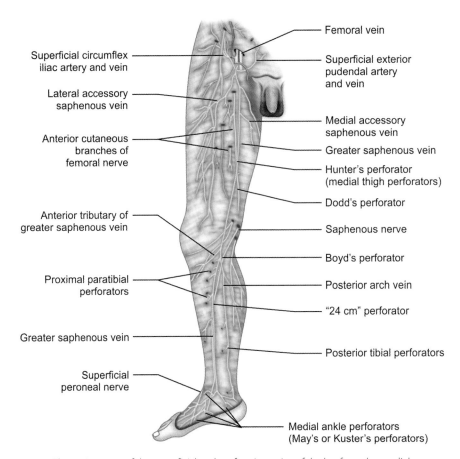

**Fig. 6** Anatomy of the superficial and perforating veins of the leg from the medial

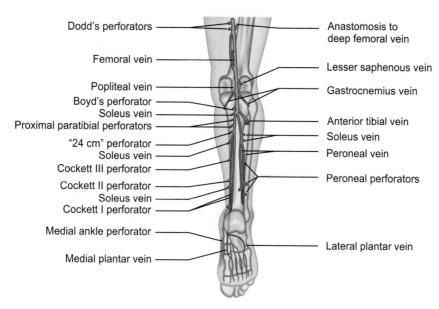

**Fig. 7** Anatomy of the deep veins and perforators of the lower extremity posterior aspect

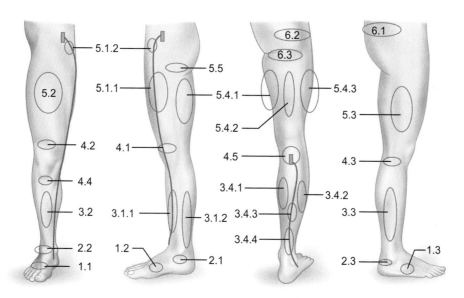

**Fig. 8** New nomenclature for perforating veins (PV). 1.1, 1.2, 1.3 are the dorsal, medial, lateral foot PVs. 2.1, 2.2 and 2.3 are medial, anterior, and lateral PVs of the ankle. Leg PVs: 3.1.1, paratibial PV; 3.1.2, posterior tibial PV; 3.2, anterior leg PV; 3.3, lateral leg PV; 3.4.1, medial gastrocnemius PV; 3.4.2, lateral gastrocnemius PV; 3.4.3, intergemellar PV; 3.4.4, para-achillean PV. Knee PVs: 4.1, medial knee PV; 4.2, suprapatellar PV; 4.3, lateral knee PV; 4.4, infrapatellar PV; 4.5, popliteal fossa PV. Thigh PVs: 5.1.1, PV of the femoral canal; 5.1.2, inguinal PV; 5.2, anterior thigh PV; 5.3, lateral thigh PV; 5.4.1, posteromedial thigh PV; 5.4.2, sciatic PV; 5.4.3, posterolateral thigh PV; 5.5, pudendal PV. Gluteal PVs: 6.1, superior gluteal PV; 6.2, midgluteal PV; 6.3, lower gluteal PV
*Source:* Caggiati A, et al. J Vasc Surg. 2002;36:416-22.

–  Bancroft's sign—tenderness on compression of anterioposterior but not lateral aspect of calf.
–  Lowenburg's sign—prompt calf pain on inflating a sphygmomanometer cuff to 80 mm Hg.

## Examination of Venous Reflux

This can be performed with a hand-held Doppler at the office or patient sent to the vascular laboratory for testing.

## ■ DIFFERENTIAL DIAGNOSIS

Unilateral swelling and pain are differentiated as below:
• Leg trauma (hematoma, muscle injury)
• Cellulitis
• Ruptured baker's cyst
• Arthritis of knee and ankle joint
• Swelling from recent knee or hip surgery
• Pelvic venous obstruction or external compression of iliac vein
• Superficial phlebitis
• Venous insufficiency (varicose veins)
• Critical limb ischemia due to PVD
• Neurological pain.
    Edema of CVI has to be distinguished from edema of heart failure, kidney failure, and cirrhosis by careful history and examination.
    Chronic lymphedema is another condition we have to distinguish. It causes thickening of the skin and firmness of the subcutaneous tissue. It extends onto the distal foot and toes, which does not happen in venous edema (square toe sign) (Fig. 9).
    Marjolin ulcer may develop in chronic inflammation or venous stasis and must be considered if healing is delayed (Fig. 10).

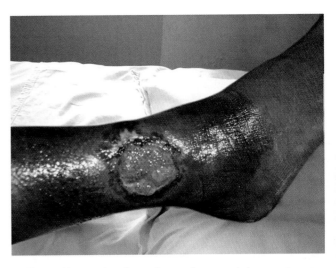

**Fig. 10** Venous ulcer due to short saphenous vein incompetence

## ■ DIAGNOSTIC EVALUATION AND APPROACH

## CVI and Varicose Veins Evaluation

The following questions must be answered by the doctor:
• Is there reflux?
• Is there obstruction?
• Are both present?
• What is the severity of both reflux and obstruction?
• Is there a calf or musculoskeletal problem?
• Are the abnormalities present enough to explain the patient's presentation or are there additional factors?
• What is the prognosis of the patient?

## Approach to CVI and Varicosities: Using the CEAP Clinical Classification

The clinical classes are C1, C2, C3 followed by subscript for symptomatic (s) and asymptomatic (a). 'E' stands for etiology which could be primary (Ep) or secondary (Es). 'A' stands for anatomy to localize the anatomic areas involved, which could be superficial (As) or deep (Ad) or perforators (Ap). 'P' stands for pathophysiology which could be reflux (Pr) or obstruction (Po) or both (Pr,o). This classification helps in deciding direct diagnostic test selection in patients presenting with CVI.

## Decision Making Based on the Clinical Class of CEAP Classification (Table 3)

Based on this classification, diagnostic testing is done at three levels.
• Level 1 testing—history, physical examination, and evaluation of venous system using a hand-held Doppler.

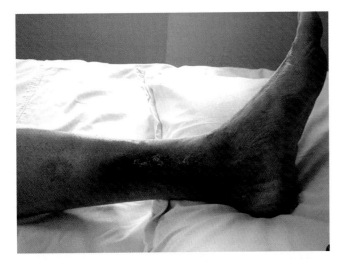

**Fig. 9** Stasis dermatitis

**Table 3** Differentiation between various types of leg ulcers

| Features | Arterial ulcers | Venous ulcers | Neuropathic ulcers | Vasculitis | Pyoderma gangrenosum |
|---|---|---|---|---|---|
| Location | Plantar surface head of 1st and 5th metatarsal | Medial aspect above medial malleolus | Over metatarsophalangeal joints | Medial aspect lower leg | Legs and trunk |
| Appearance | Round with sharply demarcated borders and pale base | Irregular margins flat or with steep elevation. Shallow base with exudate | Destructive ulcers with deep base. May have vascular insufficiency (diabetics) | Necrotic base with irregular margins | Begin with pustules and then necrosis and multiple ulcers with well-defined raised and undermined borders. Ulcers may join in reticulated patterns with intact skin in between |
| Pain | Painful | Mild pain | Painless | Painful | Painful |
| Associated features | Prolonged capillary filling and pallor on elevation | Dermatitis and indurated skin. Scar in middle and lower leg | Numb foot and paresthesia. Asymptomatic with thick callus in pressure areas | Sclerodactyly and joint deformities (rheumatoid arthritis) | 50% have ulcerative colitis, Crohn's disease, chronic active hepatitis, rheumatoid arthritis, or malignancy |
| Additional testing | Low ankle-brachial index (ABI) or toe index | History of CVI or DVT | Failure to perceive of a 10 g monofilament is a proven indicator of peripheral sensory neuropathy | Serologic testing for collagen vascular disease | Serological testing and blood cultures |

- Level 2 testing—level 1 tests and color Doppler study and air plethysmography (APG).
- Level 3 testing—level 1 tests and magnetic resonance venography or invasive tests like phlebography (ascending and descending).

Telangiectasia is always superficial with primary etiology. It is classified as C1. If symptomatic, it is C1s and if asymptomatic, C1a.

- *Testing in class 0/1*—no visible signs of venous disease—telangiectasia or reticular veins. In asymptomatic patients, no further testing is needed. In symptomatic CVI cases with aching, tiredness and heaviness color Doppler to see reflux at the saphenofemoral (SF), sapheno-popliteal (SP), superficial veins, and deep veins (femoral and popliteal) are done. Look for obstruction in the deep system. If these tests are negative then no further tests are required.
- *Testing in class 2*—varicose veins present without edema or skin changes—here color Doppler study is done to evaluate reflux at the SF or SP junctions. Also deep system is evaluated for obstruction (DVT) or reflux (CVI). Look for perforator reflux.
- *Testing in class 3*—edema with varicose veins but no skin changes—unilateral edema is mostly due to veins of the lower limb. Color Doppler study shows obstruction or reflux.
- *Testing in class 4/5/6*—skin changes and open or healed ulcers and edema and varicose veins—here thorough history and examination with color Doppler study are indicated. Most patients have venous reflux with or without obstruction. Isolated superficial venous reflux in these patients is not common. The use of venography helps identify patients for deep valve repair or transplant.

It is indicated in patients with grade 3 or 4 reflux who have recurrent symptoms of venous insufficiency after treating superficial and perforator vein incompetence. Color Doppler is recommended for all patients with skin changes. In patients for deep valve surgery, APG and venography are recommended.

- *Designating etiology (E), anatomy (A), and pathophysiology (P)*—skin changes and swelling may be due to primary, secondary, or congenital causes. Color Doppler study helps to differentiate between incompetence, obstruction, and perforators. To determine the etiology may need additional testing like ascending and descending venography. Anatomy (A) to know site of involvement as superficial or deep. Pathophysiology (P) is important to differentiate reflux from obstruction. In primary disease, there is only reflux but in secondary, there is generally a combination of obstruction and reflux. Here, additional test is needed like air plethysmograph (APG).

## Vascular Laboratory Testing in CVI and Varicose Veins

- *Ultrasound evaluation of reflux*—the purpose is to find out the presence of reflux between communication points between the deep and superficial venous systems—saphenofemoral junction, saphenopopliteal junction, and perforators in between. It is performed with the patient standing when the direction of flow is evaluated from the change in color. Compression of the calf with sudden release confirms the change in color and confirms that there is reflux due to valvular incompetence.

- *Photoplethysmography*—it is a noninvasive technique for characterizing CVI. Local blood flow changes to the skin are detected by a probe placed on the leg with infrared diode. As the sensitivity and the specificity are low, the technique has been abandoned by many.
- *Air plethysmography*—this measures venous reflux, calf muscle pump function, and outflow obstruction. It has 100% sensitivity and 90% specificity. It contains a sleeve of air filled polyurethane that surrounds the leg. The air chambers are connected to a very sensitive pressure transducer which allows pressure measurements to be made with accuracy. The advantages of APG are:
  - Air plethysmography gives the doctor information about the different components contributing to CVI (reflux versus obstruction).
  - It is useful in the preoperative and postoperative evaluation and the assessment of nonoperative therapies.
  - It can inform us that graded compression stockings are more effective in controlling reflux than improving calf muscle function for patients with less severe CVI (CEAP class 4).
  - However, those with more severe CVI (CEAP class 5 and above) benefitted more from improvement of calf muscle pump function than reflux control.
  - Air plethysmography helps in patient selection and predicting who will benefit more from surgical therapy. Patients with no obstruction and intact calf muscle pump function should benefit from surgical treatment of venous reflux.

*The technique:* First several measurements are made with APG where functional VV is recorded. The leg of the supine patient is elevated to 45° and the patient is then made to stand. The VV is not measured. The normal VV is 80–150 mL, but in patient with severe CVI, it may rise to 400 mL. The venous filling index (VFI) is a good guide for skin changes and ulceration. VFI is the ratio between 90% venous filling and the time taken to fill this 90%—venous filling time (VFT). VFI = 90% VV/VFT 90).

In normal limbs, veins fill slowly from the arterial side with VFI <2 mL/s. In patients with severe CVI, the VFI may rise sharply to 30 mL/s. Increasing VFI is associated with ankle dermatitis and ulceration.

Calf muscle pump function is also assessed. Patient is made to tiptoe and the recorded fall in pressure represents the ejected volume (EV). The ejection fraction (EF) is measured by the formula EF = [(EV/VV) × 100]. Normally EF is >60%. In severe CVI, it may be <10%. Both EF and VFI are important indices in predicting who will develop venous ulceration. The entire test is done with the patient in a supine position. A tourniquet applied to the proximal thigh and inflated to 80 mm Hg. This is then deflated suddenly and the outflow fraction at 1 s (OF1) measured. This is expressed as a percentage of the total VV. About <28% show severe venous obstruction, 30–40% suggest moderate venous obstruction and >40% show no significant venous obstruction.

## Evaluation of DVT and Superficial Thrombophlebitis

In evaluating such patients, the following questions should be answered:
- Is there a thrombus?
- Is the thrombus acute or chronic?
- What the anatomic extent of thrombus?
- Is there concomitant reflux?
- Do the abnormalities detected explain the patient's symptoms or are other factors responsible?
- What is the prognosis of the patient?

## Vascular Laboratory Testing for Diagnosis of Venous Thrombosis

### Duplex Ultrasound Testing

This is the first investigation of choice for suspected DVT. The diagnostic criteria are:
- Thrombus—presence of echogenic band is very sensitive but not specific (<50%).
- Noncompressibility with probe—sensitivity and specificity >95%.
- Absent or reduced spontaneous flow.
- Absent or reduced respiratory variation.
- Absent of incomplete color opacification of lumen.
- Increased venous diameter.
- <50% increased diameter with Valsalva maneuver.

### Duplex Differentiation of Chronic versus Acute Thrombosis (Table 4)

It is less sensitive and specific for diagnosing calf vein thrombosis. It has low sensitivity in diagnosing asymptomatic postoperative DVT.

Impedance plethysmography and ascending venography are rarely performed because they are less accurate than

**Table 4** Differentiating acute from chronic thrombosis

| Diagnostic criteria | Acute thrombus | Chronic thrombus |
|---|---|---|
| Echo characteristics | Lucent homogeneous | Dense heterogeneous |
| Lumen | Smooth | Irregular |
| Compressibility | Spongy | Firm |
| Diameter of vein | Dilated | Decreased or normal |
| Collaterals | Absent | Present |
| Flow channel | Confluent | Multiple |

Duplex ultrasound, more costly, and cumbersome for the patient.

Descending venography is also rarely done but can delineate reflux well. The catheter is placed in the distal iliac vein and the table tilted 60° head up. The dye moves down due to gravity or Valsalva maneuver. Kistner graded reflux as—0, no reflux; 1, reflux to upper thigh; 2, reflux to lower thigh; 3, reflux to below knee. The test once again is cumbersome and costly. The same result can be achieved by duplex ultrasound and therefore preferred.

Magnetic resonance venography is useful in diagnosing May–Turner syndrome, which is compression of the left iliac vein by the right iliac artery leading to edema of the left leg and the higher incidence of left iliofemoral DVT. It is the best technique in diagnosing gonadal vein thrombosis. The sensitivity and specificity for above knee clots are 97% and

95%, whereas for calf vein thrombi, they are 85% and 96%, respectively. It can differentiate acute from chronic DVT. Acute DVT shows perithrombus enhancement.

## Spiral Computed Tomography Venography

This has shown promise in diagnosing DVT and other soft tissue diseases in patients with leg swelling. It is still in the early stages and needs further studies.

## ■ CONCLUSION

History, thorough examination, and a color Duplex ultra-sound study in the clinic are carried out to determine if it is an acute or chronic process (Flow chart 1).

**Flow chart 1** Approach to venous disease

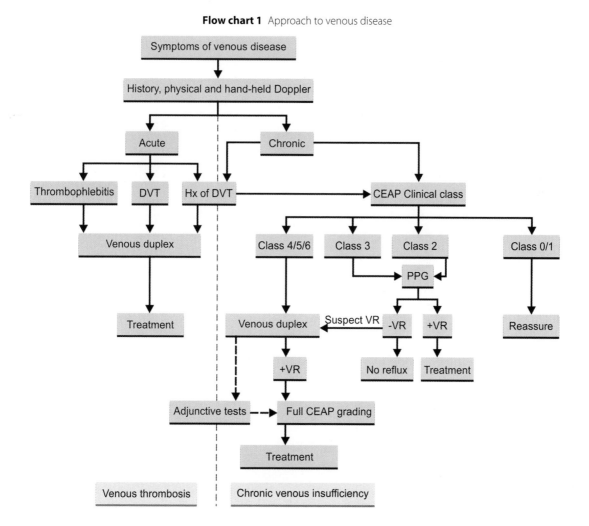

## PRACTICAL POINTS

- Toe swelling (square toe sign) typically indicates lymphedema instead of venous edema.
- Suspect May–Turner syndrome (compression of left iliac vein by right common iliac artery) when left iliofemoral DVT is present.
- Clinical signs for DVT like Homens are not specific and should not be relied upon.
- The presence of pigmentation and eczematous changes on the medial side of the lower leg (statis dermatitis) is pathognomonic of CVI.
- Lack of compressibility of vein with ultrasound probe is highly sensitive and specific of DVT (>95%).
- Air plethysmography is extremely sensitive (>95%) for reflux and provides information on outflow obstruction and calf pump function.
- CEAP classification is very helpful to guide which investigation is helpful with venous symptoms.
- Most patients with CEAP class 4/5/6 changes have deep venous reflux with or without concominant obstruction. Isolated superficial venous reflux in these patients is uncommon.

# 18

# Approach to the Management of Varicose Veins

*Jaisom Chopra*

## ■ INTRODUCTION

- Varicose veins are a common problem and affect the appearance and the quality of life.
- Varicose veins involve one-third (33%) of the adult population in the world.
- They may be asymptomatic or lead to heaviness, fatigue, and throbbing pain.
- They are the most common disorder of a group of venous disorders known as chronic venous insufficiency (CVI).
- They are common on the lower extremity but may be present in the vulva, spermatic cord (varicocele), rectum (hemorrhoids), or esophagus (esophageal varices).
- Varicose veins are tortuous, twisted, bulging in appearance. They may be truncal, reticular, or telangiectasia.

- Truncal varicose veins involve the long and short saphenous veins and their branches (Fig. 1).
- Reticular veins are smaller, superficial, greenish-blue, and flat tortuous veins.
- Telangiectasia is small blue or red veins <1 mm in diameter (Fig. 2).
- They are rare in childhood but when present one should look for other congenital vascular syndromes like Klippel–Trenaunay syndrome, Maffucci syndrome, and cutis marmorata telangiectatica congenita.
- The treatment options include sclerotherapy, endovenous saphenous vein obliteration using Laser or radiofrequency ablation (RFA) technique and ambulatory phlebectomy.
- The symptoms of varicose veins and their management have been ignored or underestimated over the years.

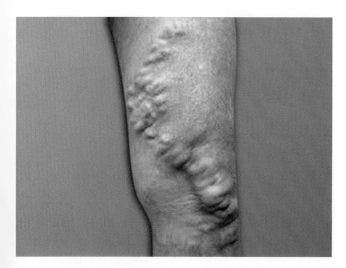

**Fig. 1** Truncal varicose veins

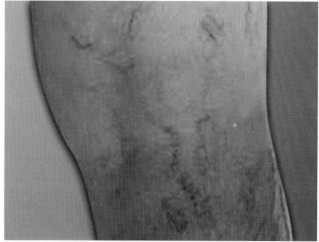

**Fig. 2** Telangiectasia

# ■ CLINICAL FEATURES

## Incidence and Prevalence

- Two years incidence in Framingham study—39.4 new cases per 1,000 men and 51.9 new cases per 1,000 women.
- Prevalence in women is 25–33% and in men 10–20%.
- Prevalence varies according to race, ethnicity, age (increases with age), gender, and nature of job (more in standing jobs like teachers).

## Risk Factors

- There is an increase in hydrostatic pressure either directly or via an increase in intra-abdominal pressure conducted via iliac veins as in pregnancy.
- It is believed that a genetic element is involved.
- People on standing jobs at one place have a higher incidence—beauticians, surgeons, teachers, pharmacists, and so on.
- Pregnancy, obesity, height, and body mass index have been blamed.
- Hematological risk factors are elevated fibrinogen, disturbed fibrinolytic system, and abnormal platelet function. Thus, the risk factors are:
  - Heredity
  - Age—increase with increasing age
  - Gender—more common in females
  - Occupation—standing jobs
  - Sedentary lifestyle and immobility (confined to bed and plasters)
  - Long flights and automobile journeys
  - Sports increasing abdominal pressure (weight lifting)
  - Obesity
  - Tight clothing and high heels
  - Pregnancy (increase with parity)
  - Heat (UV light, sunlight, and X-rays)
  - Hormones (oral contraceptives and hormone replacement therapy)
  - Diet (fiber deficient)
  - Diverticular disease, inguinal hernias, hemorrhoids, and pelvic surgery
  - Constipation.

## Pathophysiology

The venous system of the legs consists of the superficial and deep vessels. These vessels are connected by perforating veins containing one way check valves. The blood passes from the superficial to the deep veins via the perforating veins during muscle relaxation when the pressure in the deep veins falls below the superficial veins.

Varicose veins are due to CVI because of the structural and functional defect in the venous system. This leads to ambulatory venous hypertension, which may be primary or secondary.

Primary defects involve the venous wall or the venous valves leading to venous dilatation and reflux without any thrombosis (Fig. 3). This is more common in women and most patients have a strong family history of varicose veins. Secondary varicose veins are due to thrombosis of the veins leading to obstruction, reflux, or a combination.

Varicose veins are mainly primary where the venous wall is weak and the surrounding connective tissue shows abnormal distensibility. The dilatation causes separation of the valve cusps within the vein leading to valvular incompetence or reflux (Fig. 4).

Secondary defects are due to the valve cusp damage because of the previous thrombosis thus varicose veins are at sites where the deep and superficial venous systems communicate—saphenofemoral, saphenopopliteal, or where perforating veins connect the two systems.

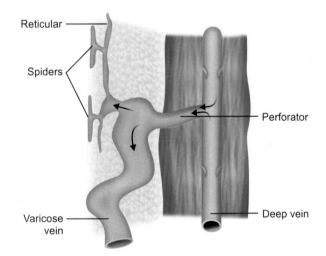

**Fig. 3** Reflux leading to varicose veins

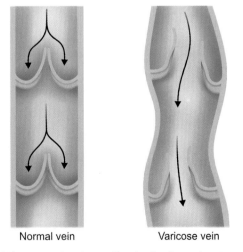

Normal vein          Varicose vein

**Fig. 4** Valve separation due to dilatation leading to incompetence

## Symptoms and Signs

### Symptoms

- The most common complaints are pain or discomfort and swelling. The pain may be an ache, cramp like, tingling, burning, fatigue, itching, or heaviness in the legs.
- Symptoms are less severe in the morning and increase as the day passes. They are aggravated by prolonged standing or sitting and relieved by leg elevation or walking.
- Women complain more than men. Mostly women complain of an ache in the legs, whereas men say cramp like pain. Varicose veins are exacerbated during menses and pregnancy.
- Symptoms do not correlate with size and the number of veins. Patients with telangiectasia may complain of severe burning, heaviness, and swelling, while grossly dilated large veins may be totally asymptomatic.
- Patients may come in as an emergency with profuse bleeding from the veins either spontaneously or after minimal trauma. It can be controlled by pressure application and leg elevation.

Thus, the symptoms are:
- Cramping pain
- Burning pain
- Heaviness
- Itching
- Fatigue
- Throbbing pain
- Restlessness
- Tingling.

### Signs

These include edema, hyperpigmentation, eczema, ulceration, lipodermatosclerosis, hemorrhage (Fig. 5), and superficial thrombophlebitis. Hyperpigmentation and ulceration are more common on the medial side above the ankle. It is a result of venous hypertension (Fig. 6). Pigmentation is due to extravasation of the RBCs into the skin over time. 0.3% of the adult population suffers from venous ulcers. They are difficult to heal and are often recurrent. They are painful and small. Superficial thrombophlebitis occurs in varicose veins, is painful, red, swollen, and tender over the varicosity. The long saphenous vein is mostly involved. Thus, the signs are:
- Dermatitis
- Hemorrhage
- Superficial thrombophlebitis
- Ulceration
- Lipodermatosclerosis.

## Classification of Varicose Veins

The most common classification is the CEAP—clinical presentation, etiology, anatomy, and pathophysiology. According to this:
- 'C'—Clinical presentation helps deciding the investigations to be ordered and the treatment required.
- 'E'—etiology—congenital, primary, or secondary.
- 'A'—anatomy—superficial or deep.
- 'P'—pathophysiology—reflux or obstruction or both.

## ■ DIAGNOSIS

### History and Physical Examination

A careful history of the present and the past illness should be taken with careful attention to the risk factors. In physical examination, the entire arterial system should be examined including the abdomen. A record should be made of the truncal varicose veins, the reticular veins, and the telangiectasia.

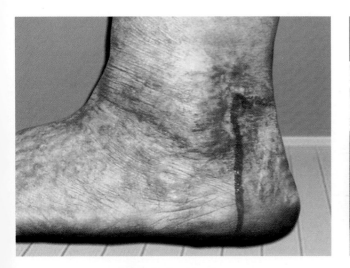

**Fig. 5** Profuse bleeding

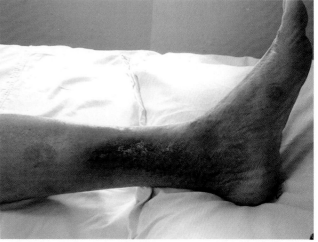

**Fig. 6** Stasis dermatitis

Skin changes due to the complications of varicose veins like dermatitis (Fig. 7), lipodermatosclerosis (Fig. 8), and ulcers (Fig. 9) should be made. The good old tests of the past like cough test, tapping test, Brodie–Trendelenburg test, and Perthes test have caused confusion among doctors and have been replaced by noninvasive laboratory testing.

## Laboratory Testing

- Color Doppler study has emerged the test of choice for varicose veins because of its high sensitivity and specificity rates, being noninvasive and patient friendly.
- Venography, once the gold standard is too cumbersome, invasive, expensive, and with a lower specificity and sensitivity than color Doppler.
- Other tests like ambulatory venous pressure measurements, photoplethysmography and air plethysmography have not justified the replacement of color Doppler study.

## ■ TREATMENT

This depends on the magnitude of symptoms and the health of the patient. The options are:
- External compression
- Sclerotherapy
- Laser therapy and light therapy
- Endovenous obliteration of the saphenous vein
- Transilluminated powered phlebectomy
- Ligation and stripping.

## Conventional Treatment

This includes graded compression stockings, limb elevation (Fig. 10), plenty of ambulation, and good skin hygiene. Patients with CEAP class 1, 2, and some in class 3 use this option.

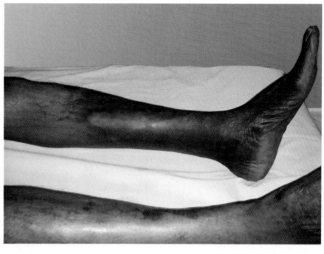

**Fig. 8** Hard dark skin

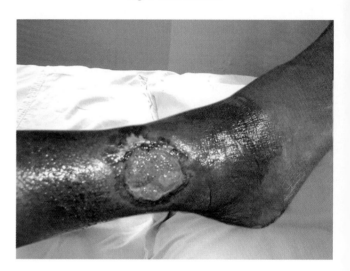

**Fig. 9** Venous ulcer

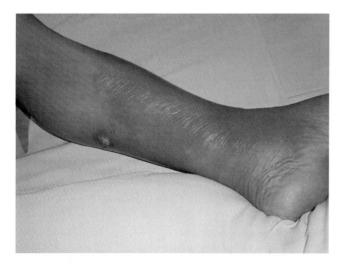

**Fig. 7** Superficial thrombophlebitis

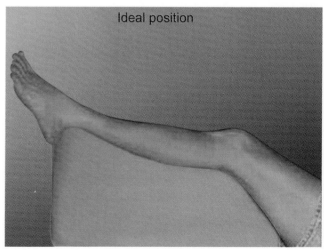

**Fig. 10** Limb elevation a vital part of treatment

## External Compression Therapy

This is the mainstay of treating most cases of CVI. This method is very sensitive in treating pain, swelling, and ulcers. Compression may be in the form of bandages, elastic stockings (Fig. 11), or intermittent pneumatic compression.

These may be used separately or in conjunction with sclerotherapy or surgery. Contraindications to compression therapy include arterial occlusive disease with an ABI < 0.6 or ankle pressure < 60 mm Hg, active skin disease or allergy to the stockings. Although it is much cheaper than other forms of treatment, but being cumbersome, the compliance by the patient is not very high. The compression varies from 20 to 50 mm Hg and used according to the requirement. They have to replace from time to time because they lose their elasticity.

## Medication

These are all of doubtful benefit.
- Diuretics helps reduce edema but does not help reduce pain or discomfort.
- Horse chestnut extract is a herbal product that decreases edema by increasing venous tone and venous flow. A trial conducted with only placebo versus horse chestnut extract found results with horse chestnut superior to placebo.
- Aesculus hippocastanum is used in Europe for varicose veins and edema.
- Daflon is a micronized purified flavonoid—a venotropic drug. It reduces the leg circumference by inhibiting inflammatory reaction and reducing capillary hyper-permeability. It is most effective when used in conjunction with compression therapy, sclerotherapy, or surgery.

## Sclerotherapy

It is used often for cosmetic reasons and common in telan-giectasia, reticular veins (Fig. 12), and small varicose veins or residual veins post-surgery. It eliminates pain and discomfort and may reduce complications like ulcers and bleeding. The agents include—sodium tetradecyl sulfate, hypertonic saline (10–23.4%), dextrose (25%), and sodium morrhuate (5%). Avoid extravasation into the surrounding tissue and so use it with color Doppler to enhance its effect and reduce the complications.

*Complications of sclerotherapy include:*
- Pain or cramping
- Hyperpigmentation
- Telangiectatic mapping
- Blistering or necrosis
- Superficial thrombophlebitis
- Deep vein thrombosis
- Urticaria
- Edema.

*Contraindications to sclerotherapy:*
- Acute DVT
- Bed-ridden or immobile patient
- Cellulitis of leg
- Allergy to sclerosant
- Uncontrolled diabetes
- Bleeding disorders or thrombophilias
- Undergoing chemotherapy for cancer
- Arterial disease
- Patients on oral contraceptives and hormone replacement therapy (HRT)
- Pregnant patients
- Breastfeeding.
  Most recommend 2–3 weeks treatment.

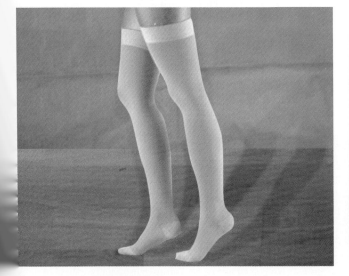

**Fig. 11** Compression stockings

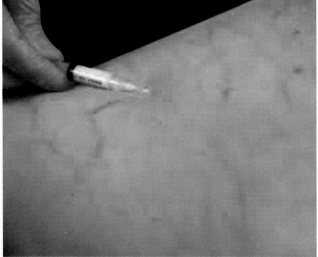

**Fig. 12** Sclerosant given into the varicose vein

## Laser Therapy and High Intensity Light Therapies

These have gained popularity over the past few years. Laser has been there since the 1970s, whereas pulsed light therapies have been there since the 1990s. They are applied indirectly over the vessel and their effectiveness depends on the depth of the vessel, its size, and flow. The results have not been very encouraging and these therapies are more expensive than sclerotherapy.

Laser is used for isolated superficial fine caliber telangiectasia and for failed sclerotherapy (Fig. 13). Because of the postoperative pain, local anesthetic cream and cooling is used in its treatment. Hyperpigmentation, blistering, and superficial erosions are seen as side effects after treatment.

## Surgical and Endovascular Therapy

Knowing the anatomical site and degree of valvular reflux, ruling out obstruction in the deep and superficial systems besides deep vein incompetence helps in planning the management. Without completely understanding the exact problem, we may worsen the venous disease despite our best efforts. All patients must be classified by the CEAP class prior to surgical intervention. Surgery and endovenous treatment are preferred in symptomatic large truncal varicose veins. Indications for surgery are:

- Skin changes
- Ulceration
- Bleeding
- Pain
- Swelling
- Cosmetic.

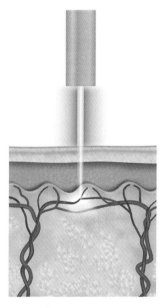

**Fig. 13** Laser therapy for dermal varicose veins

*The goals of surgery are:*

- Elimination for need for compression stockings
- Prevention of recurrent ulcers
- Prevention of skin changes
- Returning patient to near normal lifestyle.

## Saphenous Vein Ligation

High tie-ligation of saphenous vein along with all the branches at the SFJ with ablation of the thigh portion of the LSV alone correct most of the problems (Figs 14A and B). To this is added below knee sclerotherapy to give good results cosmetically and therapeutically.

## Perforator Ligation

The minimally invasive technique of subfascial endoscopic perforator surgery is shown to be effective either alone or in combination with saphenous vein surgery. The perforators are located using color Doppler study seeing bidirectional flow. A surgical endoscope using gas insufflation is performed and the perforators are identified and ligated or ligated and divided. This technique is best for CEAP class 4–6 CVI. However, new ulcers or recurrence is still a major problem, especially in post-thrombotic limbs.

## Ambulatory Phlebectomy (Stab Avulsion or Hook Phlebectomy)

This is a relatively inexpensive, effective, and easy method for removal of varicose veins. It can be used in truncal varicosities where high flow limits the use of sclerotherapy and in young where veins may be thicker and not easily torn on avulsion (Figs 15A to C). This technique is less effective where reflux is present as in saphenofemoral or saphenopopliteal junctions. The veins are drawn out of a pinhole incision and removed piecemeal. It is effective but there is bruising and hematoma formation, which slowly gets absorbed. The other complications are pain, infection, and hyperpigmentation.

## Endovenous Saphenous Vein Obliteration

This is a recent advance using radiofrequency or laser to obliterate the vein using heat at 85°C. This results in wall thickening, contraction of the lumen, fibrosis, and eventual occlusion (Figs 16A to C). This technique needs the placement of the catheter at the SF junction under duplex ultrasound. This is endovenous laser therapy (EVLT) of radiofrequency ablation (RFA).

## Steps of Endovascular Vein Therapy

*Step 1*—Use color Doppler on table to locate the vein (Figs 17A and B).

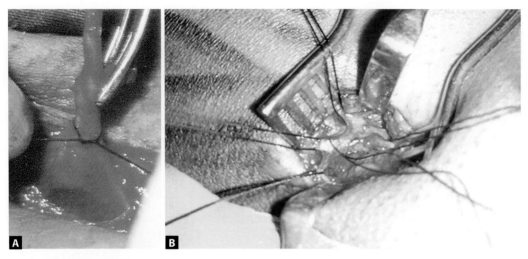

**Figs 14A and B** (A) High tie and stripping; (B) Ligation of the multiple branches prevents recurrence

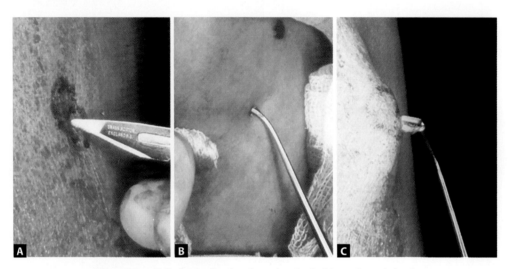

**Figs 15A to C** Perforator ligation through a tiny incision using vein hook

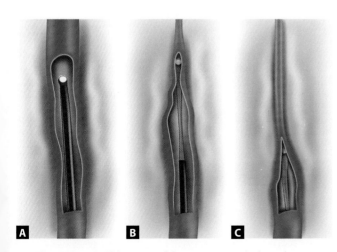

**Figs 16A to C** Obliteration of the varicose vein by heat therapy

*Step 2*—Introduce a needle into the vein using color Doppler (Figs 18A and B).

*Step 3*—Laser or RFA catheter introduced into vein (Figs 19A and B).

Many surgeons prefer high ligation (Trendelenburg operation) along with endovenous RFA as the recurrence rates are lower. However, it needs general anesthesia, longer convalescence time, and is prone to more side effects compared with RFA alone. The patient satisfaction is reported to be very high. 2-year follow-up showed success rate (defined as lack of recanalization or patient seeking further treatment) between 70% and 90%. Side effects are skin burns, paresthesia due to saphenous nerve injury, hematoma, burning or stinging pain, and deep vein thrombosis. The above procedure can be performed using a laser probe.

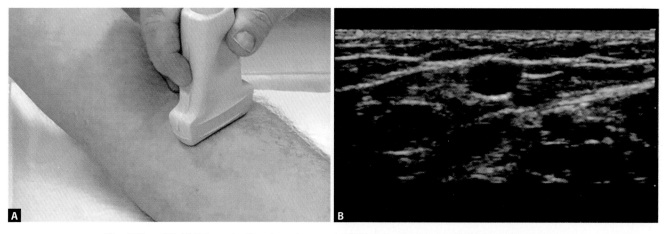

**Figs 17A and B** (A) Using color Doppler to locate vein; (B) Vein localized as rounded homogeneous area

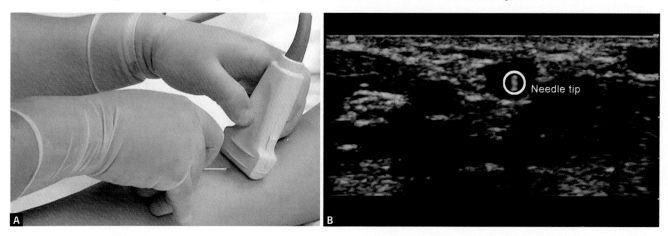

**Figs 18A and B** (A) Needle introduced into the vein using color Doppler; (B) Needle tip seen in the vein

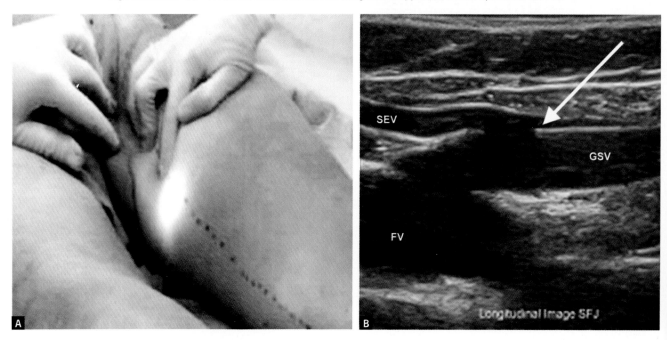

**Figs 19A and B** (A) Laser light present below skin and confirmed by color Doppler; (B) RFA fiber at the SF junction

## Complications of Endovenous Therapy

- Leg edema that slowly resolves within 6–8 weeks.
- Pain and tenderness over the ablated vein, which takes 6–8 weeks to resolve. It is much more prominent in laser therapy (EVLT).
- Skin burns is rare but more common in EVLT. Avoided by giving tumescent anesthesia around the vein guided by color Doppler.
- Rarely abscess formation at site of EVLT. More likely in patients with ulcers.
- Very rarely vein still patent due to less energy being delivered through RFA or EVLT. More due to technical reasons.

## Transilluminated Power Phlebectomy

It is a further advance in this surgery and is used to remove truncal varices. It involves endoscopic resection or ablation of superficial varices using a powered vein resector, an irrigating illuminator, and tumescent anesthesia.

## ■ SUMMARY

- Varicose veins are a common problem and present with pain, fatigue, restlessness, and heaviness in the legs.
- Symptoms are less in the morning and increase as the day progresses.
- The signs include edema, discoloration, ulceration, and lipodermatosclerosis.
- Duplex ultrasound is the investigation of choice.
- They are relieved by leg elevation, walking, or compression stockings.
- The treatment options are conservative, interventional, or surgical.

## PRACTICAL POINTS

- Physical examination must include examination of the arterial system, abdomen, and both legs sitting and standing.
- The CEAP clinical class or the 'C' in CEAP (clinical presentation) is helpful in deciding the diagnostic studies.
- It is critical to rule out DVT and deep venous reflux in patient with varicose veins.
- Small varicosities like telangiectasia and reticular veins respond best to sclerotherapy.

# 19

# Venous Thromboembolism

*Jaisom Chopra*

## ◼ INTRODUCTION

- Venous thromboembolism (VTE) comprises deep vein thrombosis (DVT) and pulmonary embolism (PE) and is a common disorder.
- Incidence is 1–2% per 1,000 persons in the general population.
- It is strongly age dependent being 0.03% below 50 years and 0.4% in those over 50 years.
- It is equally common in both sexes.
- 50% with proximal DVT in legs also have PE.
- Early diagnosis of VTE is vital because if missed, it may result in the fatal complication of PE, whereas treatment with anticoagulants can have its own serious side effects.
- Leg DVT commonly starts in the calf veins and rarely causes PE but if left untreated (1 week), it extends into the proximal veins—popliteal and proximal to it, and may cause PE.
- Deep vein thrombosis occurs because of venous obstruction and inflammation of the vein wall and perivascular tissue (Fig. 1).
- Pulmonary embolism occurs when thrombi dislodge from the legs and pass to the pulmonary veins and lodge in the lung tissue (Fig. 2).
- Venous thrombi are composed of fibrin and RBCs.
- Venous thromboembolism happens due to: (1) vessel wall damage, (2) activation of the blood coagulation, and (3) venous stasis—Virchow's triad (Fig. 3).
- Vessel wall damage is seen in hip and knee surgery, venous catheterization, and severe burns.
- Activation of the blood coagulation may be acquired like the release of tissue factor after damage to the vessel wall or the release of thromboplastin by leukocytes bound to the activated endothelium. Activation of the blood coagulation may be congenital like antithrombin III, protein C and S deficiency, factor V Leiden and prothrombin gene mutation. Both factors cause hypercoagulable states leading to thrombosis.
- Venous stasis prevents clearance of the activated coagulation factors leading to interaction of formed blood elements and the vessel wall.

Several risk factors for VTE are recognized:
- Prolonged immobility (>3 days)
- Stroke or paralysis
- Previous VTE
- Cancer
- Major surgery
- Major trauma
- Indwelling central venous catheters
- Pregnancy and puerperium
- Estrogen use.

Venous thromboembolism may be secondary (associated with one or more risk factors) or primary (idiopathic or unprovoked).

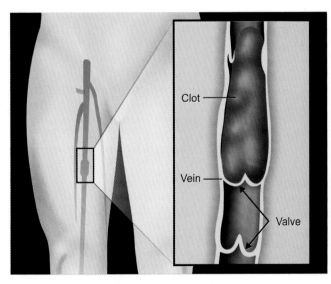

**Fig. 1** Deep vein thrombosis

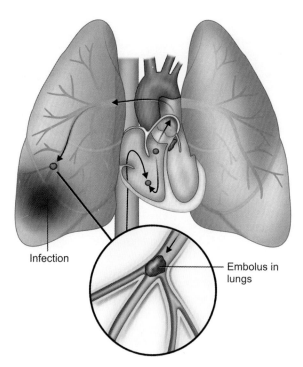

Infection

Embolus in lungs

**Fig. 2** Pulmonary embolism

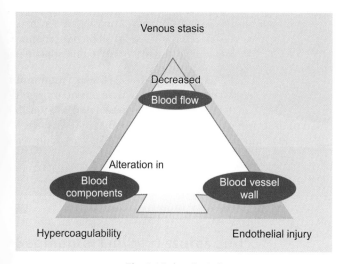

Venous stasis

Decreased
Blood flow

Alteration in
Blood components

Blood vessel wall

Hypercoagulability

Endothelial injury

**Fig. 3** Virchow's triad

Thrombophilias or hypercoagulable states refer to increased tendency to develop VTE.

Laboratory testing is interfered within:
- Heparin therapy, acute thrombosis, hepatic dysfunction, and nephrotic syndrome as they cause reduction in the antithrombin plasma concentrations.
- Coumarin derivatives, acute thrombosis, and hepatic dysfunction cause reduction in protein C and S plasma concentrations.

Testing for thrombophilia should be considered in patient with one or more of the following:
- First episode of unprovoked VTE in patients over 60 years
- Strong family history of thrombosis (first degree relatives)
- Venous thrombosis involving unusual sites (portal, mesenteric or cerebral veins)
- Patients with extensive VTE
- Patients with recurrent VTE
- Venous thromboembolism in women on birth control pills, hormone replacement therapy (HRT), or during pregnancy.

# ■ CLINICAL FEATURES

These are most unreliable. Symptoms are uncommon and nonspecific unless the proximal veins are involved. Presentation of PE depends upon:
- Size of thrombus
- Location in the pulmonary tree
- Presence of pulmonary infarction
- Patient's underlying pulmonary reserve.

## Clinical Features of Deep Vein Thrombosis

### Symptoms
- Leg pain—isolated calf pain with or without medial thigh discomfort
- Swelling of leg.

### Signs
- Leg swelling especially with following features:
  - Entire leg swollen (Fig. 4)
  - 3 cm or more increase in circumference of symptomatic leg 10 cm below tibial tuberosity

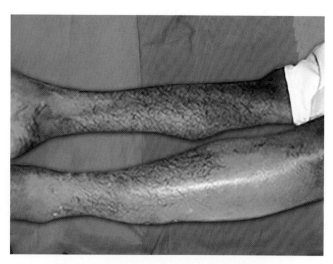

**Fig. 4** Swelling left leg due to deep vein thrombosis

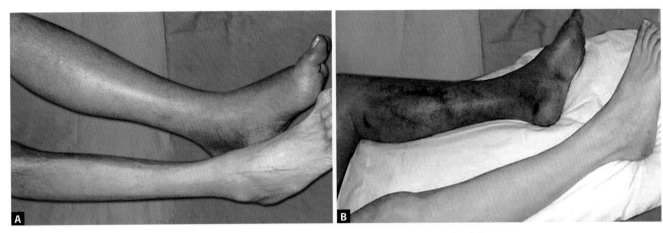

**Figs 5A and B**  (A) Phlegmasia alba dolens; (B) Phlegmasia cerulea dolens

- Localized tenderness along distribution of deep venous system
- Redness and warmth
- Phlegmasia alba dolens—white and cold leg due to iliofemoral thrombosis with arterial spasm (Fig. 5A)
- Phlegmasia cerulea dolens—markedly swollen leg with cyanosis due to iliofemoral thrombosis (Fig. 5B).
  Homen's sign is neither sensitive nor specific for DVT though commonly performed.

### Differential Diagnosis

- Leg trauma (hematoma or muscle injury)
- Cellulitis
- Ruptured baker's cyst
- Arthritis of knee or ankle joint
- Swelling following recent hip or knee surgery
- Pelvic venous obstruction or external compression of iliac vein
- Superficial phlebitis
- Venous insufficiency
- Occlusive arterial disease
- Neurogenic pain.

## Clinical Features of Pulmonary Embolism

### Symptoms

- Chest pain or discomfort (pleuritic)
- Unexplained dyspnea
- Hemoptysis
- Cough
- Symptoms of DVT
- Shock or loss of consciousness due to obstruction of right ventricular outflow.

### Signs

- Tachypnea
- Tachycardia
- Cyanosis
- Fourth heart sound
- Increased pulmonic sound
- Inspiratory crackles
- Pleural rub
- Clinical signs or pleural effusion
- Signs of right heart failure.

### Differential Diagnosis

- Chest pain
- Dyspnea
- Pleural effusion
- Hemoptysis
- Right heart failure
- Cardiovascular collapse.

A combination of:
- Signs and symptoms of VTE
- Risk factors of VTE
- Exclusion of alternative diagnosis.
  The above three help us to classify DVT or PE into low, moderate, or high probability.

## ■ DIAGNOSIS

## Clinical Assessment

A thorough history and physical examination based on symptoms and signs, risk factors for VTE, and presence of an alternative diagnosis is taken. Based on the resultant score, the patients are classified as low, moderate, and high probability of DVT and PE (Tables 1 and 2).

**Table 1** Predicting probability of deep vein thrombosis

| Clinical feature | Score |
|---|---|
| Active cancer—ongoing or within 6 months | 1 |
| Paralysis, paresis, recent plaster immobilization | 1 |
| Bedridden over 3 days or major surgery within 4 weeks | 1 |
| Tender along deep vein system | 1 |
| Entire leg swollen | 1 |
| Calf swelling >3 cm compared with asymptomatic leg (10 cm below tibial tuberosity) | 1 |
| Pitting edema greater in the symptomatic leg | 1 |
| Nonvaricose superficial veins | 1 |
| Alternative diagnosis likely or greater than DVT | -2 |
| Total | |

**Table 2** Predicting probability of pulmonary embolism

| Variable | Score |
|---|---|
| Immobilization or surgery in last 4 weeks | 1.5 |
| Malignancy (ongoing or in previous 6 months) | 1.0 |
| Previous DVT or PE | 1.5 |
| Hemoptysis | 1.0 |
| Heart rate >100 beats/min | 1.5 |
| Clinical signs and symptoms of DVT ( leg swelling and pain with palpation of deep veins) | 3.0 |
| An alternative diagnosis less likely than PE | 3.0 |
| Total | |

In deep vein thrombosis, if patient has symptoms in both legs then more symptomatic leg is used. The probability is high ≥3; moderate 1 or 2; and low ≤0.

In pulmonary embolism, low probability <2.0; moderate probability 2.0–6.0; high probability ≥6.0.

## Diagnosis of Deep Vein Thrombosis

### Compression Venous Ultrasonography

If not compressible, it is diagnostic of DVT but is more valuable for proximal veins like femoral, popliteal, and till the calf trifurcation veins (Figs 6A and B).

The specificity is 96% and sensitivity is 95%. It is not very reliable for calf veins because they are too small and variable. Because ultrasound for calf veins thrombus is so unreliable, it should be repeated after 7–10 days to see any extension into the larger veins. If extension is positive then venography is performed to confirm the diagnosis.

### D-Dimer Assay

It is the degradation product of cross-linked fibrin occurring in acute thrombosis. It is not specific to DVT and may be found in infection and malignancy. Negative results exclude DVT especially, if ultrasound is also negative.

### Contrast Venography

This shows an intraluminal filling defect and can reliably detect calf vein, iliac vein, and inferior vena cava (IVC) DVT. It is not performed routinely because it is cumbersome, expensive, and invasive. Besides it, there may be side effects of contrast.

### Magnetic Resonance Venography (Fig. 7).

Approach to the management of first episode of DVT is shown in Flow chart 1.

## Diagnosis of Pulmonary Embolism

### Diagnostic Tests

*Pulmonary angiography (Fig. 8):* It is the gold standard in the diagnosis of PE but is invasive, expensive, contraindicated in renal impairment patients, and not possible in unstable cases. Persistent intraluminal filling defect or sharp cutoff of a vessel 2.5 mm diameter is diagnostic of PE.

*Ventilation perfusion (V/Q) lung scanning:* It is the first test performed in suspected PE. Normal perfusion scan found in 30% rules out PE. Segmental perfusion defects found in 10% show high probability of PE.

Nondiagnostic scans like:
- Segmental perfusion defects with matched ventilation defects
- Subsegmental perfusion defects with or without ventilation defects
- Perfusion defects with corresponding abnormalities on CXR.

These occur in two out of three cases with clinically suspected PE and need further testing to exclude or diagnose PE.

*Spiral CT:* It is minimally invasive and allows visualization of pulmonary vessels, parenchyma, pleura, and mediastinum. It allows alternative diagnosis in 25%. Intraluminal filling defects in main pulmonary arteries or lobular arteries shows high probability for PE but if filling defects are seen segmental pulmonary arteries, they are of low probability (Fig. 9).

*D-dimer assay:* It is evaluated in suspected PE but are of doubtful value. SimpliRED D-dimer and Vidas D-dimer are more in PE.

*Testing for DVT using bilateral proximal compression ultrasonography or venography:* It is an indirect way to diagnose PE. If DVT is present, anticoagulation is indicated and provided other etiologies are excluded. It is safe to withhold anticoagulation and is suspected DVT if initial ultrasound is normal and serial ultrasounds are performed after 1 week.

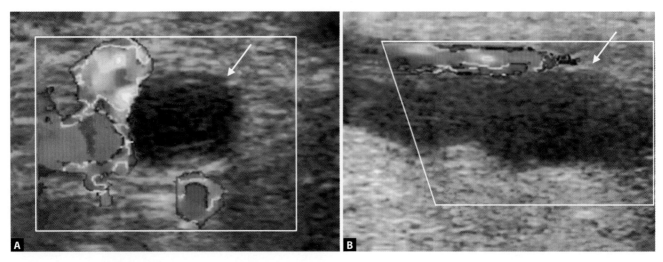

**Figs 6A and B** No flow in vein and not compressible—transverse section (A) and longitudinal section (B)

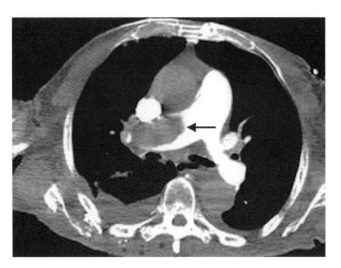

**Fig. 7** Magnetic resonance venography showing thrombus in the IVC

These are low to moderate risk patients with nondiagnostic V/Q scan and CT scan.

The tests used to exclude other conditions but should not be used to diagnose PE are:
- Chest X-ray—to exclude atelectasis, parenchymal abnormalities, pleural effusion, and pleural-based densities
- ECG—S-T or T wave changes are not specific to PE
- Alveolar-arterial gradient is not very helpful with PE.

### Approach to Diagnosis of First Episode of PE

There is no single test sensitive enough to diagnose or exclude PE with surety. The approach is given in Flow charts 2A and 2B.

## ■ MANAGEMENT OF PATIENTS WITH ACUTE VENOUS THROMBOSIS

The goal of the treatment is:
- Prevent embolization of thrombus
- Minimize long-term complications of VTE—post-thrombotic syndrome and chronic thromboembolic pulmonary hypertension.

Anticoagulation is the mainstay for the treatment of acute VTE. The anticoagulation regimen for DVT and PE are similar and includes intravenous unfractionated heparin or subcutaneous low-molecular weight heparin (LMWH) followed by oral anticoagulation along with oxygen, leg elevation, and compression bandages to the legs. Studies have shown that subcutaneous LMWH is as effective as intravenous unfractionated heparin.

Low-molecular weight heparin as outpatient treatment is indicated in:
- Hemodynamically stable patients
- Patients with low bleeding risk
- Good renal function
- Practical system for administering LMWH and monitoring it
- Practical system for evaluating recurrent VTE and bleeding.

Thrombolytic therapy is indicated patients with:
- Low bleeding risk
- Massive PE causing hemodynamic instability
- Extensive iliofemoral DVT.

Before giving anticoagulation, assess the risk—contraindications for anticoagulation (Table 3).

Baseline blood tests like complete blood count, activated partial thromboplastin time (aPTT), and International

**Flow chart 1** Diagnostic approach in patients with suspected first DVT

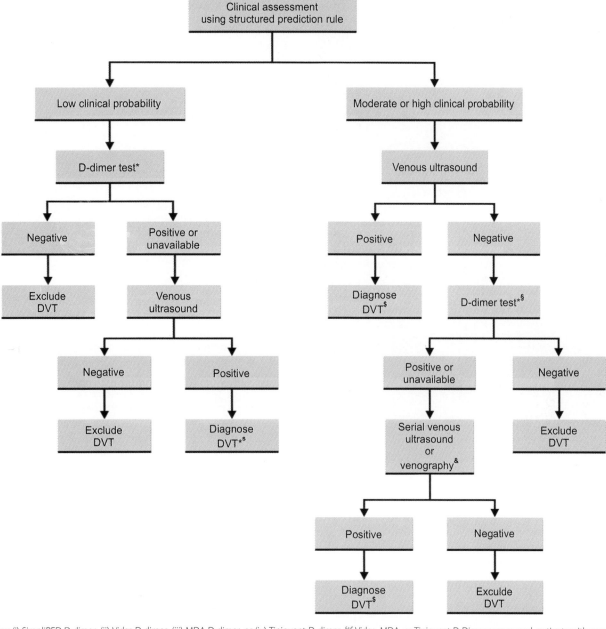

*, Using (i) SimpliRED D-dimer, (ii) Vidas D-dimer, (iii) MDA D-dimer, or (iv) Tiniquant D-dimer, §If Vidas, MDA, or Tiniquant D-Dimer assays used, patients with moderate clinical probability can be managed similarly to patients with a low clinical probability of DVT, #Venography should be considered to exclude possibility of false-positive (positiive predictive value of positive ultrosound in patients with low pretest probability is 65%§, If isolated calf thrombus on ultrosound, consider venography to confirm diagnosis, &Consider venography if patient is unable to return for serial ultrosound or clinical probability is high

Normalization Ratio (INR) are performed but anticoagulation should not be delayed.

IVC filter is indicated in:
- Anticoagulation is contraindicated
- Recurrent PE despite adequate anticoagulation.

# Anticoagulants

## Unfractionated Heparin

It is a glycosaminoglycan with molecular weight 15,000 Da. It acts by catalyzing the effect of antithrombin III, a natural

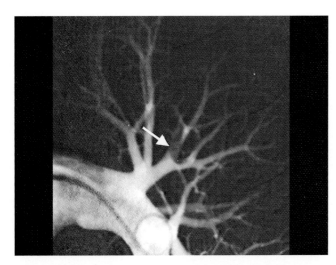

**Fig. 8** Pulmonary angiography showing thrombus

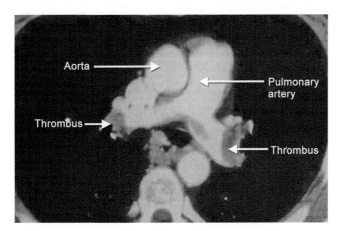

**Fig. 9** Spiral CT showing clots in the pulmonary tree

inhibitor that inactivates factors IIa (thrombin), Xa, and IXa. Unfractionated heparin (UH) is given IV with a loading dose of 80 IU/kg or fixed dose of 5,000 IU, followed by continuous infusion of 18 IU/kg/h or a fixed dose of 30,000–35,000 IU/24 h and monitored via aPTT 6 hourly, which is maintained between 2 and 3.5 times control. With UH, platelet count is done daily to see for heparin-induced thrombocytopenia (HIT), which can occur in the first week of therapy. Long time use can give rise to osteoporosis.

## Low-Molecular Weight Heparin

This is a fragment of UH obtained from chemical or enzymatic depolarization. The mean molecular weight is 4,000–5,000 Da and it catalyzes antithrombin III but is less active against factor IIa than against factor Xa. Thus, the advantages of LMWH over UH are:
• Longer half-life and dose-independent clearance mechanism due to reduced binding to macrophages.

• Less binding to endothelium and plasma proteins increasing its bioavailability and predictability of anti-coagulant response.
• Less bleeding for an equivalent antithrombotic effect.

Low-molecular weight heparin is cleared via kidneys and used in caution in renal failure. The risk of bleeding, HIT, and osteoporosis appears to be lower in LMWH than UH. Monitoring factor Xa assay, 3–4 h after injection is recommended in:
• Patients with renal insufficiency
• Body weight <50 or >100 kg
• Pregnancy.

Dose schedule for LMWH in various preparations in the treatment of VTE:
• Dalteparin (fragmin)—200 U/kg once daily or 100 U/kg twice daily
• Enoxaparin (lovenox)—1 mg/kg twice daily or 1.5 mg/kg once daily
• Tinzaparin (innohep)—175 U/kg once daily.

## Oral Anticoagulation

Coumarin derivatives (warfarin and acenocoumarol) are oral anti-Vitamin K antagonists are used for long-term treatment of VTE. It can be commenced within 24 h of parenteral anticoagulation with heparin or LMWH in a dose of 5–10 mg. Lower starting doses 2–4 mg are recommended in elderly, low body weight, and malnourished. The doses are adjusted according to the INR, which is done after 2–3 doses and adjusted to a target range of 2.0–3.0. The schedule for INR is:
• Twice weekly for first 1–2 weeks
• Weekly for another 4 weeks
• Every 2 weekly for another 1 month
• Then once a month.

More frequent INR is recommended if the patient becomes unstable or his medication changes.
• Warfarin decreases the functional activity of Vitamin K-dependent coagulation factors—II, VII, IX, X, and protein C and S. The plasma concentration of factor VII and protein C fall rapidly due to their short half lives (6–8 h), whereas a decrease in other clotting factors is delayed for 24–48 h. That is why, an increase in INR due to reduced factor VII only occurs about 24 h before the antithrombotic effect due to reduced factor II. During this hypercoagulable state occurring due to low protein C levels, we should continue UH or LMWH for 5 days to prevent propagation of the thrombus. It is only stopped when the INR is in therapeutic range for 2 consecutive days. Complications of warfarin therapy are—bleeding, alopecia, and skin-induced necrosis. This occurs in patients with inherent protein C and S deficiency who are started on anticoagulation therapy with warfarin alone. It can be prevented by starting with parenteral heparin and followed by warfarin. Coumarin derivatives cross the placenta and can cause spontaneous abortion and a specific embryopathy if administered during the first trimester of pregnancy (between 6 and 12 weeks of gestation).

**Flow chart 2A** Diagnostic approach in patients with suspectd first PE

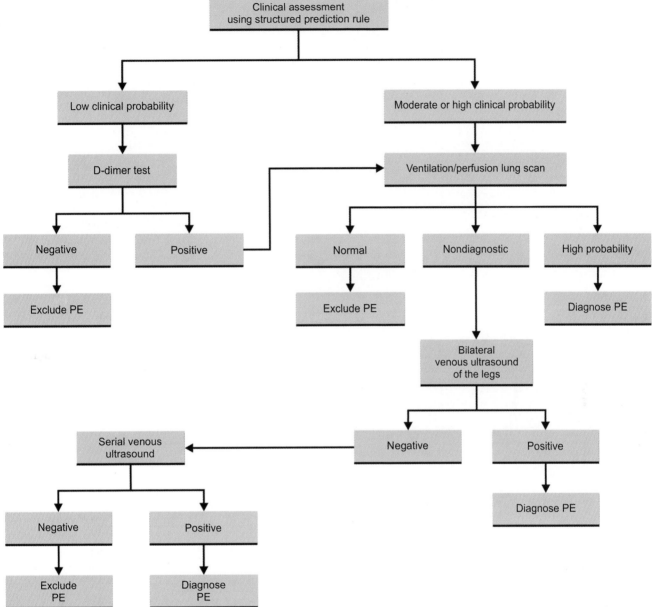

**Table 3** Contraindications to anticoagulation (absolute and relative)

| Absolute | Relative |
|---|---|
| Active hemorrhage | Recent GI hemorrhage or stroke (<14 days) |
| Neurosurgery or intracranial bleeding within 7 days (including hemorrhagic stroke) | Recent major surgery (<1–2 days) |
| Severe thrombocytopenia (<20 × 10$^9$/L) | Moderate thrombocytopenia (20–50 × 10$^9$/L) |
| History of heparin-induced thrombocytopenia within 90 days | Uncontrolled hypertension |
| | Brain metastasis |
| | Inherited coagulopathy |

**Flow chart 2B**   Diagnostic approach in patients with suspected first PE

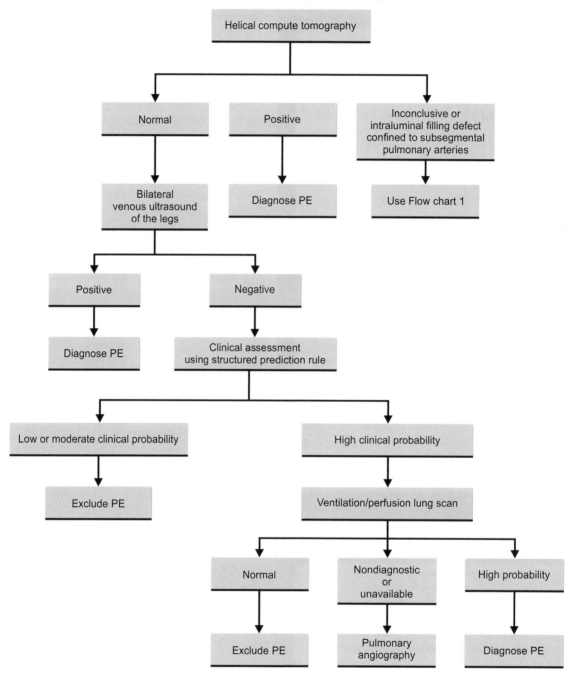

## Duration of Anticoagulant Therapy

- Parenteral anticoagulation (UF and LMWH) is administered for 5 days and on day 2, warfarin is started. In massive PE, or severe iliofemoral DVT heparin is continued for 10 days. Heparin therapy is discontinued when the INR reached 2 times control on two consecutive days.
- For first episode of VTE duration of anticoagulation is individualized.

- Oral anticoagulation is given for 3 months in proximal DVT or PE or symptomatic calf vein DVT.
- Indefinite anticoagulation is considered for recurrent idiopathic VTE or continuing risk factors like cancer or antiphospholipid syndrome.
- Six months of oral anticoagulation is recommended in first episode of idiopathic VTE.

# SPECIAL ISSUES

## Management of Bleeding Associated with Anticoagulation

Morbidity and mortality associated with this depends on the severity and the site of bleeding. Evaluate if the bleeding is life threatening or into a critical site like intracranial or pericardial, adrenal, or intraocular space. Evaluate for contributing risk factors like antiplatelet agents and nonsteroidal anti-inflammatory agents, lab tests like antiplatelet and aPTT results and risk of recurrent VTE.

### Unfractionated Heparin

If a patient is on UH and has life-threatening bleeding or bleeding into a critical space the following steps are taken:
- Stop heparin infusion
- Replace volume loss
- Give IV protamine sulfate
  - 1 mg protamine sulfate reverses 100 U of UF
  - Maximum dose of 50 mg in any 10 min period
  - In severe cases, infusion 10 mg/h is given
  - S/E includes hypotension, flushing, bradycardia, bronchospasm, and anaphylaxis
  - Slow infusion minimizes hypotension
- Consider IVC filter in recent VTE.

Management of patients with non-life-threatening bleeding include:
- Stop heparin in aPTT is >80 s and start when lower
- Local measures to control bleeding.

### Low-Molecular Weight Heparin

The management is like for UH but protamine sulfate only partially reverses the effect of LMWH by neutralizing the antithrombin activity but partially reverses the anti-Xa activity. It is however recommended in severe bleeding with LMWH.

### Warfarin

Management of life-threatening bleeding or into a critical space with warfarin:
- Stop warfarin
- Replace volume loss
- Administer fresh frozen plasma (FFP) or prothrombin complex concentrate (PCC)
  - FFP 15 mL/kg
  - Prothrombin complex concentrate preferred if worried about volume overload
  - Specific dose for each PCC
  - Potential thrombogenicity reported with PCC.

- Administer Vitamin K
  - Slow infusion after dilution of 5 mg
  - Severe reactions and anaphylactic death can occur and so it is only given where there is life-threatening bleeding
- Consider IVC filter for recurrent VTE.

In asymptomatic patients with high INR stop warfarin and monitor PT/INR till suitable levels have been reached. If needed 1–3 mg of oral Vitamin K is given.

### Heparin-induced Thrombocytopenia

It is an immune-mediated thrombocytopenia occurring between 5 and 10 days of UH or LMWH therapy. It can develop earlier if the patient has had the treatment before or may occur after completion of the therapy. It is suspected when the platelet count falls below 50% or <100,000/mm³. It is due to the formation of an antibody against the platelet/factor 4 (PF4) complex. The heparin PF4/IgG immune complexes activate platelets resulting in release of procoagulant platelet-derived microparticles. Thus, recurrence or extension of existing VTE and arterial thromboembolism may occur. The diagnosis is difficult because the platelet-activation assay and ELISAs are not readily available. Treatment includes:
- Stopping UH or LMWH
- Danaparoid, lepirudin, or argatroban therapy
- Warfarin delayed till the platelet count is >100,000/mm³.

### Indications for Inferior Vena Cava Filter

The primary indications are:
- Contraindications to anticoagulation and complications of anticoagulation
- Recurrent PE despite anticoagulation
- Chronic pulmonary hypertension and reduced cardiac reserve.

Relative indications:
- Free floating emboli in pelvic veins or IVC
- Deep vein thrombosis and planned orthopedic surgery
- Surgical therapy for PE
- Recurrent septic emboli or PE in cancer patients.

# CONCLUSION

- The clinical diagnosis of DVT and PE is unreliable as many conditions mimic DVT.
- It is essential to assess the clinical probability.
- Only one of the three of the clinically probably cases are confirmed DVT or PE on diagnostic testing.
- About 80% VTE cases can be safely treated at home with LMWH.
- The duration of anticoagulation varies but is generally for 3–6 months.
- Bleeding is the main complication of anticoagulation and needs to be monitored closely and treated.

## PRACTICAL POINTS

- If D-dimer assay is used to evaluate VTE, ensure it has been validated in this setting.
- Never use abnormal D-dimer result to diagnose VTE.
- If we have to test for thrombophilia, draw blood for antithrombin measurement before heparin is given.
- Draw blood for protein C and S measurement before anticoagulation.
- If clinical suspicion for VTE is high and tests are negative continue further testing.
- Patients must avoid antiplatelet drugs with warfarin and must inform the doctor of any change in diet or medication or of acute illness.
- The use of high doses of Vitamin K to reverse supratherapeutic INR may cause warfarin resistance when it is restarted (use higher dose of warfarin).
- Repeat testing for recurrence at regular intervals, even after anticoagulation has stopped, because 50% of DVT have residual thrombus on ultrasound and 33% of PE patients have residual perfusion defects on lung scanning after 1 year of treatment.

# 20

# Approach to the Management of Chronic Venous Insufficiency

*Jaisom Chopra*

## ■ INTRODUCTION

- Chronic venous insufficiency (CVI) is due to lower extremity venous hypertension and is caused by abnormalities in the venous wall and/or venous valves.
- Generally, previous deep venous thrombosis (DVT) is responsible but can be idiopathic.
- Rare causes are arteriovenous (AV) fistulas, cavernous hemangiomas, and pelvic tumors.
- Varicose veins are the most common cause of CVI and affect 10–30% of the adult population.
- Other symptoms include edema, skin changes with hyper-pigmentation, lipodermatosclerosis, and ulceration.
- The incidence of venous stasis syndrome is 76/100,000 person/year and rises as age increases.
- Stasis venous ulcers are a big drain on the state and therefore prevention, early diagnosis, and treatment is very relevant.

## ■ CLINICAL FEATURES

### History and Physical Examination

The symptoms of CVI are variable and include:
- Leg tiredness
- Itching
- Burning
- Cramping
- Swelling.

Physical examination may show:
- Prominent dilated superficial veins
- Edema
- Skin changes
- Ulceration.

## Presenting Features

The typical presentation is:
- Bilateral or unilateral lower limb edema above the ankles without involving the foot or toes. It responds to elevation and is worse in the evenings after the day's standing (Fig. 1)
- Hyperpigmentation (Fig. 2)
- Eczema (Fig. 3)
- Lipodermatosclerosis (scarring to skin and fat) (Fig. 4)
- Varicose veins (Fig. 5)
- Skin ulceration is large and irregular with shallow moist granulation base. They are painful and located above the malleoli (Fig. 6).

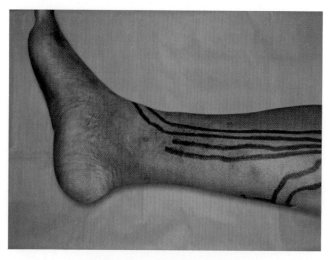

**Fig. 1** Ankle edema sparing foot

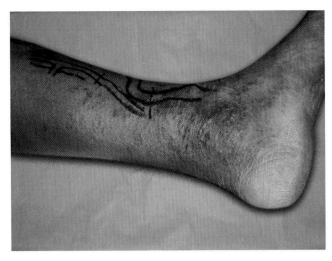

**Fig. 2** Hyperpigmentation

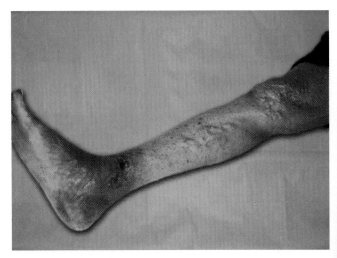

**Fig. 5** Varicose veins and stasis dermatitis

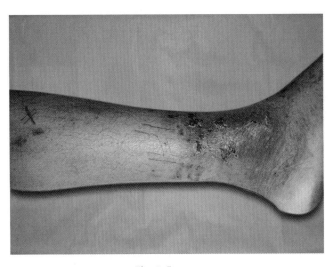

**Fig. 3** Eczema

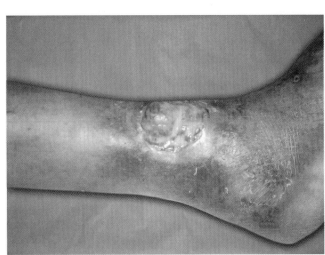

**Fig. 6** Venous ulcer

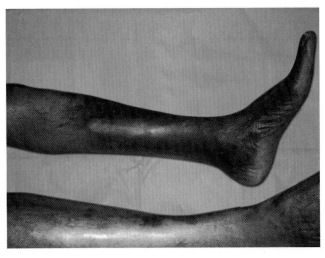

**Fig. 4** Lipodermatosclerosis

## Pathophysiology

This can be broken down into changes that involve:

- Large venous vessels
- Microvasculature
- Tissue.

There is valvular dysfunction in the large veins of the legs resulting in a standing column of blood leading to venous hypertension (Fig. 7).

Venous hypertension is defined as end exercise venous pressure at the ankle more than 30 mm Hg (normal pressure is 15 mm Hg). This leads to capillary dysfunction and tissue injury. The most common cause of valvular dysfunction is DVT. If this is not present, then we suspect valvular agenesis or aplasia. Thirty percent of patients with DVT develop CVI within 8 years. The incidence of CVI rises if there is a delay in the treatment of DVT or proximal veins are involved such as

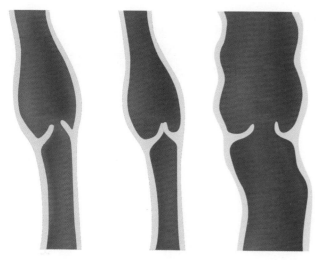

**Fig. 7** Vein dilatation with valve dysfunction

**Table 1** Risk factors for deep vein thrombosis

| Inherited | Acquired | Mixed |
|---|---|---|
| Antithrombin deficiency | Venous instrumentation | Hyperhomocysteinemia |
| Protein C deficiency | Age | Increased factor VIII levels |
| Protein S deficiency | Immobilization | Increased fibrinogen levels |
| Factor V Leiden | Surgery | Increased factor IX levels |
| Prothrombin G20210A | Pregnancy | Increased factor XI levels |
| Blood group (non-O) | Oral contraceptives | |
| | Hormone replacement | |
| | Antiphospholipid syndrome | |
| | Myeloproliferative disorders | |
| | External compression (May-Turner syndrome, pelvic tumors) | |
| | Trauma | |
| | Malignancy | |

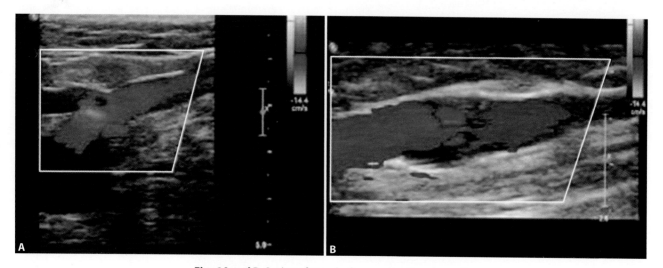

**Figs 8A and B** Saphenofemoral reflux on color-Doppler study

iliofemoral veins and inferior vena cava (IVC). Skin ulceration is more common in patients with recurrent DVT. The risk factors for DVT are listed in Table 1.

Once valvular dysfunction occurs, venous hypertension that follows has profound effects at the microvascular level. Capillaries dilate and become tortuous followed by extravasation of red blood cell (RBC), macromolecules and fluid occurs. White blood cell (WBC) adheres to the endothelium and becomes activated. This leads to capillary thrombosis and tissue hypoxia. The tissue RBC breakdown leading to pigmentation is caused by hemosiderin deposition. The perivascular space becomes surrounded by intravascular matrix proteins. The chronic inflammation leads to scarring and fibrosis of the subcutaneous tissue. Macrophages,

mast cells, and T lymphocytes cause tissue destruction and reduced perfusion causing ischemia, skin breakdown, and ulceration.

## ■ DIAGNOSIS

The tests may be noninvasive or invasive.

Noninvasive tests are performed on every patient after a detailed history and examination including the arterial system and venous system using a bed-side hand-held Doppler. They include:
- Ultrasound testing (Fig. 8)
- Photoplethysmography (PPG)
- Air plethysmography (APG).

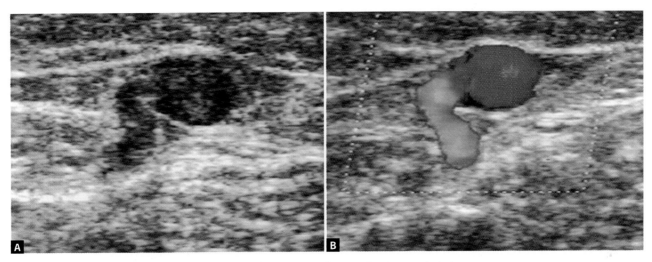

**Figs 9A and B** Color Doppler showing perforator reflux due to valvular incompetence

The invasive tests include:
- Magnetic resonance venography (MRV)
- Phlebography.

The latter two are used only when surgery is contemplated.

Duplex evaluation helps localize specific perforators contributing to the varicose veins and helps differentiate between venous obstruction and valvular incompetence (Fig. 9).

## Duplex Ultrasound

It can diagnose both acute and chronic DVT and incompetence. Compression maneuvers along with augmentation and flow patterns shows saphenofemoral and saphenopopliteal reflux, deep, and superficial veins and perforator reflux. Incompetence at the saphenofemoral junction (SFJ) and saphenopopliteal junction (SPJ) is manifest by Valsalva maneuver and patient in reverse Trendelenburg (15°) position. The incompetent perforators are located by holding the transducer over the perforator and looking for bidirectional flow by compressing and releasing the calf. The limitations are:
- Operator dependent
- Inability to accurately localize lesion above the groin.

## Photoplethysmography

It is performed for screening CVI but cannot quantify the severity and site of CVI. If it is positive, then further tests are needed, but if negative for CVI, then no further testing is necessary.

## Air Plethysmography

It is helpful in:
- Measuring venous reflux
- Calf muscle pump function
- Presence or absence of outflow obstruction.

This consists of a sleeve worn on the leg containing air chambers that are connected to a very sensitive pressure transducer. It measures the functional venous volume, which normally is 80–150 mL but in CVI may increase to 400 mL. The patient is supine and the leg elevated to 45° with the knee slightly flexed. Now, the patient is made to stand and the venous filling index (VFI) measured, which is the ratio between 90% venous volume (VV) and the time taken to fill this 90% (VFT90). Thus, VFI = 90% VV/VFT90. Normally, veins fill from the arterial side with VFI less than 2 mL/s, but in CVI with severe reflux, it may increase to more than 30 mL/s. Increasing VFI is associated with skin changes and ulceration.

Calf muscle pump function is also assessed. The patient now does tip-toe movements and the recorded decrease in pressure represents the ejected volume (EV). Thus, the ejection fraction (EF) is measured by EF = EV/VV × 100. A normal EF is more than 60% while in severe CVI it may be less than 10%. Like VFI, EF is also an important predictor if the patient will develop venous ulcer. The evaluation of venous outflow is also studied with APG. With the patient supine, a proximal thigh tourniquet is inflated to 80 mm Hg. It is then suddenly deflated and the venous outflow fraction at 1 second (OF$_1$) measured. It is expressed as a percentage of the total venous volume. An OF$_1$ less than 28% indicates severe venous obstruction. OF$_1$ between 30% and 40% suggests moderate obstruction and more than 40% absence of significant venous outflow obstruction.

The air plethysmography (APG) gives us a good idea of the various competent contributing to overall severity of CVI. It can be used to assess the effects of treatment like compression stockings are more effective in controlling reflux than improving the calf muscle pump function. It can help us to pick patients for surgical therapy—who would benefit and who will not. So, patients with no outflow obstruction and intact calf muscle pump function will surely benefit with surgical treatment of venous reflux.

## Phlebography

Ascending and descending phlebography, once considered the gold standard, is no longer used because it is invasive, cumbersome, and expensive. It has been replaced by the kinder, patient friendly, noninvasive, and equally effective duplex scanning. By descending phlebography, we can grade the reflux from the saphenofermoral junction:

- Grade I—to upper thigh
- Grade II—till lower thigh but not popliteal vein
- Grade III—till the popliteal vein below the knee
- Grade IV—till the mid-calf.

## ■ MANAGEMENT

### Nonoperative Management of CVI

The goals are:

- Relieving the symptoms
- Preventing ulcer formation
- Promoting ulcer healing.

### Ways to Achieve These Goals

- It is extremely important to prevent edema, as it promotes ulcer formation due to skin breakdown and increases morbidity.
- Patients are taught the importance of leg elevation, exercise to improve the calf muscle pump function, and hygiene (Fig. 10).
- There are no drugs to prevent ulcer formation, therefore the mainstay is compression therapy (Fig. 11).
- Before subjecting the patient to compression, always evaluate for arterial disease. Palpable ankle pulses with no complaint of claudication need no further tests. If the ankle pulses are not palpable or there is a strong history

if intermittent claudication then ankle–brachial index measurement is a must followed by duplex ultrasound.

The recommended compression at the ankle is 30–40 mm Hg with graded compression up the leg. A study conducted for the first episode DVT treated with compression versus no compression stockings showed 60% developed post-phlebitic syndrome within 2 years, if stockings were not worn, whereas half of these developed the complications if stockings were worn.

## Management of Venous Ulcer

Adequate compression is the cornerstone of healing ulcers. The combination of wound covering and compression allows healing of ulcers within 5 months. Multilayer compression therapy helps 80% of the ulcers to heal in 12 weeks and include:

- Bandage of cotton that absorbs the wound exudates and protects bony prominences
- Crape bandage that helps absorb exudates and compresses cotton to shape
- Light compression bandage to maintain pressure and the shape of the limb
- Cohesive flexible bandage that applies pressure, maintaining effective levels of compression.

Once the ulcer has healed, recurrence is prevented compression and methods to reduce the edema.

## Endovascular Treatment of Chronic Venous Occlusion

In May-Turner syndrome, repetitive pulsatile trauma by the right common iliac artery crossing the left common iliac vein causes venous obstruction especially in young pregnant women. A percutaneous venoplasty is performed and stent placed. The results are gratifying (Fig. 12).

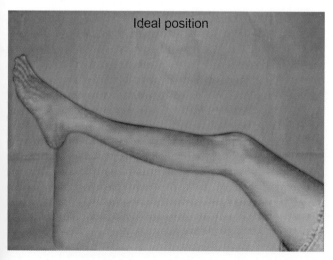

**Fig. 10** Leg elevation

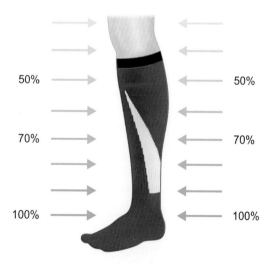

**Fig. 11** Percentage of graduated compression

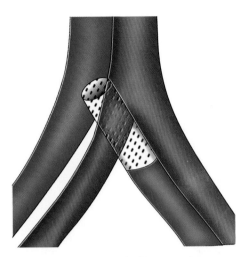

**Fig. 12** Stenting in May-Turner syndrome

## Surgical Management

### General Principles

The most difficult in patient selection is determining who will benefit and what procedure is to be performed. We have to determine the exact site of obstruction, the site of incompetent valve, and the degree of reflux. Without a complete understanding of the pathology, the outcome can go horribly wrong (Flow chart 1).

All patients must be evaluated by CEAP classification (clinical presentation, etiology, anatomy and pathophysiology) prior to surgery (Table 2).

Also, the venous clinical severity scoring system helps assess changes in the venous condition with therapy (Table 3).

Varicose veins must be more than 4 mm in diameter.

### Sclerotherapy

Good technique for treatment of telangiectasia and varicosities (1–3 mm diameter). Sodium tetradecyl sulfate (STDs) 0.5–3% is commonly injected into the veins (0.25–0.5 mL). External compression is applied to produce apposition of the inflamed wall and avoid thrombus formation (Fig. 13).
The likely complications include:
- Pigmentation
- Pain
- Skin necrosis
- DVT (rarely)
- Anaphylactic reaction (very rarely).

### Superficial Vein Resection

The short and mid-term results are good and they help limit the gravitational reflux. High tie and stripping are performed along with stab avulsions through 2–3 mm incisions (Figs 14 and 15).

As most perforating veins are located by duplex study, the need to strip the long saphenous vein (LSV) below the knee does not arise. Also, most perforators below the knee enter into the posterior arch vein rather than the LSV. The complications include:
- Early and late recurrences
- Hematoma formation
- Lymphocele
- Wound infection
- Transient numbness.

Radiofrequency ablation and laser therapy are becoming popular along with foam therapy.

### Perforator Ligation

Subfascial endoscopic perforator surgery (SEPS) alone or with LSV surgery is being performed. The identification of bidirectional flow and localization of the perforators is done by duplex and they are marked. The endoscope is introduced via a single small port and gas insufflation is done. The perforators are ligated and divided. This is used for class 4–6 CVI. Despite this, the recurrence and new ulcer development is a major problem in post-thrombotic limbs.

### Valvuloplasty

The incompetent valves are treated and provided that there is no venous obstruction. This could be by venotomy (internal valvuloplasty) (Fig. 16A) or by taking an external suture (external valvuloplasty) (Fig. 16B).

The purpose is to bring the valve attachments closer by suturing the valve attachments alone or including the valve cusp edges in the repair (Fig. 17).

The long-term follow-up showed success of 60–75%. Postoperative complications occur in only 10% and include thrombosis and bleeding.

### Venous Segment Transfer

The diseased femoral vein is divided and the proximal limb sealed off, while the distal limb anastomosed to the long saphenous vein or the profunda femoris vein with competent valves. The anastomosis may be end to end or end to side. The ulcer recurrence rate stands at 35%, while ulcer-free interval is shorter than primary valvuloplasty.

### Vein Valve Transplantation

Here, a segment of the axillary vein of proven competence by Doppler ultrasound is taken. Either the incompetent popliteal vein or the femoral vein is exposed. A short segment of the vein is excised and the competent axillary vein interposed with interrupted sutures (Fig. 18).

**Flow chart 1** Diagnostic and therapeutic approach to a patient with venous symptoms

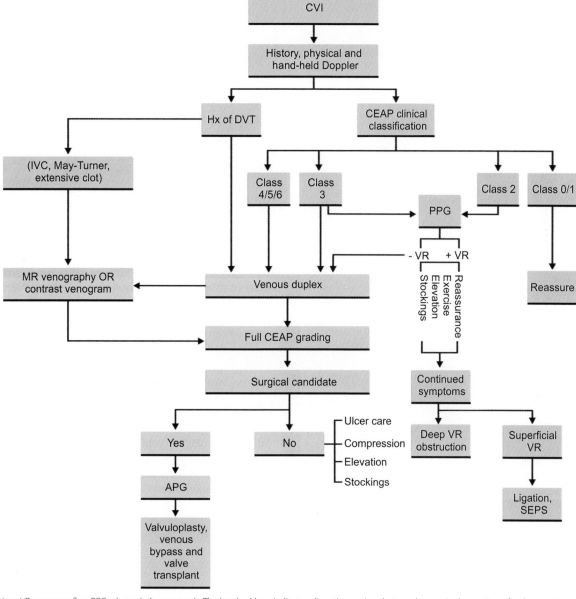

*Abbreviations:* VR, venous reflux; PPG, photoplethysmograph. The hatched bars indicate adjunctive testing that may be required sometimes for diagnostic purposes and for full CEAP classification and may include the following studies: contrast venography, APG, and MR venography.

The patency and the competency of the interposed axillary vein is noted with duplex scanning, and if still defective, then additional valvuloplasty performed. By this method, 80% ulcers heal but the recurrence rate is 30%.

## Venous Bypass

This is an important technique in patient with failed medical treatment. The cross-over femorofemoral bypass is used for iliac vein occlusion, while saphenopopliteal bypass is used for femoral vein occlusion (Fig. 19).

Both surgeries need a single veno-venous anastomosis. Both these procedures need a saphenous vein that is not varicosed and patent. For femorofemoral bypass, the contralateral LSV is used, while for femoropopliteal bypass, the ipsilateral LSV is used (Fig. 20).

The success rate can be 70–80% and long-term patency is 70% with femorofemoral bypass and 50% with femoropopliteal bypass. The morbidity is 5–10% while the mortality is negligible. Recently, iliac vein venoplasty and stenting for the occluded segment is being performed.

**Table 2** Different classifications for venous reflux

| | |
|---|---|
| Clinical classification (add "a" for asymptomatic and "s" for symptomatic) | 0–no visible or palpable signs of venous disease<br>1–telangiectasias or reticular veins<br>2–varicose veins<br>3–edema<br>4–skin changes: dermatitis, eczema, or lipodermatosclerosis<br>5–skin changes—healed ulceration<br>6–skin changes—active ulceration |
| Etiological classification | $E_c$–congenital<br>$E_p$–primary with cause not known<br>$E_s$–secondary with known cause (post-thrombotic, post-traumatic) |
| Anatomical classification | Superficial veins ($A_s$)<br>1–telangiectasias/reticular veins<br>2–long saphenous vein above the knee<br>3–long saphenous vein below the knee<br>4–short saphenous vein<br>5–non-saphenous veins<br>Deep veins ($A_d$)<br>6–inferior vena cava<br>7–common iliac vein<br>8–internal iliac vein<br>9–external iliac vein<br>10–pelvic veins (gonadal, broad ligament)<br>11–common femoral<br>12–deep femoral vein<br>13–superficial femoral vein<br>14–popliteal vein<br>15–crural veins (anterior tibial, posterior tibial and peroneal veins)<br>16–muscular veins (gastrocnemius and soleus)<br>Perforating veins (Ap)<br>17–thigh veins<br>18–calf veins |
| Pathophysiological classification | $P_r$–reflux<br>$P_o$–obstruction<br>$P_{r,o}$–reflux and obstruction |

**Table 3** Grades of chronic venous insufficiency depending upon the clinical presentation

| Attribute | Absent = 0 | Mild = 1 | Moderate = 2 | Severe = 3 |
|---|---|---|---|---|
| Pain | None | Occasional, not restricting activity or needing analgesics | Daily, moderate activity limitation, occasional analgesics | Daily severe, limiting activity or needing regular use of analgesics |
| Varicose veins | None | Few scattered or branch VVs | Multiple: LSV varicosed and confined to calf or thigh | Extensive in thigh and calf involving thigh and calf |
| Venous edema | None | Evening ankle edema only | Afternoon edema above ankle | Morning edema above ankle needing elevation and activity change |
| Skin pigmentation | None or focal, low intensity (tan) | Diffuse but limited in area and old (brown) | Diffuse over lower 1/3 leg or recent pigmentation | Distribution above lower 1/3 and recent pigmentation |
| Inflammation | None | Mild cellulitis around ulcer area | Moderate cellulitis involving lower 1/3 | Severe cellulitis lower 1/3 and above or significant venous eczema |
| Induration | None | Focal circum-malleolar (<5 cm) | Medial or lateral < lower 1/3 leg | Entire lower 1/3 leg or more |
| No. of active ulcers | 0 | 1 | 2 | >2 |
| Active ulceration duration | None | <3 months | >3 months, <1 year | Not healed >1 year |
| Active ulcer size | None | <2 cm diameter | 2–6 cm diameter | >6 cm diameter |
| Compressive therapy | Not used or not compliant | Intermittent use of stocking | Wears elastic stocking most days | Full compliance: stocking and elevation |

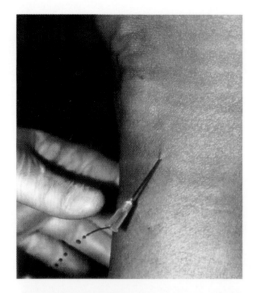

**Fig. 13** Sclerotherapy–drug is inserted into the diseased vein

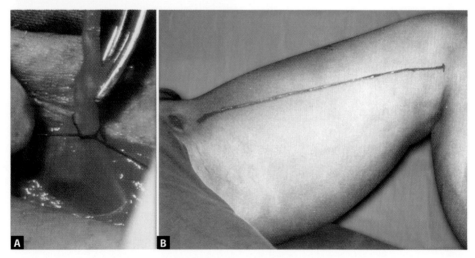

**Figs 14A and B** High tie and stripping

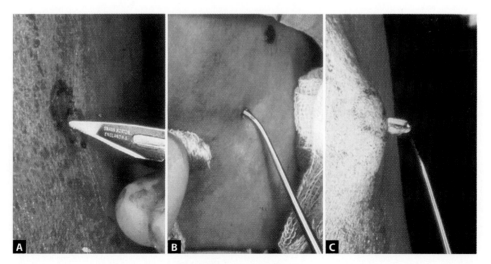

**Figs 15A to C** Stab avulsions

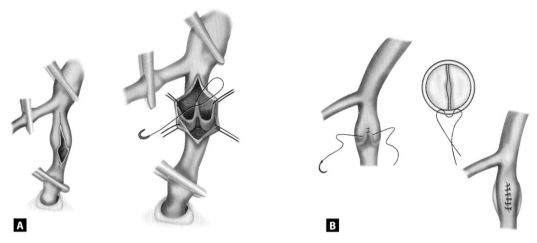

**Figs 16A and B**  (A) Longitudinal incision for internal valvuloplasty; (B) External valvuloplasty

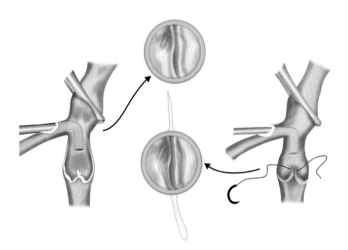

**Fig. 17**  External valvuloplasty under angioscopic guidance

## ■ CONCLUSION

Chronic venous insufficiency (CVI) is a common disorder due to chronic venous reflux and venous hypertension. Varicose veins are the most common manifestation of CVI. Untreated lower limb edema in CVI is a prelude to venous ulceration. The goals of management of CVI are:

- Patient education
- Symptoms control
- Preventing ulcers
- Promoting ulcer healing.

Graded compression stockings help treat CVI in initial stages. Always grade CVI using the CEAP classification and venous clinical scoring system prior to any surgical intervention.

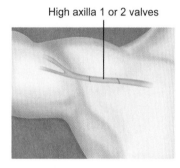

High axilla 1 or 2 valves

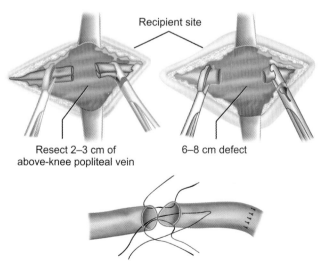

Recipient site

Resect 2–3 cm of above-knee popliteal vein

6–8 cm defect

**Fig. 18**  Axillary vein transposition to defective popliteal vein in the leg

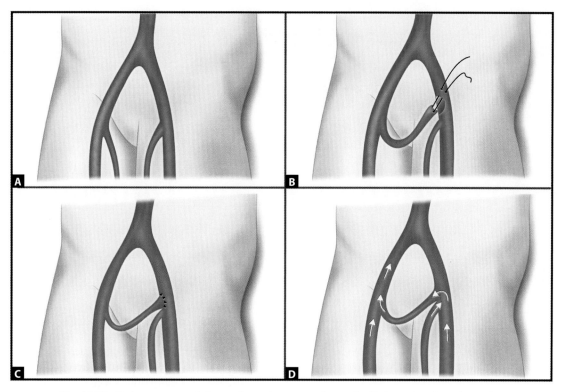

**Figs 19A to D**  Autogenous vein femorofemoral cross-over bypass for iliofemoral outflow obstruction

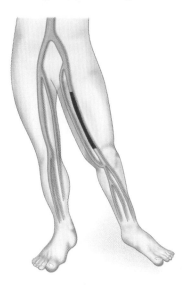

**Fig. 20**  Autogenous vein saphenopopliteal venous bypass for SF vein obstruction

## PRACTICAL POINTS

- CVI occurs in patients with DVT but could occur as a primary idiopathic phenomenon.
- Varicose veins are the most common manifestation of CVI.
- Chronic venous ulcers occur typically above the medial malleolus and less rarely above the lateral malleolus.
- Venous hypertension is the end-exercise venous pressure at the ankle above 30 mm Hg (normal is 15 mm Hg).
- A rare cause of non-healing venous ulcers is squamous cell carcinoma (Marjolin's ulcer).
- APG has high sensitivity and specificity for diagnosing any reflux.
- CEAP clinical class is helpful in deciding the diagnostic tests.
- Full CEAP classification is needed prior to any invasive treatment approach.

# 21

# Upper Extremity Deep Vein Thrombosis and Superior Vena Cava Thrombosis

*Jaisom Chopra*

## ■ INTRODUCTION

- Upper extremity deep vein thrombosis (UEDVT) is an increasing common clinical problem responsible for considerable morbidity.
- UEDVT involves the subclavian and axillary veins and may be primary or secondary.
- UEDVT presents as swelling and pain.

Upper extremity deep vein thrombosis may be either primary or secondary:

- *Primary (idiopathic) DVT*
  - Effort thrombosis of axillary and subclavian veins (Paget-Schroetter syndrome)
  - Occult cancer
  - Thrombophilia.
- *Secondary*
  - Central venous catheters
  - Pacemakers and defibrillators
  - Local head and neck malignancy.

## ■ CLASSIFICATION OF UPPER EXTREMITY DEEP VEIN THROMBOSIS

This typically involves the axillary, subclavian, and brachiocephalic veins and is becoming increasingly common due to use of indwelling catheters in the upper extremity.

### Primary Upper Extremity Thrombosis

- This may arise de novo or may be effort induced (Paget–Schroetter syndrome).
- It may be a presentation of undetected cancer.
- Repeated micro-trauma may be responsible for the thrombosis.
- Stricture of the axillo-subclavian vein due to chronic compression of the hypertrophied scalene muscle/subclavius

tendon and the first rib. This is seen in the dominant arm after strenuous exercise such as weight lifting, rowing, or baseball pitching in healthy young persons. This repeated trauma activates the coagulation cascade.
- Seen also in thoracic outlet syndrome (TOS) where compression of the neurovascular bundle along with brachial plexus, subclavian artery and vein.

### Secondary Thrombosis

- Due to indwelling catheters, pacemakers and external compression from malignancy.
- There is generally swelling and discomfort. However, there may be no symptoms at all and detected accidently on incidental imaging.
- High fever suggests septic thrombophlebitis and infectious cause should be found.

### Central Venous Thrombosis Associated with Long-term Central Venous Instrumentation

- Central lines are responsible for partial thrombosis in 30–45% and complete thrombosis in 5–10%. The common procedures causing thrombosis are hemodialysis catheters, chemotherapy, total parenteral nutrition (TPN), and repeated transfusions (Fig. 1). The incidence of thrombosis is same for catheters placed for short or long-term. The determinant for clot formation is:
  - Size of catheter used
  - Use of subclavian access route
  - Underlying central venous stenosis.
  - Hemodialysis patients are more prone due to multiple catheter insertions and formations of ipsilateral AV fistulas.

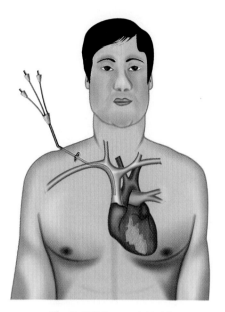

**Fig. 1** CVP line on right side

**Table 1** Symptoms and signs of UEDVT

| | Symptoms | Signs |
|---|---|---|
| Axillary or subclavian vein thrombosis | Vague shoulder/neck discomfort<br><br>Arm or hand edema | Supraclavicular fullness<br>Arm or hand edema<br>Extremity cyanosis<br>Dilated cutaneous veins<br>Jugular vein distension<br>Cannot introduce central venous pressure (CVP) catheter |
| Thoracic outlet syndrome | Pain radiating to arm or forearm<br><br>Hand weakness | Brachial plexus tenderness<br>Arm and hand atrophy<br>Positive Adson or Wright maneuver |
| Superior vena cava syndrome | Fullness and ache in head and neck aggravated by dependency and stretching neck (increase venous return)<br>Swelling of face, neck, and eyelids | Engorged neck and upper extremity veins |

# ■ CLINICAL FEATURES

## Symptoms and Signs (Table 1)

- Axillary and subclavian vein thrombosis may be totally asymptomatic.
- Superior vena cava (SVC) occlusion leads to facial and arm edema, head fullness, blurred vision, and shortness of breath.
- In TOS, pain radiates to the fourth and fifth digits due to injury to the brachial plexus.
- In TOS, symptoms worsen with abduction and lifting of shoulder.
- Adson's maneuver—arm is extended on the affected side and the neck is extended and head rotated to the same side (Fig. 2). A positive test is weakening of the radial pulse on the affected side on deep inspiration, which shows compression of the subclavian artery.
- Wright's maneuver—the shoulder abducted and the humerus externally rotated. A positive test is weakening of the radial pulse (Fig. 3).

## Diagnostic Imaging (Table 2)

- Duplex ultrasound is noninvasive and highly sensitive and specific. However, it has limitations that include:
  - Overshadowing by the clavicle that may impair seeing a short segment of the subclavian vein leading to false negative result
  - Extension of SVC clot may be inadequately seen.

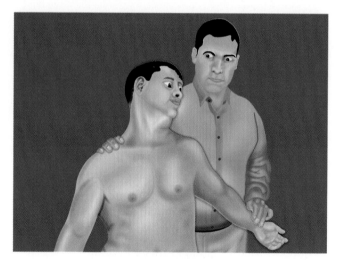

**Fig. 2** Adson's test

- Magnetic resonance venography (MRV)—visualizes clot in the thoracic veins, noninvasively.
- Contrast venography—is gold standard and performed prior to surgical intervention, catheter-directed thrombolysis, or venoplasty. It has the following limitations:
  - Iodine contrast reaction
  - Difficult to cannulate vein in an edematous arm
  - Exposure to radiation in pregnant females.

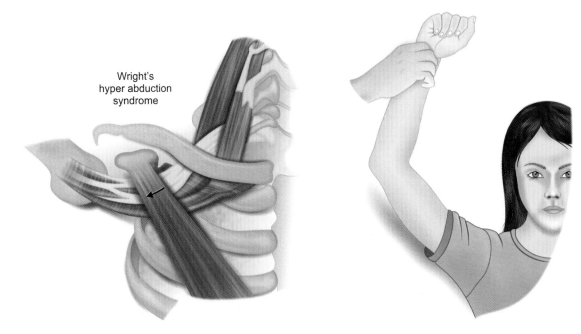

Wright's
hyper abduction
syndrome

**Fig. 3** Wright's manuever

**Table 2** Advantages and disadvantages of the imaging modalities

| | Advantages | Disadvantages |
|---|---|---|
| Ultrasound | Inexpensive, noninvasive, and reproducible | May fail to detect central thrombus lying directly below clavicle |
| CT scan | Detects central thrombus and presence of external vessel compression | Reaction to contrast dye |
| Magnetic resonance venography | Accurately detects central thrombus, collaterals, and blood flow | Limited availability<br>Claustrophobia<br>Unsuitable for patients with metal implants |

## ■ MANAGEMENT OF PATIENT

This depends upon the etiology being primary or secondary. The goals are:
- Prevention of further progression of thrombus
- Improvement in venous blood flow
- Prevention of recurrent thrombus
  The treatment options are tabulated in Table 3.

### Anticoagulation

- Initially, unfractionated heparin or low molecular heparin is given followed by warfarin or its substitute for at least 3 months keeping International Normalized Ratio (INR) between 2 and 3. Thrombophilia needs prolonged anticoagulation.
- Venous catheter responsible for UEDVT must be removed and anticoagulation given.
- Swelling is reduced by limb elevation and graduated compression sleeve.

- About one-third of patients with UEDVT have pulmonary embolism (PE), which could be fatal.
- Catheter removal may cause fibrin sheath to peel off from the catheter and embolize to the lungs. So, patients should be observed for PE after removal of catheter.

### Thrombolytics

- Unless contraindicated, all patients with acute or subacute UEDVT proven venographically should undergo CDT with or without percutaneous mechanical thrombectomy.
- Early lysis minimizes scarring and fibrosis.
- Patients presenting before 7 days have best response, while after 7 days the response reduces.
- Thrombolytic agents used are urokinase and recombinant tissue plasminogen (rTPA). CDT using rTPA as a continuous infusion 1–2 mg/h for 8 h with serial venograms to see response of treatment. A pulse wave catheter placed in the thrombus delivers rTPA over 15 minutes.

**Table 3** Treatment options for UEDVT

| *General measures* |
| --- |
| Limb elevation |
| Graduated compression arm sleeve |
| Physiotherapy |
| Diuretics |
| Anticoagulants |
| Heparin as bridge to warfarin |
| Low-molecular weight heparin (LMWH) as bridge to warfarin |
| LMWH as monotherapy |
| *Endovascular approaches* |
| Catheter-directed thrombolysis (CDT) |
| Suction thrombectomy |
| Angioplasty with or without stenting |
| *Surgical therapy* |
| Surgical thrombectomy |
| Thoracic outlet compression |
| SVC filter |

Heparin is given with thrombolytic agents to reduce clot formation around the catheter.

- Mechanical thrombectomy reduces the bulk of thrombus thus helping the clot to dissolve using lower dose of thrombolysis. Research is underway to use combination of ultrasound and thrombolysis for early thrombus dissolution.

## Endovascular Treatment

This has largely replaced surgical treatment in symptomatic primary and secondary UEDVT (Flow chart 1).

All types of secondary UEDVT and recurrences are treated by endovascular means with good results and patency rates. Hemodialysis patients with repeated subclavian punctures have a high restenosis rate after stenting. In such cases, repeated balloon dilatation or surgical bypass is indicated. Recurrent stenosis after stenting may also be treated with brachytherapy or drug-eluting stent.

## Surgery

- It is only for patients with vein compression causing recurrent thrombosis and post-thrombotic syndrome.
- The assessment is made after successful thrombolysis using ultrasound or venogram in the shoulder abducted position.
- Surgical thrombectomy is rarely done in refractory cases and carries the risk from general anesthesia, pneumothorax, and brachial plexus injury.

- Before surgical therapy, a conservative approach is indicated including physiotherapy to reduce muscle compression of subclavian vein, weight loss if indicated, and nonsteroidal anti-inflammatory drugs.

### Timing of Surgical Decompression

If after successful thrombolysis there is significant stenosis, then early surgical correction is indicated, whereas if the stenosis is minimal and good flow is achieved, then surgical correction is not urgent.

### Prophylaxis

This reduces the chances of UEDVT in cancer patients with indwelling CVP catheters. Warfarin is administered in minidose of 1 mg daily that does not prolong PT or cause bleeding. This low therapy is avoided in patients with advanced liver disease, liver metastasis, poor nutrition, or receiving broad-spectrum antibiotics, as it may cause bleeding from prolonged PT. The alternative is LMWH in once-daily dose of 2500 U dalteparin. There is no bleeding even with chemotherapy that causes bone marrow depression. It is avoided in patients with renal dysfunction.

## ■ SPECIAL ISSUES

## Post-thrombotic Syndrome (Fig. 4)

- This is caused by venous hypertension secondary to outflow obstruction and valvular injury.
- It may cause mild edema without much trouble or it may present with incapacitating limb swelling with pain and ulceration.
- Graded compression sleeve is recommended.
- The results of conventional anticoagulation therapy are doubtful and a large majority develops long-term complications and therefore initial thrombolysis is recommended in primary UEDVT especially the young.
- In secondary UEDVT, surgery or thrombolysis is seldom needed and anticoagulation is recommended.
- The short-term mortality is high and is from causes such as cancer, infection, and multisystem organ failure rather than UEDVT.

## ■ SUPERIOR VENA CAVA THROMBOSIS

Malignancy accounts for more than 85% and the causes are given in Table 4.

## Clinical Features

- Fullness in the head and neck worsened by lying and exercise
- Patient may have a throbbing headache
- There is accompanying venous hypertension responsible for confusion, dizziness, and orthopnea

**Flow chart 1** Management of patients with UEDVT

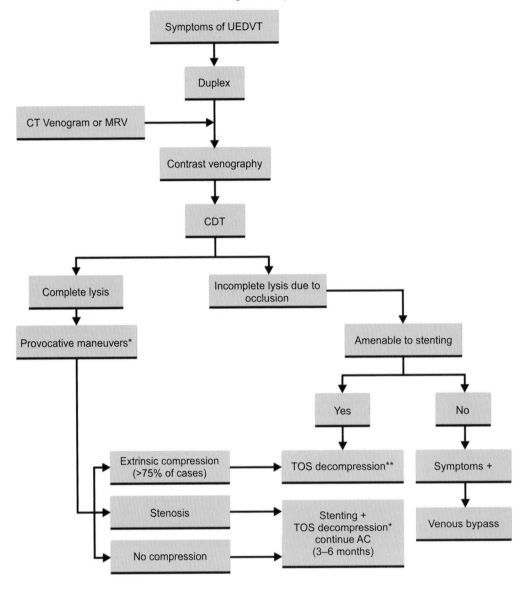

* done on repeat venography at conclusion of lytic protocal
** typically done 2–4 weeks later

- There is swelling of the face, eyelids, and upper extremity
- There is venous engorgement in the neck and dilated veins over the chest wall (Fig. 5)
- In lung cancer, there may be malignant SVC syndrome (SVS) causing hemoptysis, hoarseness (recurrent laryngeal nerve involvement), weight loss, and lymph node swelling.

## Diagnostic Imaging

- The diagnosis is made on contrast computed tomographic (CT) chest. There is non-opacification of SVC along with extensive collaterals
- Duplex ultrasound is not very helpful
- MRV is an alternative to contrast CT chest.

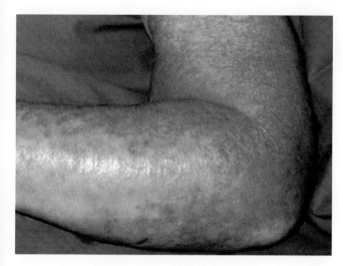

**Fig. 4** Post-thrombotic syndrome

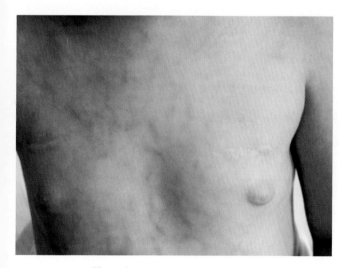

**Fig. 5** Superior vena cava syndrome

## Management of SVC Syndrome

### General Measures

- Sleep with pillows
- Avoid heavy exercise
- Avoid tight fitting garments
- Diuretic if edema is severe
- Thrombolysis for acute SVC syndrome.

**Table 4** Causes of malignancy

| Malignancy |
| --- |
| Adenocarcinoma lung |
| Thyroid carcinoma |
| Mediastinal lymphoma, thymoma or teratoma |
| Non-malignant (benign) |
| Mediastinitis and mediastinal fibrosis |
| Indwelling lines such as CVP catheters |
| Pacemakers and defibrillators |

### Approach to SVC Thrombosis (Flow chart 2)

- Radiation therapy with or without chemotherapy for malignancies reduces the tumor bulk and gives relief.
- These patients present several months with chronic SVC syndrome.
- Venography is done bilaterally via the basialic vein to see the extent of the thrombosis and for catheter-directed thrombolysis (CDT).
- This therapy is contraindicated in metastatic disease to the brain and the spinal cord.

### Endoscopic Approach to SVC Syndrome

Venoplasty and stenting is indicated wherever possible. Primary patency rates for 1 year are 50–75% while secondary patency rates range from 25% to 85%. In 25%, adjuvent CDT is done with success of over 95%.

### Surgical Approach

Indicated in those with life expectancy more than 1 year. Bypass graft using PTFE from left innominate to right atrium is used.

## ■ CONCLUSION

- UEDVT is a common problem due to the increased use of CVP catheters for chemotherapy, bone marrow transplant, dialysis, and TPN.
- Concern about PE but fortunately fatal PE is rare.
- Duplex ultrasound is noninvasive with high sensitivity and specificity.
- Anticoagulation with warfarin is key to treatment in UEDVT.
- Endovascular therapy has replaced surgery.
- Low-dose warfarin is effective in patients with CVP catheters.

**Flow chart 2** Approach to SVC syndrome

## PRACTICAL POINTS

- Seen in 25% with CVP catheters.
- Coagulation disorders in these patients is uncertain.
- Testing for hypercoagulable states should be done in idiopathic cases, family history of DVT, history of recurrent miscarriage, or prior personal history of DVT.
- Endoscopic venoplasty and stenting is primarily done in patients with UEDVT and SVC syndrome.
- Endovascular techniques are also helpful to prolong patency of PTFE grafts for SVC occlusions.

# 22

# Management of Vasculogenic Impotence

*Jaisom Chopra*

## ■ INTRODUCTION

- Erectile dysfunction (ED) is the persistent inability to attain or to maintain penile erection sufficient for sexual performance.
- The incidence increases with age and affects 30% males between 40 and 70 years. In US, there are 30 million sufferers.
  Risk factors are the same to that of atherosclerosis and listed in Table 1.
- ED often coexists with coronary artery disease (CAD) and is found in patients with myocardial infarction (MI) and chronic heart failure (CHF). Drugs such as antihypertensives, diuretics, and antianginal also affect ED. Though not proven, possibly oxidative stress resulting in vascular endothelial dysfunction results in ED.

**Table 1** Risk factors of vasculogenic impotence

| |
|---|
| Hypertension |
| Trauma or surgery to the pelvis or the spine |
| Vascular surgery |
| Hyperlipidemia |
| Coronary or peripheral artery disease |
| Diabetes |
| Hypogonadism |
| Peyronie's disease |
| Endocrine disorder |
| Smoking |
| Depression |
| Alcohol and drug abuse |

## ■ CLINICAL FEATURES

### Physiology and Pathophysiology of Erection

#### Vascular Supply and Innervations of the Penis

- Erection is a hemodynamic event as a result of multiple influences on the penile smooth muscle. It requires adequate blood flow to the paired corpora cavernosa surrounding the penile urethra and the corpora spongiosum at the glans penis (Fig. 1).
- The central nervous system (CNS) plays a vital role in penile erection. The hypothalamus is the integration point for central control of erection, as it receives rich sensory supply of impulses from other brain areas. Auditory stimuli, visual stimuli, and fantasy initiate impulses that project to the hypothalamus and then travel via the spinal cord to the peripheral nerves that supply the penile vasculature, initiating erection (Fig. 2).

Penis is innervated by sympathetic (T11–L2), parasympathetic (S2–S4), and somatic (S2–S4) nerves. Sympathetic input is anti-erectile, while parasympathetic and somatic inputs are pro-erectile. Both the sympathetic and parasympathetic fibers reach the inferior hypogastric plexus in the pelvis where the autonomic input to the pelvis is integrated and penile innervations via the cavernous nerves originate. The lesser cavernous nerves travel along the penis to supply the penile urethra and the erectile tissue of the corpora spongiosum, whereas the greater cavernous nerves innervate the helicine arteries in the erectile tissue. The somatic component, the pudendal nerve through the dorsal nerve branches, is responsible for the penile sensation and the contraction and relaxation of the extracorporeal striated muscles (bulbocavernosus and ischiocavernosus).

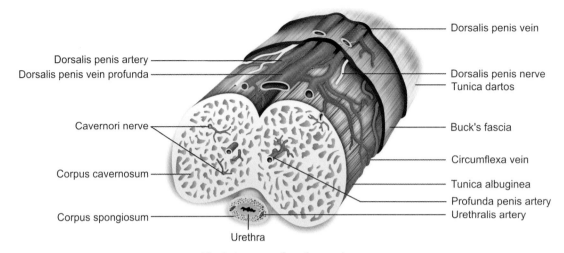

**Fig. 1** Anatomy of penile vasculature

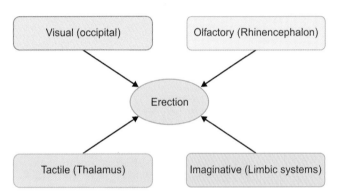

**Fig. 2** Stimuli for erection

## Erection Phase

- In response to sexual stimulus, parasympathetic neural activity predominates causing increased blood flow to cavernous sinuses and erection due to smooth muscle relaxation. Smooth muscle relaxation is mediated by the neurotransmitter nitric oxide released from the endothelium of corpus cavernosa during nonadrenergic, noncholinergic neurotransmission.
- Nitric oxide activates a soluble guanylyl cyclase that increases intracellular concentration of cyclic guanosine monophosphate (cGMP). cGMP helps accumulate cGMP-dependent protein kinase, which in turn phosphorylates specific proteins and ion-channels (potassium). This results in hyperpolarization of smooth muscle cell membrane with resultant sequestration of intracellular calcium in the endoplasmic reticulum and blocking the calcium influx by calcium channel inhibition. Thus, decrease of the intracellular calcium concentration and smooth muscle relaxation takes place. The rapid filling of the penile sinusoids expands the sinuses and in turn compresses the subtruncal venular plexuses causing

near-total occlusion of the venous outflow. This traps the blood within the corpus cavernosum raising the penis from a dependent to erectile position. The intracavernosal pressures may exceed 90 mm Hg during full phase of penile erection. During intercourse or masturbation, the bulbocavernosus reflux results in forcible compression of the base of the blood filled corpora cavernosae causing the penis to become even harder with transcavernous pressures exceeding several hundred mm Hg. During the maintenance phase of penile erection, blood flow into and leaving the penis temporarily stops (Fig. 3).

## Detumescence Phase

There is sudden suppression of the neurotransmitter release, breakdown of the second messenger products, or discharge of sympathetic stimuli during ejaculation. Constriction of the trabecular smooth muscles reopens the venous channels causing the expulsion of the trapped blood and return of the flaccid state.

Erectile dysfunction (ED) may be due to abnormalities in one or several steps involved in the initiation or maintenance of the erection.

## Differential Diagnosis of ED

This may be psychogenic, organic, or mixed etiologies (Table 2).

## Psychogenic Erectile Dysfunction

Depression, anxiety, and schizophrenia are common psychiatric disorders associated with ED secondary to decreased libido and treatments that may have undesired effects on ED. There may be no medical problem but may represent performance anxiety that may be triggered by:

- Anger and feel isolated from partner
- Separation/divorce

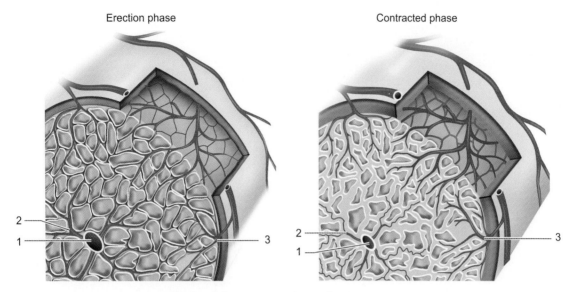

Erection phase                    Contracted phase

**Fig. 3** 1. Helicine arteries 2. Sinusoids 3. Emissary veins

**Table 2** Differential diagnosis of ED

|  | Common disorder | Pathophysiology |
|---|---|---|
| Psychogenic | Depression<br>Anxiety disorder<br>Relationship conflict<br>Schizophrenia<br>Stress | Decreased libido<br>Treatment side effects |
| Organic<br>Neurogenic | Cerebrovascular accident<br>Alzheimer's or Parkinson's<br>Spinal cord injury<br>Diabetic neuropathy<br>Radical pelvic surgery | Failure to initiate or<br>transmit nerve impulses |
| Hormonal | Hypogonadism<br>Thyroid disease<br>hyperprolactinemia | Decreased libido<br>Endothelial dysfunction |
| Vascular | Atherosclerosis<br>Peyronie's disease<br>Trauma | Endothelial dysfunction<br>Decreased arterial blood<br>flow<br>Impaired veno-occlusion |
| Drug induced | Antidepressants<br>Antihypertensives<br>Diuretics<br>Alcohol and cigarette abuse | Central suppression<br>Decreased libido |
| Multifactorial<br>systemic<br>diseases | Diabetes mellitus<br>Chronic renal failure<br>Coronary artery disease | Vascular dysfunction<br>Neural dysfunction |
| Mixed<br>psychogenic<br>and organic | Mixed of above | Multifactorial |

- Guilt
- Illness in self or partner
- Job failure or great disappointment with self.

## Organic Causes of Erectile Dysfunction

- Neurogenic—damage to CNS from cardiovascular accident (CVA) or degenerative processes such as Alzheimer's or Parkinson's disease may lead to ED. Peripheral nerve damage due to spinal cord injury, diabetic neuropathy, aortic, or prostate surgery may also lead to ED.
- Endocrine—testosterone deficiency causes reduced libido and inability to maintain erection secondary to low levels of nitric oxide synthase. Besides hyperprolactinemia, hyperthyroidism and hypothyroidism can cause ED. If the cause is determined, then correction leads to correction of ED.
- Vasculogenic—anatomic defects in arterial and venous systems may be responsible for ED. Arterial stenosis or inability to vasodilate arteries due to atherosclerosis prevents adequate blood flow into the penis for erection and is the most common of ED. Aortoiliac occlusive disease causing claudication, reduced femoral pulses, and flow along with ED is called Leriche's syndrome. Venous dysfunction causing failure of veins to close during erection may prevent maintenance of erection. Causes of abnormal venous drainage include Peyronie's disease, aging, and diabetes mellitus.
- Medications (Table 3).
- Mixed—systemic diseases such as diabetes, chronic renal failure, coronary artery disease, and aging can contribute to ED secondary to neurogenic and vascular dysfunction.

**Table 3** Medications for ED

| Category | Class |
|---|---|
| Antihypertensives/ heart failure | β-blockers—atenolol, metoprolol, and pro-panolol |
| | Diuretics—thiazide agents and loop diuretics |
| | Vasodilators—hydralazine, diazoxide, and minoxidil |
| | Spironolactone |
| Antidepressants | Selective serotonin uptake inhibitors—fluoxetine, fluvoxamine, paroxetine, sertraline |
| | Tricyclic antidepressants—amitriptyline, imipramine, nortriptyline |
| | Monoamine oxidase inhibitors—phenelzine, isocarboxazid, tranylcypromine |
| | Selective serotonin and norepinephrine reuptake inhibitors—venlafaxine |
| | Lithium |
| Antipsychotics | Phenothiazines—chlorpromazine, thioridazine, fluphenazine |
| Antiepileptics | Diphenylhydantoin, carbamazepine, valproic acid |
| Lipid lowering | Gemfibrozil |
| Ulcer healing | H2 antagonists |
| Anti-gout | Allopurinol |
| | Indomethacin |
| Anti-Parkinson's | L-dopa |
| Miscellaneous | Antihistamines—phenothiazine |
| Hormonal agents | Estrogen, androgen, cyproterone acetate, luteinizing hormone-releasing hormone analogs |

**Flow chart 1** Initial approach to ED and differentiating psychogenic from organic ED

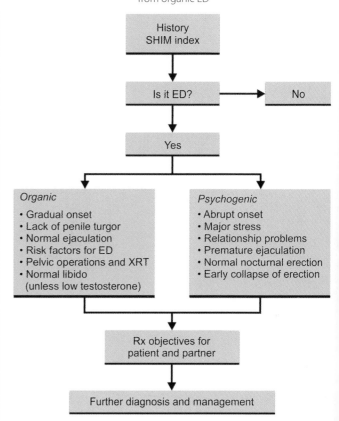

## ■ DIAGNOSIS

## History

- It is important to take a complete history and understand what the patient means by ED, as this may prevent much testing (Flow chart 1).
- It is often helpful to have a clear picture of the cycle of event involved leading up to ED and working one's way downwards from CNS. One has to distinguish psyco-genic causes from organic causes. A sensitive sexual history is needed to record changes in sexual desire and disturbances in orgasm or ejaculation. The questions enlisting in Table 4 may be helpful.
- One must ask about the nature of onset of ED, frequency, duration, and quality of erections; presence of morning or night erections; and ability to achieve sexual satisfaction. The Sexual Health Inventory for Men (SHIM) is a questionnaire to help screening ED patients in vascular patients (Table 5).
- There is a scale of 1–5 with 1 being the least functional response. The SHIM score lies between 5 and 25. More than 22 show normal erectile function, while less than 11 show moderate to severe ED.

**Table 4** Screening for erectile dysfunction (ED): evaluating the phases of male sexual cycle

| Sexual phase | Question | Information |
|---|---|---|
| Desire | Do you feel in the mood, have desire, sexual thoughts? | ED preceded with loss of desire signals hormonal problems, relationship problems, medication side effect, depression |
| Arousal | Do you have trouble getting or keeping an erection? Do you wake up with an erection? Can you get an erection with self stimulation? | Distinguishes psychogenic from organic ED. Indicates stress or anxiety as a trigger |
| Orgasm | Do you feel you ejaculate too quickly? Do you ever have difficulty reaching orgasm or ejaculating? | Anxiety over quick or delayed (retrograde) ejaculation may lead to psychogenic ED |
| Resolution | Do you have pain after sex? Do you light up a cigarette after sex? | Reveals Peyronie's disease or pain disorder. Reveals risk factor for ED |

**Table 5** Sexual health inventory for men

| Over the past 6 months | Very low | Low | Moderate | High | Very high |
|---|---|---|---|---|---|
| How do you rate your confidence to get and keep an erection? | 1 | 2 | 3 | 4 | 5 |
| When you had erection with sexual stimulation how often were your erections hard enough for penetration? | Never or almost never 1 | A few times (much less than half the time) 2 | Sometime (about half the times) 3 | Most times (much more than half the time) 4 | Almost always or always 5 |
| During sexual intercourse how often were you able to maintain your erection after penetration? | Never or almost never 1 | A few times (much less than half the time) 2 | Sometime (about half the times) 3 | Most times (much more than half the time) 4 | Almost always or always 5 |
| During sexual intercourse how difficult was it to maintain your erection till completion? | Extremely difficult 1 | Very difficult 2 | Difficult 3 | Slightly difficult 4 | Never difficult 5 |
| On attempting sexual intercourse how often was it satisfactory for you? | Never or almost never 1 | A few times (much less than half the time) 2 | Sometime (about half the times) 3 | Most times (much more than half the time) 4 | Almost always or always 5 |

- ED may be a manifestation of systemic disease so all patients must be screened for diabetes and CAD. History of alcoholism, cigarette smoking, and hypogonadism should be sought, as it may cause decrease libido.

## Physical Examination

Look for hormonal imbalance as in atrophic testis, reduced peripheral pulses as in peripheral vascular disease (PVD), and neuropathy as detected on sensory examination (Flow chart 2).

## Laboratory Testing

Routine testing in ED consists of:
- Fasting blood sugar or glycosylated hemoglobin
- Renal function tests
- Liver function tests
- Lipid profile
- Testosterone or androgen index
- Prolactin levels
- Sickle screen in African-American patients.

## Specialized Testing

- Vascular testing is generally not indicated unless PAD is severe
- Penile blood pressure index is done to show resting blood flow to penis.
- Nocturnal penile tumescence testing (NPT) in psychogenic cause to ED. It measures spontaneous night time erections. Patients with night time erection on NPT are more likely to have a psychogenic cause while patients with no night time erections are likely to have an organic cause.
- If PVD is suspected as a cause of ED, then color Doppler study and penile angiography are considered before revascularization.

**Flow chart 2** Recommended diagnostic approach to ED

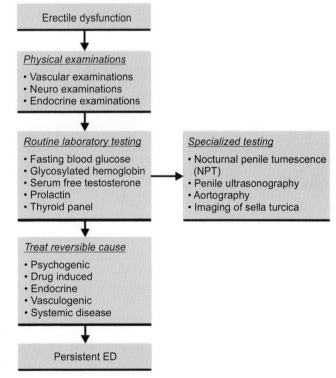

## ■ MANAGEMENT

- The first step is to assess for reversible causes. Patients with hyperprolactinemia, hypothyroidism, or hyperthyroidism should be treated for the causes.
- If neurological causes (brain and spinal cord) are suspected, then neurological consultation is sought.

- Patients with psychological ED should have psychosexual therapy.
- If medication is responsible, then alter or stop the offending drug.
- The patient progresses to the staged therapy choosing the options with which he and his partner are most comfortable.
- Various lifestyle modifications are suggested, as they have a positive impact on the patient's health. These include diet, exercise programs, stress reduction, reduce alcohol, and drug abuse and stop smoking (Flow chart 3).

## Androgens in Erectile Dysfunction

- This is for patients with well-documented hypogonadism because if this is not present and the patient receives androgens, his sexual behavior is activated without improving ED
- Testosterone stimulates libido at the CNS level
- Androgen replacement therapy includes oral therapy, intramuscular injection, or subcutaneous implants
- Testosterone therapy does not improve ED unless free testosterone levels are very low (<8 pg/mL)
- Oral testosterone is less effective than intramuscular

- Testosterone has an, increased incidence of liver toxicity, prostatic hypertrophy and cancer
- Digital rectal examination, baseline PSA, and lipid profile are done before starting testosterone therapy and repeated every 6–12 months to monitor patients receiving androgen therapy.

## First Line of Treatment of ED

- *Phosphodiesterase Type 5 (PDE 5) inhibitors:* This constitutes first line of treatment, as PDE 5 have been isolated in the human tissue and it inhibits PDE 5 found in the tissue of the corpora cavernosum of the penis. By blocking the degradation of cGMP by nitric oxide, PDE inhibition promotes vasodilatation and erectile function in ED. The available PDE 5 inhibitors are listed in Table 6.
- Nitrates and α-blockers for benign prostate hypertrophy interfere with these drugs and are best avoided.

## Second Line Treatment Approaches

*Intraurethral therapy:* Alprostadil or prostaglandin $E_1$ is a medicated urethral system for erection (MUSE) and helps vasodilate penile vasculature locally. By this, 60–70% have long enough erection to engage in sexual intercourse. The side effects are:
- Discomfort of application
- Penile pain
- Urethral bleeding
- Urinary tract infection (UTI)
- Dizziness.
It is contraindicated in:
- UTI
- Urethritis
- Priapism.

**Flow chart 3** Treatment options in ED

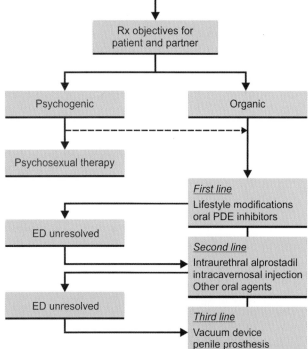

**Table 6** Pharmacology of phosphodiesterase type 5 inhibitors

| PDE 5 inhibitors | Doses | Half life | Common side effects | Notes |
|---|---|---|---|---|
| Sildenafil (viagra) | 25, 50, 100 mg starting with 50 mg empty stomach | 4 h-peak plasma levels 1 h | Headache, abnormal color vision, flushing | Efficacious, safe, longest clinical experience |
| Vardenafil (levitra) | 2.5, 5, 10, 20 mg starting with 5 mg empty stomach | 4–5 h peak plasma levels in 0.7 h | Headache, flushing and rhinitis | Same as sildenafil but higher potency |
| Tadalafil (cialis) | 5, 10, 20 mg starting with 10 mg after meals | 17.5 h peak plasma levels in 2 h | Headache, myalgia, dyspepsia | Longest half-life. Fewer visual side effects. Back-pain and myalgia |

*Intracavernous injection of vasodilators:* Using $PGE_1$ is effective in those who fail to respond to PDE 5 inhibitors. This treatment is more efficacious, better tolerated and preferred over transurethral application. Tri-mixture consists of $PGE_1$ and papaverine and phenolamine. The mixture has:
- High efficacy
- Low pain incidence
- Lower cost per dose
- It is given to those with failed PDE 5 therapy and have penile pain with $PGE_1$ injection.

Side effects include:
- Penile hematoma
- Penile edema
- Fibrotic changes within tunica albugeniea in form of plaques and nodules.

*Other oral agents:* Apomorphine a dopamine agonist causes penile erection within 20 minutes when given sublingually. The efficacy is less than PDE. It is avoided in those on bromocriptine and side effects include—nausea, headache, and dizziness. Other oral agents not FDA approved are:
- Yohimbine, an $\alpha_2$ adrenergic receptor antagonist
- Oral phentolamine
- Trazodone—serotonin antagonist.

## Third Line of Treatment

*Vacuum devices:* These create negative pressure increasing penile blood flow and placing compression rings at the base of the penis to prevent venous drainage. The side effects are:
- Difficult to use
- Compression prevents ejaculation.

*Penile prosthesis:* It is the surgical implantation of penile prosthesis. The technical success rate is high with revision rate of 2.5% at 2 years and removal rate 4.4% at 2 years. Patient and partner satisfaction is 80%.

Side effects are:
- Risk of surgical procedure
- Infection
- Chances of mechanical failure needing reimplantation.

## ■ CONCLUSION

- ED is common in vascular patients.
- ED has multiple etiologies.
- Differential diagnosis of ED—psychogenic and organic causes like neurologic, vascular, hormonal, and iatrogenic.
- Risk factors for ED are the same for cardiovascular disease.
- Evaluation for ED includes history, physical examination, laboratory tests, and screening for cardiovascular disease.
- First line of treatment in the management is PDE 5 inhibitors.
- Nitrates are contraindicated with PDE 5 inhibitors.

**Table 7** Therapeutic choices in ED

| | Advantages | Disadvantages |
|---|---|---|
| Drugs PDE 5 inhibitors | Effective, minimal side effects, oral | Contraindicated in patients taking nitrates, liver failure, hypotension, angina, and retinal disorders. Slow onset of action |
| Intracavernosal injections of PGE₁ | Quick onset. Good response in 60–70%. 80–90% patient and partner satisfaction | Invasive and needs patient education may develop hematoma, penile pain, fibrosis and priapism |
| Transurethral alprostadil (MUSE) | Proven efficacy in erections adequate for intercourse. Lower risk of priapism than intracavernosal injections | Slow acting, lower efficacy, and higher side effect than intracavernosal injection. Mild penile pain (10–29%). Needs manual dexterity, good eyesite, and insertion after micturition |
| *Devices* | | |
| Vacuum devices | Low side effect and suitable for side range of patients | Cumbersome with loss of spontaneity, 'cold penis' for partner, erections are uncomfortable and ejaculation impaired |
| Penile prosthesis | Technical success rates are high with low revision rates (2.5%) and removal rate (4.5%) at 2 years. High partner satisfaction | Invasive operative procedure. Infection in 2–16%. Long-term complications—erosion, migration and penile necrosis |

- Sildenafil (viagra) is safe with no additional risk with cardiovascular disease.
- Second line of treatment—oral medications, transurethral delivery and penile self injection.
- Third line of treatment—vacuum-assisted devices and penile prosthesis.
- The personal preference of patient and partner is improtant in therapeutic decision making (Table 7).

## ■ SPECIAL ISSUES

## Safety and Cardiovascular Effects of PDE 5 Inhibitors

Its use may lead to MI and cardiac arrest in cardiovascular patients. It may be that the physical demand of sex may be responsible for the event especially in those who have always lived a sedentary life. Drug interactions with nitrate lead to hypotension. Sildenafil inhibits platelets, vascular smooth muscles, and heart with cardiovascular risk. Recent studies have suggested that there is no increased risk of cardiovascular events with viagra.

## Selected Studies in Patients at Risk with Sildenafil

Three large studies were carried out to see the effects of sildenafil on coronary artery disease. The studies concluded that there was a reduction in the systolic and diastolic pressures at rest but at peak exercise there was a similar increase in systolic and diastolic pressures with no difference in the placebo and sildenafil group patients with congestive heart failure. Several cases of sudden death in patients on sildenafil raising the possibility of arrhythmia in addition to ischemia. Studies, however confirmed that in patients on double the recommended dose no changes in ECG parameters including QT interval.

## PRACTICAL POINTS

- Sexual Health Inventory for Men should be filled in prior to examination as a quick way to screen ED.
- Normal nocturnal erections or erections in response to masturbation suggest a psychogenic cause.
- Hypogonadism is an uncommon cause of ED in vascular clinic. When evaluating hypogonadism always ask for free testosterone as total testosterone may be low.
- ED is generally vasculogenic in origin, a true vascular stenosis causing reduced blood flow is suspected in patients with claudication and absent femoral pulses (Leriches's syndrome).
- PDE 5 is the effective first line of treatment but nitrates are contraindicated.
- Transurethral $PGE_1$ has low risk of priapism as compared to intracavernosal injections.
- Tri-mixture of papaverine and $PGE_1$ and phentolamine is used there is failure of:
  - PDE 5 inhibitor therapy
  - Intraurethral alprostadil
  - Papaverine/phentolamine combination
  - Severe penile pain with $PGE_1$ injection.
- Mechanical options for treatment of ED are vacuum-assisted devices and penile prosthesis.

# 23

# Approach to and Management of Inflammatory Vasculitis

*Jaisom Chopra*

## ■ INTRODUCTION

- Primary vasculitis is idiopathic and presents with constitutional features, limb, or organ ischemia with tissue inflammation.
- Multiorgan dysfunction may increase the suspicion of systemic vasculitis. However, multisystem diseases may result from nonvasculitic causes.
- Single organ dysfunction may be a result of inflammatory vasculitis.

*Even if one suspects vasculitic disorders, it is very difficult to prove it because of:*
- Difficulty of obtaining tissue for "gold standard" histopathological diagnosis
- Lack of diagnostic serological tests
  - Thus, the diagnosis depends on relative clinical findings along with consistent biopsies. Angiography is not diagnostic unless we excluded the possibility of infection or malignancy.

## ■ CLASSIFICATION OF PRIMARY VASCULITIDES (FIG. 1)

The classifications are based on:
- Distinction between primary and secondary vasculitis
- Recognition of dominant blood vessel size
- Presence or absence of antineutrophil cytoplasmic antibodies (ANCA).

## ■ LARGE VESSEL VASCULITIS

### Takayasu Arteritis

- It is a chronic granulomatous panarteritis affecting large elastic arteries such as aorta and its main branches,

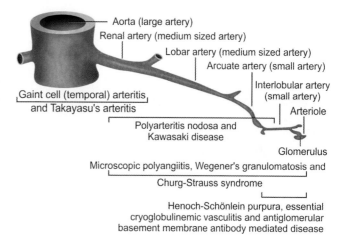

**Fig. 1** Classification of systemic vasculitides

coronary, and occasionally pulmonary. This inflammation causes stenosis, occlusion, aneurysm, and secondary thrombosis. This disorder progresses in three stages:
- Pre-pulseless phase having nonspecific inflammatory symptoms
- Painful arteries
- Burnt out disease with vessel occlusion and distal ischemia.

### Epidemiology

Prevalence rates and distribution differ in different ethnic groups. The highest rates are in Asian countries—Japan, Korea, China, and India—being less common among the whites. The disease peaks in the third decade and is more common in females.

## Clinical Features

- Musculoskeletal and constitutional symptoms are present in 30–40%. The patient may be asymptomatic with bruit, diminished pulses, claudication of the arms or legs, cardiovascular accidents, myocardial infarction, or aortic insufficiency.
- Ischemic symptoms with stenosis or occlusion are the hallmark of the disease.
  The American College of Rheumatology (ACR) criteria for diagnosis of Takayasu arteritis (TA) are listed in Table 1.

*TA is suspected in any:*
- Young patient with bruit
- Atypical distribution of ischemic symptoms such as upper limb
- Age-inappropriate vascular disease such as myocardial infarction (MI), congestive heart failure (CHF), abdominal aortic aneurysm (AAA), or aortic insufficiency.

**Table 1** Criteria for diagnosis of Takayasu arteritis

| Criterion | Findings |
|---|---|
| Age of onset | Present at about 40 years |
| Blood pressure difference >10 mm Hg | Difference between the two arms is >10 mm Hg (systolic BP) |
| Claudication of extremities | Fatigue or muscle discomfort while in use in the upper limbs |
| Decrease brachial artery pulse | Reduced pulses of one or both radial arteries |
| Bruit over subclavian arteries or aorta | Audible bruit over subclavian arteries or aorta |
| Aortogram abnormalities | Stenosis or occlusions in the arteries—entire aorta, its prominent branches, or large arteries in the extremities. This is not caused by atherosclerosis, fibromuscular dysplasia. The changes are focal or segmental |

*The angiography findings in TA are typical (Fig. 2):*
- Type I—branches from the aortic arch
- Type IIa—ascending aorta, aortic arch and its branches
- Type IIb—same as IIa and thoracic descending aorta
- Type III—thoracic descending aorta and abdominal aorta and renal arteries
- Type IV—abdominal aorta and renal arteries
- Type V—combined features of type IIb and IV.

## Diagnosis

- Acute phase reactants such as erythrocyte sedimentation rate (ESR) and C-reactive protein (CRE) is elevated in more than 50% of the TA patients.
- Every suspected TA case should have blood pressure (BP) recorded in all four limbs because subclavian artery stenosis is very common in TA and the BP measurements are unreliable.
- Renal artery stenosis may cause uncontrolled hypertension, and in cases of bilateral subclavian artery disease, this may not be recognized till the patient lands up with cerebrovascular accident (CVA), MI, or CHF.
- Confirmation of the diagnosis or staging is carried out by angiogram or magnetic resonance angiography (MRA). Three-dimensional (3-D) contrast-enhanced MRA evaluates the anatomy, vessel wall thickening as a potential sign of inflammation.

## Treatment

- Glucocorticoids are mainstay of treatment in patients with TA having a resolution of 25–100%. An initial dose of 30 mg prednisolone with active arteritis—51% had improved quality of life; 37% had no change while 12% worsened. In another large study, prednisolone was given at 1 mg/kg/day in the acute phase of TA for 1–3 months and then tapered to alternate days and further tapered

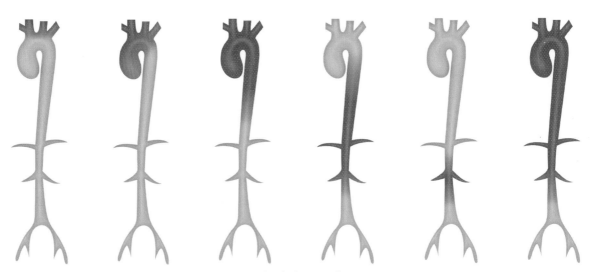

**Fig. 2** Angiographic findings in Takayasu arteritis

according to demand. By this method, there was a 52% remission.

*Cytotoxic therapy is considered when:*
- There is progression of disease despite a high dose of glucocorticoids
- Relapse upon tapering of the glucocorticoid
- High rate of complications with glucocorticoids
- Major organ at risk.

- The most common used cytotoxic drugs are methotrexate and cyclophosphamide. They induce remission and minimize glucocorticoid toxicity.
- The use of statins has been advocated because of their anti-inflammatory effect that increased immunity.
- The role of antiplatelet drugs such as aspirin and dipyridamole remains unclear.
- Angioplasty with or without stenting has not shown much promise because of the high incidence of restenosis and thrombosis.
- Vascular tissue samples should be obtained whenever possible.

## Giant Cell Arteritis of the Elderly

- Giant cell arteritis (GCA) is also called temporal arteritis or cranial arteritis and is an inflammatory vasculopathy affecting the medium and large vessels (Fig. 3).
- Activated macrophages and CD4+ T-cells are found in all vessel layers probably entering through the vasa-vasorum. Giant cells may or may not be found in the vessel wall.

### Epidemiology

It is fairly common in the whites compared with the others affecting persons over 50 and peaking by 70 years. It is two times more common in females.

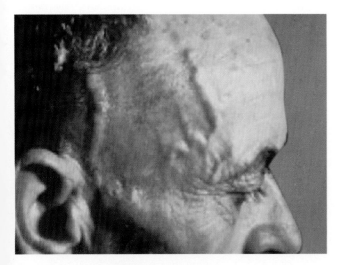

**Fig. 3** Temporal arteritis

### Clinical Features

- Jaw claudication
- Diplopia
- Prominent or enlarged temporal artery
- Synovitis
- Headache of sudden onset
- Erythrocyte sedimentation rate is markedly elevated
- Polymyalgia rheumatica (PMR) is a clinical syndrome closely related to GCA in which there is symmetrical proximal aching and morning stiffness due to low-grade proximal synovitis, bursitis, and tenosynovitis. PMR is present in 40% GCA patients.
- Loss of vision is the most dreaded complication being secondary to ischemia of the optic nerve due to arteritis of branch of the ophthalmic or posterior ciliary arteries or retinal arterioles. Permanent loss of vision takes place in 20%.
- TIA or stroke is the most common neurological finding in 30% of GCA cases.
- Occlusion of the large proximal extremity arteries in 15% cases affecting subclavian, axillary, or brachial arteries leads to claudication of the arm with reduced wrist pulses.
- GCA patients are 20 times more likely to develop thoracic aorta aneurysms.
- Temporal artery biopsy may be positive in GCA cases.

### Diagnosis

- Seen in patients over 50 years of age with abrupt onset of headache, visual loss, and fever of unknown origin. It is necessary to exclude atherosclerosis of aorta and its branches and carotid. Elevated acute phase reactants such as ESR and CRP with the clinical features go in favor of GCA rather than atherosclerosis (Flow chart 1).
- Biopsy of temporal artery under local anesthesia (LA) is performed and treatment with glucocorticoids does not alter the biopsy results. The diagnosis is confirmed by presence of inflammatory cells in the arterial wall with destruction of inner elastic membrane (Fig. 4).

### Treatment

- GCA is extremely sensitive to steroids and reduces the chances of vascular complications. Most respond to 40–60 mg prednisolone orally once daily within 3–5 days of treatment. Rarely is the dose needed to be increased by 10–20 mg. In those with immediate threatening symptoms such as visual loss, IV prednisolone is given followed by oral therapy.
- After the initial response, the dose can be reduced every 2 weeks by 10%. Once the daily dose is 20 mg, then it is decreased every 4 weeks to below 10 mg once daily.
- Follow-up by blood tests is recommended doing the ESR, CRP, and interleukin-6 levels.

**Flow chart 1** Diagnostic approach to gaint cell arteritis

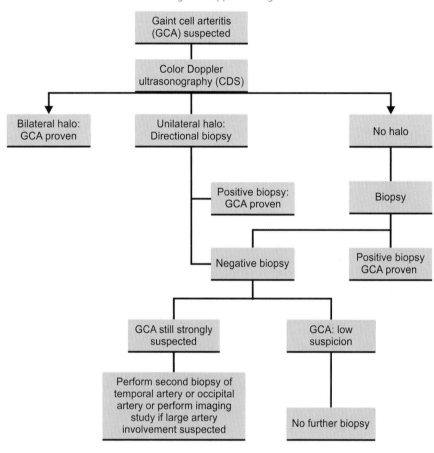

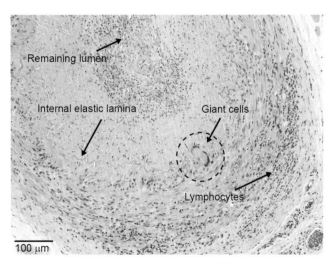

**Fig. 4** Histopathology of gaint cell arteritis

- The role of aspirin and statins shows some benefit against ischemic cardiovascular events.
- Role of immunosuppressants is unclear.
- Osteoporosis is a major concern in patients on long-term steroids.

## ■ MEDIUM VESSEL VASCULITIS

### Polyarteritis Nodosa

Polyarteritis nodosa (PAN) is necrotizing vasculitis of the medium muscular arteries. Inflammatory cells destroy the vessel wall leading to necrosis and aneurysmal formation.

### Epidemiology

It can affect any age group but mostly 40–60 years. Males being twice as commonly involved as females. The association with viral hepatitis B and C is well known.

### Clinical Features

- Malaise, fever, myalgia, arthralgia occur commonly in PAN.
- It has prelection for peripheral nerves, GI tract, and muscular renal arteries.
- Mononeuritis or polyneuropathy is common.
- Gastrointestinal manifestation may present as ischemia—intestinal angina mainly after meals. Intestinal perforation due to ischemia is a devastating complication of PAN.

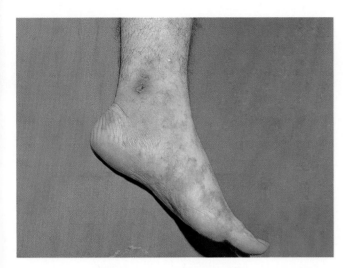
**Fig. 5** Ulcers in polyarteritis nodosa

- Hypertension—renin mediated may occur as well as renal infarction.
- There may be subcutaneous nodules, ulcers, and digital gangrene (Fig. 5).

## Diagnosis

- Documenting necrotizing vasculitis in the affected organ
- Biopsy
- Angiograms show microaneurysms.

## Treatment

Glucocorticoids are an important part of the treatment and increased survival in PAN. Immunosuppressants such as cyclophosphamide are added in severe refractory cases.

## Kawasaki Disease

Kawasaki disease (KD) is a mucocutaneous lymph node syndrome. There is necrotizing vasculitis involving the medium-sized muscular arteries mainly pediatric coronary arteries.

## Epidemiology

It affects children below 12 years and is very rare.

## Clinical Features

An acute febrile illness presenting with fever, conjunctivitis, cervical lymphadenopathy, erythematous rash, oral mucositis, and arthritis.

## Diagnosis (Fig. 6)

- Fever more than 5 days
- Conjunctivitis
- Dry fissured lips and strawberry tongue and red oral and pharyngeal mucosa
- Red palms and soles and edema
- Macular polymorphous rash on trunk
- Swollen cervical lymph nodes.
  Five of the above six criteria must be present along with fever for diagnosis.

## Treatment

- Intravenous gamma globulin (IVGG) reduces coronary artery aneurysm formation, subsides the fever, and reduces myocardial inflammation.
- IVGG is given in a single infusion 2 g/kg with aspirin 80–100 mg/kg/day till fever subsides and then aspirin is reduced to 3–5 mg/kg/day sufficient for antiplatelet effect for 6–8 weeks if there is no evidence of coronary artery abnormalities but indefinitely if there is evidence.

## ■ SMALL TO MEDIUM VESSEL VASCULITIS (FLOW CHART 2)

These include:
- Wegener's granulomatosis (WG)
- Churg–Strauss syndrome (CSS)
- Microscopic polyangiitis (MPA)
- Henoch–Schönlein purpura (HS).

## Wegener's Granulomatosis

It is a systemic vasculitis involving medium and small vessels with nectotizing and granulomatous inflammation in selected organs.

## Epidemiology

Incidence is one in 30,000 people.

## Clinical Features

- Mainly involves upper and lower respiratory tracts and kidneys with necrotic inflammation.
- In 25%, upper respiratory tract and lungs are involved, while in 80% there is kidney involvement.
- Involvement of the lungs, heart, gastrointestinal tract (GIT), and central nervous system (CNS) may be life-threatening.
- Moreover, any system in the body could be involved.
- Frequent urine analysis is needed to know about the renal involvement from glomerulonephritis, which is a silent process.

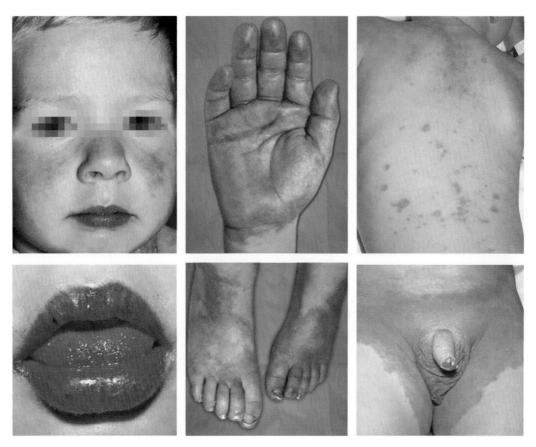

**Fig. 6** Myocarditis and coronary aneurysms may develop

## Diagnosis

Confirmed by tissue biopsy (necrotizing granulomatous inflammation) at the site of active disease.

## Treatment

- Aggressive therapy with prednisolone (1 mg/kg/day) and cyclophosphamide (2 mg/kg/day) has dramatically improved survival from 15–50% to 85%.
- Methotrexate given weekly in addition of glucocorticoid is an alternative if the patient does not have life-threatening disease.
- Once there is remission of the disease induced by cyclophosphamide for several months, converting to methotrexate or azathioprine has helped remission to continue in 60%.
- Educate patients about importance of nasal and sinus hygiene.
- Subglottic stenosis is treated by intralesion injection of long-acting glucocorticoids.

# Churg–Strauss Syndrome

It is allergic granulomatosis and angiitis in a multi-system disorder characterized by rhinitis or asthma, peripheral blood eosinophilia along with small and medium sized vessel vasculitis.

## Epidemiology

The annual incidence of Churg–Strauss syndrome (CSS) is four cases per million involving all ages.

## Clinical Features

- More common in the second and third decades of life and present with allergic rhinitis, asthma, and atrophic disease.
- Eosinophilic phase—peripheral blood eosinophilia and eosinophilic infiltration of lungs and GIT.
- Vasculitic phase—vasculitis of medium and small vessels along with extravascular granulomatosis.

**Flow chart 2** Algorithmic approach of small vessel vasculitis

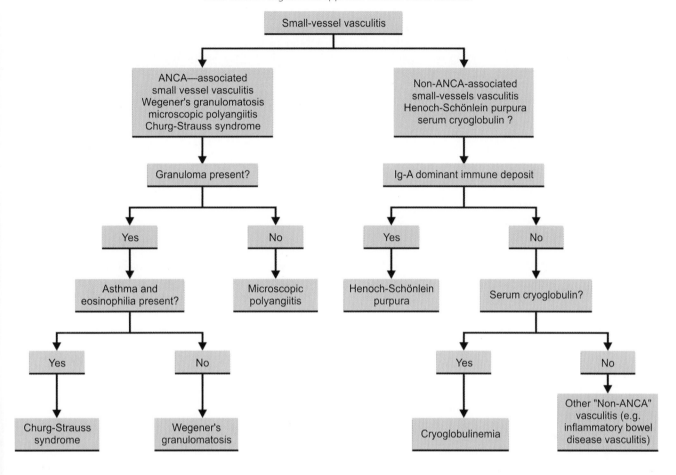

- Asthma is a cardinal feature of CSS and precedes vasculitic phase by a decade.
- Skin lesions such as palpable purpura, macular, or papular erythematous rash, hemorrhagic lesions, and tender nodules.
- Heart involvement leads to pericarditis, CHF, or MI.
- CNS involvement—mononeuritis multiplex and polyneuropathy.
- Almost any organ could be involved.

## Diagnosis

- Depends on clinical findings and confirmed by biopsy
- Biopsy findings—eosinophil infiltrates, necrosis, eosinophilic giant cell vasculitis, and necrotizing granuloma
- The main laboratory findings—eosinophilia more than $1,500/mm^3$
- ANCAs are present in 50–85% and are perinuclear.

## Treatment

- Glucocorticoids 1 mg/kg/day and tapered according to the need

- The effectiveness or remissions are monitored by eosinophil counts.

## Microscopic Polyangiitis

It is necrotizing vasculitis affecting medium and small arteries mainly involving the kidney and pulmonary capillaries.

## Epidemiology

Annually three to five cases per million. It is more common in whites and has a slight predilection for males.

## Clinical Features

- Patients present with pulmonary–renal syndrome
- Skin involvement—purpura, subcutaneous nodules
- Neurological involvement—mononeuritis multiplex.

## Diagnosis

- Focal thrombosis with fibrinoid necrosis of capillaries—characteristic.

- Renal biopsy—15–20% crescentic formation with few glomerular immune deposits.
- ANAC in 85% usually perinuclear pattern and myeloperoxidase specific.

### Treatment

- A serious disease with risk of death or end-stage renal failure
- Is active and aggressive on the same lines as Wegener's granulomatosis (given above).

## Henoch-Schönlein Purpura

Henoch–Schönlein purpura (HSP) is systemic vasculitis with prominent cutaneous component. It affects small-sized vessels with immunoglobulin A dominant immune deposits.

### Epidemiology

Twenty per 100,000 children with upper respiratory tract infection.

### Clinical Features

- Fever with palpable purpura on the legs and buttock (Fig. 7)
- There may be arthritis and abdominal pain.
- Complications include bowel ischemia (intussusception in children) and glomerulonephritis.

### Diagnosis

- The classical triad of nonthrombotic thrombocytopenic purpura and knee arthritis and abdominal pain along with miscroscopic hematuria seals the diagnosis.

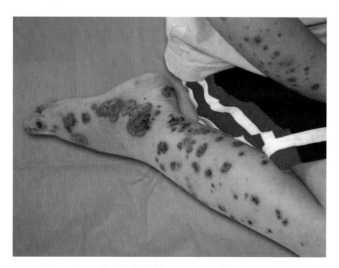

**Fig. 7** Palpable purpura on legs

- The diagnosis is confirmed by deposition of IgA in the skin and kidney tissues by immunofluorescence microscopy.
- Biopsy of the skin lesion shows inflammation of small blood vessels, leukocytoclastic vasculitis.

### Treatment

- Low to moderate doses of prednisolone provides complete recovery in more than 90% cases.
- Recurrences occur in one-third of the cases mainly in patients with nephritis. More aggressive treatment is done in these patients.

## Cutaneous Leukocytoclastic Angiitis

- It may be part of the other syndromes listed above or isolated.
- Immune complexes and cutaneous vasculitis are associated with bacterial or viral infections, systemic autoimmune disease, or malignancies. Thus, these associated conditions have to be excluded.
- Other manifestations include peripheral neuropathy, arthralgias, malaise, fatigue, Raynaud's phenomenon, and glomerulonephritis.
- Leg ulcers may form and must be distinguished from other causes.

### Diagnosis

- Clinical findings and skin biopsy showing leukocytoclastic vasculitis on skin biopsy confirm the diagnosis.
- Immunofluorescence on skin biopsy to recognize HSP.
- It is classified as primary only when other etiologies are excluded.

### Treatment

- Therapy depends on disease severity.
- Antihistaminics are first line of treatment.
- Nonsteroidal anti-inflammatory drugs are beneficial in some.
- Pentoxifylline is helpful in occlusive vasculopathy.
- Glucocorticoids are helpful but are not needed in non-threatening disease.
- Immunosuppersive drugs such as azathioprine and methotrexate are used in low doses to reduce prednisolone dose in difficult cases.

## Microaneurism

### Diagnosis

*Approach to diagnostic testing:* There are no specific blood tests to clinch the diagnosis (Table 2).

**Table 2** Selected laboratory tests in the evaluation of patients with possible primary vasculitis

| Test | Comments |
|---|---|
| Platelet count | Thrombocytosis during acute phase. Thrombocytopenic not expected. Consider systemic lupus erythematosus (SLE), marrow infilteration, hairy cell leukemia, thrombocytopenic purpura (TTP), disseminated intravascular coagulopathy (DIC), hypersplenism, antiphospholipid syndrome (APLS), HIV scleroderma renal crisis, heparin-induced thrombocytopenia |
| WBC count | Leukopenia is not expected in autoimmune vasculopathy. Consider SLE, lukemia, hypersplenism, sepsis, myelodysplasia, or HIV |
| ESR and CRP | Nonspecific acute phase response and is usually high in autoimmune vasculopathies. Elevated in infection and malignancy but not in Takayasu's arteritis and coronary artery disease (CAD) but is low in HSP |
| Transaminases | Elevated aspartate transaminase (ALT) and alanine transaminase (AST) in liver diseases, myositis, rabdomyolysis, hemolysis, and MI |
| Anti-glomerular basement membrane (GBM) | Elevated in alveolar hemorrhage with or without glomerulonephritis |
| Antinuclear antibody (ANA) | Only on suspicion of SLE not otherwise |
| Antineutrophil cytoplasmic antibody (ANCA) | Only on suspicion of Wegener's granulomatosis and microscopic polyarteritis |
| Drug screen | Unexplained CNS symptoms, myocardial ischemia, vascular spasm, panic attacks with systemic features and tachycardia. Screen urine |
| Blood cultures | Febrile, multisystem or wasting illness, pulmonary infiltrates, focal ischemia or infarction |
| Antiphospholipid antibody (APLA) | Unexplained arterial or venous thrombosis, thrombocytopenia |
| Purified protein derivative (PPD) (± anergy) | Anyone needing steroid therapy, unexplained sterile pyuria or hematuria, granulomatous inflammation, chronic meningitis |
| Examination of fresh urinary sediment | Unexplained febrile or multisystem illness |
| Hepatitis serologies | Abnormal transaminases, elevated hepatic alkaline phosphatase, portal hypertension, PAN. Unexplained cryoglobulinemia, polyarteritis, cutaneous vasculitis |

## Urinalysis

Crucial test with multisystemic disease. Fresh urinary sedimentation for screening of glomerular disease should be done more than once with unexplained febrile or multisystem disease to look for glomerulonephritis, which is generally clinically silent.

## Radiographic Evaluation

According to the needs of the patients, chest X-ray (CXR) is must in pulmonary cases. Computed tomography (CT) if malignancies are expected.

## Angiography

- Only done where MRA is unavailable.
- It is only of value if there is arterial stenosis or aneurysms otherwise it cannot rule out vasculitis (Fig. 8).
- It may detect clinically silent aneurysms that occur in 60% of PAN patients.
- Microaneurysms are also found in arterial myxoma, bacterial endocarditis, peritoneal carcinomatosis, and severe arterial hypertension.
- In large vessel vasculitis (TA and GCA), there is the classic appearance of elongated tapering of vessels.
- Accurate measurements of true arterial pressures are carried out and are of value.

## Magnetic Resonance Imaging

- It is helpful in large vessel vasculitis such as TA and GCA and may be of value in medium-size vessel vasculitis—renal, mesenteric and extremity vessels.
- It can assess arterial wall thickening and edema, which is a marker of arterial inflammation.

## Pathologic Diagnosis

This is the gold standard. One must consider:
- Vasculitis may not be uniformly involved and may be patchy. So, a large sample of the vessel is desirable.

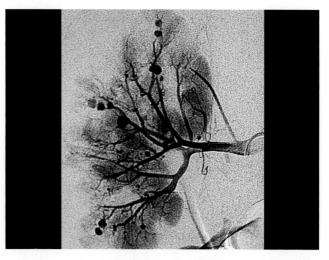

**Fig. 8** Microaneurysms on angiography

- Excision biopsy is preferred over needle, endoscopic, or bronchoscopic biopsies.
- In multiple organ involvement—which organ to biopsy depends on sensitivity of obtaining positive result and the morbidity and the mortality of the organ biopsied.
- Sampling size and the accessibility of the tissue to be biopsied.
- Avoid biopsy of the asymptomatic tissue when dealing with medium and small size vessels.

## General Management Principles

Treatment of primary vasculitis syndromes depends upon:
- Specific forms of vasculitis
- Severity of disease
- Type of organ involved.

Glucocorticoids are the first line of treatment as a standard dose or a high dose 1 mg/kg/day. They may be given as IV dose of methylprednisolone 1 g per day in severe life-threatening organ involvement.
- Immunosuppressive therapy given as cyclophosphamide or methotrexate in combination with glucocorticoids is now generally used with good advantage.
- Plasmapheresis can be life-saving in cryoglobulinemic crisis.
- With steroids, bone health, glaucoma, and proper anti-biotic prophylaxis is important. Monitoring and screening for cardiovascular disease is vital.

## ■ SPECIAL ISSUES

## Takayasu Arteritis

### Medical Management

This has two goals:
1. Management of hypertension
2. Prevention of thrombosis.

Hypertension may be difficult to detect due to subclavian stenosis and can be hard to treat.
- Renal function must be monitored and use of angiotensin receptor blockers may be used.
- Patients with unilateral renal artery stenosis are medically managed.

- Kidney size and glomerular filtration rate (GFR) should be monitored by duplex ultrasound, and if there is reduction in size, then intervention is indicated.
- Statins and aspirin are given due to their inflammatory nature.

### Percutaneous Therapy

Angioplasty and stenting are indicated if medical treatment fails. Renal artery stenosis is treated by angioplasty and stenting. PTA of subclavian and axillary is being performed more often. The indications are:
- Arm claudication
- Failure to monitor BP
- Subclavian steal
- Long-term results are superior in bypass surgery rather than PTA and stenting in patients with TA.

### Surgical Management

*Indications for surgery:*
- Reversible cerebrovascular ischemia
- Critical stenosis of three or more cerebral vessels
- Moderate aortic regurgitation
- Coronary ischemia with confirmed coronary artery involvement.

*Complications of surgery include:*
- Restenosis
- Anastomotic failure
- Aneurysms
- Thrombosis
- Infection
- Hemorrhage.

Repair of thoracic and abdominal aneurysms is indicated if over 5 cm diameter. At surgery, tissue must be obtained to assess disease activity.

## ■ CONCLUSION

- Before treating vasculitis, always try to confirm the diagnosis by tissue biopsy.
- Serological tests and markers cannot supplement tissue diagnosis.
- The diagnosis initially depends on index of suspicion.

## PRACTICAL POINTS

- Three forms of vasculitis are likely to lead to loss of pulse—TA, GCA, and Buerger's disease.
- Jaw claudication and scalp tenderness in over 50 years is specific for GCA.
- On suspecting systemic vasculitis, mainly cutaneous purpura, first exclude infection, malignancy, and thrombosis.
- ESR and CRP are not accurate gauges of disease activity in TA and GCA. In 50% of TA cases, there is no elevation, while in elderly there is no elevation of ESR.
- Vasculitis patients must be treated specifically and with monitoring of the side effects. Treatment for osteoporosis, hypertension, infection prophylaxis, hyperglycemia, and atherosclerotic vascular disease should be started.

# 24

# Lymphedema

*Jaisom Chopra*

## ■ INTRODUCTION

- It is due to lymphatic vascular insufficiency.
- It happens due to excessive, typically regionalized, interstitial accumulation of protein-rich fluid.
- This happens when there is an imbalance between the lymph load produced and the transport capacity. Either one or both these may contribute to lymphatic edema.
- It may occur due to hereditary poor development of the lymphatic channels (primary) or could be acquired (secondary) due to traumatic disruption of the structural or functional integrity of the lymphatic circulation.
- Mostly lymphedema occurs due to poor lymphatic drainage of the extremity, but respiratory and gastrointestinal (GI) involvement is commonly seen along with it.
- There is excess chronic lymph volume in the extremities. Over time, irreversible structural changes occur in the skin and soft tissue of the affected regions.
- This condition produces a detrimental psychological effect on the patient's quality of life, which may reduce his compliance to therapeutic interventions.

## ■ CLINICAL FEATURES (FIG. 1)

### Clinical Classification

The primary and secondary causes must be differentiated first (Table 1).

- Primary lymphedema can be present at birth or arise at predictable points in a patient's life. That is why primary classification is according to age—*congenital* being within the first 2 years of life. *Lymphedema precox* begins at puberty, while *lymphedema tarda* begins after 35 years and is present in only 10%.
- Primary lymphedema is autosomal dominant and is due to mutations in the domain encoding the tyrosine kinase signaling function of vascular endothelial growth factor receptor 3 (VEGFR 3) and the lymphatic endothelial receptor that mediates the effect of VEGF C and VEGF D.

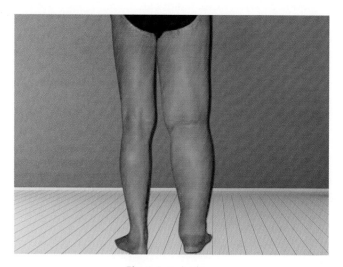

**Fig. 1** Lymphedema

**Table 1** Differences between primary and secondary causes of lymphedema

| Primary | Secondary |
|---|---|
| Congenital | Benign |
|    Familial (Milroy's disease) | Idiopathic |
|    Syndrome associated | Post-traumatic |
|    Sporadic | Postinfectious |
| Lymphedema precox | Postsurgical (axillary lymph node dissection) |
|    Familial | |
|    Sporadic | Filariasis |
| Lymphedema tarda | Malignant |
| | Tumor encroachment |
| | Primary lymphatic malignancies |

- Lymphedema precox accounts for 94% cases and is the most common primary lymphedema. It is 10 times more common in females and is commonly unilateral affecting the foot and calf.

- Secondary lymphedema is more common than primary type and is due to destruction of the lymph channels or blockage of the lymph nodes by other processes—infection, radiation, surgery, or trauma.
- The most common cause of lymphedema all over the world is filariasis in which there is destruction of the lymphatics leading to elephantiasis.

## Physiology and Pathology (Table 2)

- Lymphatic vasculature starts in the skin as blinded sinuses—initial lymphatics—where rapid flow of extracellular fluid, macromolecules, and cells occurs through the porous basement membrane. These initial lymphatics join into the lymphatic conduits having unidirectional valvular structures, prominent smooth muscle layer with autocontractility properties. Lymph flow depends on lymphatic vascular contraction influenced by neural and humoral factors. Lymph flow and contractility increase in the presence of increased tissue turgor, upright position, mechanical stimulation, and exercise. The conduit lymph vessels carry lymph to the lymph nodes where lymphovenous fluids are exchanged (Figs 2A and B).
- In the extremities, superficial (epifascial) system collects fluid from the skin and subcutaneous system, whereas the deep (subfascial) system collects fluid from the muscle, bone, and blood vessels. The superficial and the deep systems merge in the pelvis and the axilla.
- Functional and structural disruption of any competent in this intricate drainage mechanism leads to accumulation of protein-rich fluid in the interstitium leading to lymph stasis. Primary lymphedema may be due to lymphatic hypoplasia, insufficiency, anatomic absence of valves leading to lymphangiectasia, or poor contractility of the lymphatic musculature. Secondary lymphedema is due to trauma, infection, surgery, radiation, and cancer. Primary lymph cancer may cause lymphedema. When there is disruption of the lymphatic vasculature, lymphedema may take months to years to develop.
- In chronic lymph stasis, there is extracellular accumulation of proteins and cellular metabolites such as hyaluronan and glycosaminoglycans. The increased tissue colloid pressure leads to accumulation of water leading to increased hydrostatic pressure. With lymph stagnation, there are increased fibroblasts, adipocytes, and keratinocytes. Also, there is an increase in macrophages showing chronic inflammation. There is excessive tissue overgrowth in skin and subcutaneous tissue. Thus, in chronic lymphatic obstruction, there is histologically—thickening of lymphatic basement membrane, degeneration of elastin, ingress of inflammatory cells, and fibroblasts along with an increase of ground substance and pathological collagen fibers. There is progressive cutaneous and subcutaneous fibrosis.

**Table 2** Physiology and pathology of lymphedema

| Anatomic derangements | Pathology |
| --- | --- |
| Impaired lymphatic contractility, lymphatic vascular underdevelopment | Lymph stasis—accumulation of protein, fluid, and glycosaminoglycans |
| Primary valvular incompetence | Lymphatic hypertension |
| Lymphatic vascular disruption or obliteration | Secondary contractile impairments. Secondary valvular insufficiency |

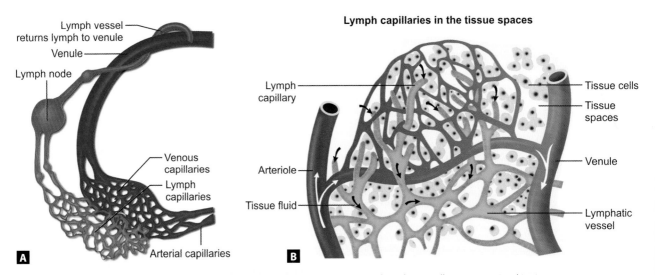

**Figs 2A and B** (A) Lymph draining into venous system; (B) Lymph and AV capillaries intertwined in tissue

## Presentation and Common Clinical Signs and Symptoms

### Natural History of Lymphedema (Fig. 3)

Patient has a long lag phase of the disease during which he remains asymptomatic and only starts to have symptoms when the compensatory mechanism starts to become inadequate to cope with the requirement of lymphatic flow. The chance of recurrent infections (cellulitis) is a common manifestation. Bacterial growth is encouraged by protein enriched interstitium and impaired immune responses. These recurrent cellulitis attacks further damage the lymphatics in skin, worsen the skin quality, and aggravate the edema.

### Signs and Symptoms of Lymphedema

In the late stages, it is apparent clinically, but in the primary stages, it poses a challenge for diagnosing. The intermittent swellings may not be enough to explain that it is due to lymphedema. One important sign is the *stemmer sign*, which is the inability to tent the skin on the dorsum of the digits. It is due to the inelastic skin because of the high collagen content and cutaneous edema that occurs due to lymphatic blockage. Subcutaneous fibrosis leads to *peau d'orange*, which is thick skin with prominent pores resembling an orange peel. There is always swelling of the dorsum of the foot with *squared off toe sign*.

## Differential Diagnosis

- Chronic venous insufficiency and post-phlebitic syndrome.
- This may be confused with lymphedema and the distinguishing features are aching pain in the legs on standing or sitting and chronic pruritis over the perforators. On examination, there may be ankle discoloration, eczema, swelling dermatosclerosis, and ulceration around the ankle area.
- *In contrast to lymphedema, here, the feet and digits are saved.* Unless there is a lymphatic element, there is never cutaneous fibrosis or thickening.

### Lipidemia

- Occurs exclusively in females and there is a deposit of fatty substances in subcutaneous tissue between pelvis and ankle.
- The feet are always spared and it arises 1–2 years after puberty and stammer's sign is negative (the skin over the dorsum of the digit can be lifted).
- There is generally a life-long history of heavy hips and thighs and there is a painful swelling.
- There is an increased tendency to bruising.

### Malignant Lymphedema

- There is blockage of the lymphatic channels by active malignant cells.
- This may point to recurrence of cancer due to intrinsic or extrinsic obstruction of the lymph flow.
- The lymphedema arises rapidly and progresses relentlessly.
- Pain is a presenting feature.
- Malignant lymphedema starts centrally and lacks the early soft consistency seen in benign lymphedema.

### Myxedema

- This is seen in association with thyroid disease and is due to the deposit of abnormal mucinous substance in the skin. Hyaluronic acid rich protein deposition in dermis produces edema that destroys the structure of the skin and reduces the elasticity of the skin. In thyrotoxicosis, it is focal limited to the pretibial region, while in hypothyroidism, it is more generalized.
- On examination, there is:
  - Roughing of the skin of the palms, soles, elbows, and knees
  - There are brittle uneven nails
  - Dull, thinning hair
  - Yellow orange discoloration of the skin
  - Reduced sweat production.

### Factitious Edema

This is due to the habitual application of tourniquet. If sufficiently chronic, it may acquire some of the cutaneous findings of lymphedema.

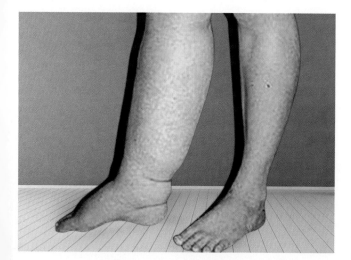

**Fig. 3** Chronic lymphoedema

## ■ DIAGNOSIS (FLOW CHART 1)

This is mostly made on history and examination findings, but where it is multifactorial, tests are needed to be sure of the cause. The available tests are:

- Isotopic lymphoscintigraphy
- Direct and indirect lymphography
- Magnetic resonance imaging (MRI)
- Computed tomography (CT) scan
- Ultrasonography
- Direct lymphography is limited to those undergoing lymphatic surgery.

Most commonly employed is isotopic lymphoscintigraphy. A subcutaneous injection of appropriate radiolabeled tracer—$^{99m}$Tc – antimony sulfide colloid, $^{99m}$Tc – sulfur colloid, and $^{99m}$Tc – albumin colloid is given. Images are recorded by a dual-detector instrument using high-resolution parallel-hole collimators in the whole body scanning mode. Injection is given into the web space and imaging done for 30–60 minutes. By this, we can:

- Differentiate lymphatic from nonlymphatic causes of leg swelling
- Know of a lymphatic mechanism of established edema
- Identify patients at a high risk of future development of lymphedema
- Know criteria for lymphatic dysfunction—delayed, asymmetric, and absent visualization of the regional lymph nodes.

- Dermal back flow—extravasation of lymph into the interstitium that accompanies the incompetence of lymphatics in this condition.
- Additional criteria—asymmetric visualization of the lymphatic channels, collateral lymphatic channels, interrupted vascular structures, visible lymph nodes of deep lymphatic system such as popliteal lymph node (LN) after web space injection into the lower extremity.

*MRI and CT scan show structural changes of lymphedema:*
- Characteristic absence of edema within the muscular compartment helps distinguish lymphedema from other forms of edema.
- Honeycomb distribution of edema within the epifascial planes along with thickening of the skin is a characteristic of lymphedema.
- These findings complement the findings on lymphoscintiscan.

Newer techniques under research are tissue tonometry and biomedical impedance analysis. These may help to detect changes in tissue turgor, which is a subclinical state.

*Direct contrast lymphography is rarely recommended because:*
- Cannulation of lymphatic channels is very difficult.
- Iodinated contrast agent is toxic to lymphatic vasculature and may contribute to extravasation.
- It is mainly used when surgical intervention is contemplated.

## ■ MANAGEMENT OF PATIENTS

### Conservative Approach

#### *Physiotherapy*

- Lymphedema is a chronic condition needing life-long management. These therapeutic interventions may retard the disease process and reduce soft tissue infections. Physiotherapy is the mainstay of the treatment and is known as complex decongestive physiotherapy (CDPT) that brings about:
  - Reduction of limb volume (Fig. 4)

**Flow chart 1** Evaluation of lymphedema

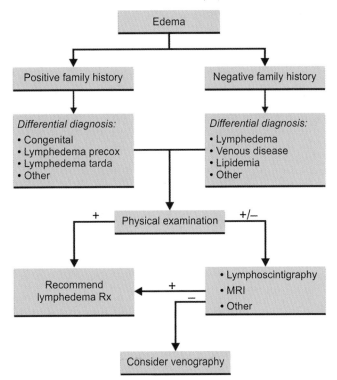

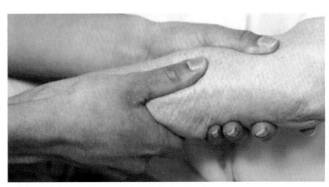

**Fig. 4** Reduction of limb volume

- Acceleration of lymph transport
- Dispersal of accumulated proteins.

This is done by:
- Massage
- Meticulous skin care
- Exercise
- Compressive elastic garments (Fig. 5).

  Massage helps in manual lymphatic drainage (MLD) by gentle stimulation of the lymphatic afferents that enhances the lymphatic contractility to augment and redirect the lymphatic flow through the unobstructed cutaneous channels. The mild tissue compression causes better filling of the initial lymphatics increasing the transport capacity through lymphatic dilatation and development of accessory lymph collectors.

- Volume reduction in a previously untreated patient is done with MLD along with nonelastic multilayered compression bandage applied after the massage and worn during exercise to prevent reaccumulation of fluid and promote lymph flow during exercise. On achieving maximum volume reduction that takes 10–15 such sessions, the patient is given a compression garment delivering a pressure of 40–80 mm Hg. These garments are proper fitting and changed every 6 months when they lose their elasticity. This is all accompanied with meticulous skin care and gentle muscular exercise to increase lymphatic pump. Intermittent pneumatic compression is helpful but contraindicated in ischemic limbs.

- Low level lazer therapy, local hyperthermia, and intra-arterial injection of autologous lymphocytes.

## Pharmacotherapy

- The only class of drugs with proven efficacy is antibiotics in soft tissue infection.

- This infection may be very subtle with skin changes but no fever or could be skin infection with high-grade fever and systemic toxicity.
- Mostly getting cultures is impossible.
- Broad-spectrum antibiotics are generally necessary for long-term—months to years.
- No other drugs have made a mark in this disease.

## Surgical Approaches

- It is mostly palliative because it may cause damage the cutaneous lymphatics and worsen the lymphedema causing further skin damage and ulceration with fistula formation.
- Surgery may be needed with an unacceptable increase in adipose tissue and fibrosis. Here, the epifascial tissue is all removed and split skin grafting done (Fig. 6).
- Microsurgical techniques such as lymphatico-lymphatic or lymphaticovenous or lymph node to venous anastomosis have been attempted with poor results.
- Other techniques attempted are transfer of omental pedicle or interposition of vascular pedicle flap to serve as a lymphatic wick.
- Recently, liposuction has been advocated with encouraging results in chronic post-mastectomy lymphedema with sustained reduction of excessive volume. This is followed by decongestive compression therapy with even better results.

## Emerging Therapies

Lymphedema currently lacks cure. The mainstay of treatment is physiotherapy but is long drownout with deterioration in the quality of life because of the slow progress. If some treatment is to emerge, it has to be on a molecular level.

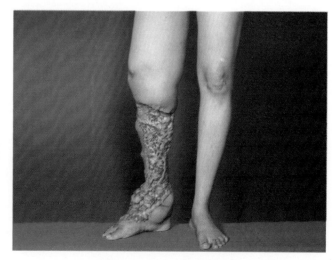

**Fig. 5** Leg support          **Fig. 6** Surgery for lymphedema

## ■ CONCLUSION

- Lymphedema produces chronic painless swelling when primarily there is poor lymphatic formation or secondary trauma.
- Lymphatic damage may precede lymphedema by weeks, months, or even years.
- The hallmark is progressive induration with inelasticity of the skin and subcutaneous tissue.
- The pathognomic signs are Stammer's sign and peau d'orange changes in the skin.

- When the diagnosis is in doubt, lymphedema can be confirmed with radioisotopic lymphoscintigraphy.
- The mainstay of therapy is complex decongestive physiotherapy (CDPT) comprising skin care, manual lymphatic drainage (MLD), bandaging, compressive garments, and exercise.
- Avoid surgery unless an unacceptable degree of subcutaneous hypertrophy hinders the patient's limb function.

## PRACTICAL POINTS

- Leg swelling with pitting edema over the dorsum of foot and "squared off" appreance to the toes is almost a sign of lymphatic involvement.
- Cellulitis is difficult to recognize in lymphedema. Start antibiotics when in doubt.
- Antibiotics must be given for a minimum of 4 weeks, the dose being at the high end of the spectrum.
- When lymphedema abruptly worsens or stops responding to usual treatment, it is invariable due to soft tissue infection or recurrent cancer.

# 25

# Hemodialysis Access

*Jaisom Chopra*

## ■ INTRODUCTION

- Patients with end-stage renal disease (ESRD) have gone up dramatically in the last several decades.
- There are 8% new cases added to the list every year.
- Of the newly diagnosed patients, 40% are diabetic individuals, 30% hypertensive, and the rest due to glomerulonephritis, polycystic kidney disease, or obstructive uropathy.
- The lifespan of the hemodialysis is limited and so many attempts have to be made to revive the existing sites.

### Indications for Hemodialysis

- Acute renal failure
- Chronic renal failure
- Medically refractory volume overload
- Hyperkalemia
- Acidosis.

## ■ ANATOMIC CONSIDERATIONS

The choice of access for hemodialysis depends upon:
- Timing (when the dialysis is to be started)
- Duration (how long will it continue)
- Stability of the patient's vasculature.

The ideal site should depend upon:
- Easy access to circulation
- Durability
- Limited complications
- Provide effective dialysis.

The material used for fistula is:
- Autogenous vein for arteriovenous (AV) fistula
- Synthetic material (polytetrafluoroethylene, PTFE).

Despite all the advantages of autogenous vein, PTFE is used in two-third of the cases because:
- Delayed usage after AV fistula placement—maturation time
- Unsuitable veins

- Greater technical expertise needed for AV fistula placement
- Catheters and ports are the other types of access.

AV fistulas can be:
- Side to side
- End to side
- End to end
- The basilic or cephalic veins are most important for AV access because they are superficial and more accessible than deep veins
- Examination is vital to determining the right sight for access placement. The following points must be considered:
  - The inflow artery and the outflow vein must be examined.
  - The inflow artery must provide adequate blood without rendering the limb ischemic.
  - The brachial, radial, and ulnar pulses are palpated and blood pressure recorded in both arms that should be within 20 mm Hg of each other.
  - Allen test is performed in all patients (Fig. 1).
  - While examining the venous system, the blood pressure cuff is inflated to 5 mm Hg above the diastolic pressure and left for about 5 minutes.
  - The cephalic vein should be relatively straight from the wrist to the anticubital fossa.
  - Accessory veins are identified and ligated during surgery, as they delay the maturation of the fistula by siphoning blood from the outflow vein.

## ■ CLINICAL ASPECTS OF FISTULA/GRAFT PLACEMENT

- The normal maturation time for AV fistula is 2–4 months. The fistula should be prepared 6–12 months before the anticipated dialysis, as there is always a likelihood for delay or failed maturation. On deciding to make a fistula, the cephalic vein in the nondominant arm is protected.
- Synthetic grafts are normally ready within 2–4 weeks and so are preferred. They are also less likely to fail early.

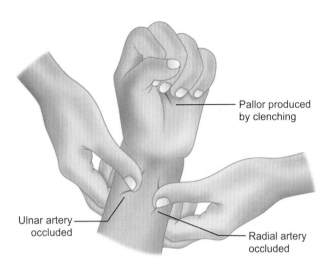

**Fig. 1** Allen test

## Arteriovenous Fistula Placement Considerations (Fig. 2)

The clinical variables that predict the chances of failure are:
- Anatomic considerations
- Advanced age
- Females
- Diabetes
- Obesity
- Preoperative color Doppler study can predict the chances of failure.

The favorable factors are:
- Arterial diameter above 2.5 mm and venous over 2 mm
- No stenosis of the artery
- Continuity of the vein with the deep system
- Absence of the calcification of the artery.

One study revealed:
- Fifty-four percent AV fistulas and 79% synthetic grafts were ready for use at 6 months.
- Forty-four percent AV fistulas and 48% synthetic grafts survived at 1 year.

Thus, AV fistuals mature late and can fail early, but once formed they do well.
- The first choice is that AV fistula is created most distally so that further fistulas can be created higher. The radiocephalic is the most common site for the first AV fistula, though the caliber is less than the proximal vessels (Fig. 3). Initially, side-to-side anastomosis was done but leads to venous congestion in the hand. To avoid this, an end-to-side fistula is carried out with distal ligation of the vein (Flow chart 1).
- The second choice is a proximal forearm fistula. A prosthetic graft can be placed so that if and when this fails,

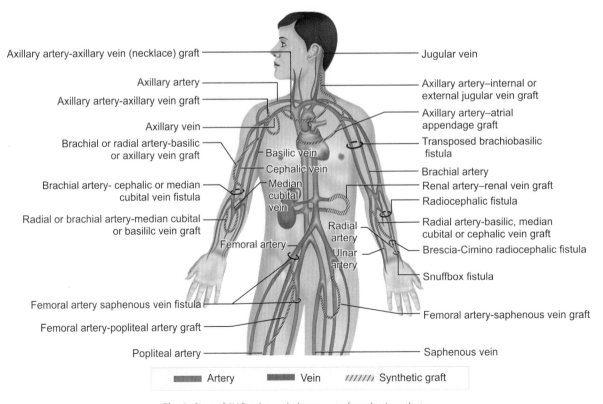

**Fig. 2** Sites of AV fistulas and placement of synthetic catheters

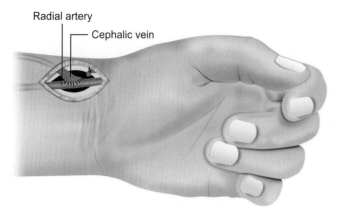

Radial artery

Cephalic vein

**Fig. 3** Radiocephalic fistula

the proximal veins are adequately dilated to form an AV fistula. The risk of this strategy is proximal vein stenosis that causes failure. A brachiobasilic fistula is more time-consuming and has a higher rate of thrombosis than a brachiocephalic fistula.

- If the fistula does not show signs of maturation within 1 month, it must be investigated to know the cause of delay.
- Color Doppler study is used to identify the presence of accessory veins.
- Stenosis at the anastomosis and central vein must be ruled out.
- Many causes for failure can be corrected by percutaneous intervention.

**Flow chart 1** Vascular access education

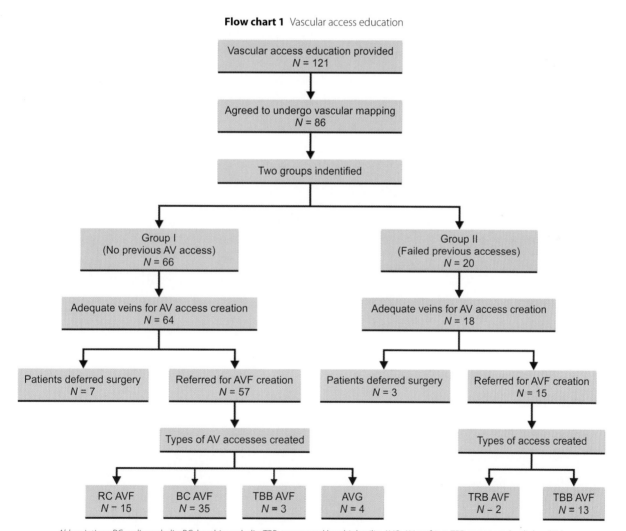

Vascular access education provided
N = 121

Agreed to undergo vascular mapping
N = 86

Two groups indentified

Group I
(No previous AV access)
N = 66

Group II
(Failed previous accesses)
N = 20

Adequate veins for AV access creation
N = 64

Adequate veins for AV access creation
N = 18

Patients deferred surgery
N = 7

Referred for AVF creation
N = 57

Patients deferred surgery
N = 3

Referred for AVF creation
N = 15

Types of AV accesses created

Types of access created

RC AVF
N - 15

BC AVF
N = 35

TBB AVF
N = 3

AVG
N = 4

TRB AVF
N - 2

TBB AVF
N = 13

*Abbreviations:* RC, radiocephalic; BC, brachiocephalic; TBB, transposed brachiobasilic; AVG, AV grafting; TRB, transposed radiobrachial.

## Prosthetic Graft Placement Considerations

- A polytetrafluoroethylene (PTFE) graft is put if conditions are unfavorable for AV fistula.
- It must be put as distally as possible first time.
- After upper extremity vessels, the neck and lower extremity are considered.
- Chest wall grafts may erode through the skin because of the thin subcutaneous tissue over the chest wall.
- Thigh grafts can be a problem in patients with atherosclerosis. With flows over 4 L/min, cardiac function must be considered.

## Arteriovenous Fistula: Physical Examination

- The AV fistula and the extremity must be monitored regularly.
- Extremity must be examined for ischemia.

New fistulas may not have adequate flow because of:

- Inadequate arterial flow.
- Accessory vein siphoning off blood flow.
- The presence of accessory vein is sought by compressing the fistula with a finger and occluding it.
- Stenosis is suggested by a strong pulse stream proximal to the stenosis and almost disappears distal to the stenosis.
- A functional fistula has a continuous thrill with a soft compressible pulse.
- The direction of flow is determined by occluding the fistula and feeling for a pulse on either side. The inflow side is the one with the pulse.
- Stenosis is more common in synthetic grafts than AV fistulas.
- Stenosis occurs in the outflow veins or venous anastomosis.
- In stenosis, there is a localized systolic thrill rather than a continuous thrill.
- If the stenosis is severe, the blood may recirculate from the venous to the arterial needle during dialysis.
- If stenosis is very critical, then venous pressure may be high enough to stop the pump.

## Duplex Evaluation of Hemodialysis Grafts and Fistulas (Table 1)

This noninvasive investigation is very helpful to assess:
- Inflow
- Venous runoff
- Measurement of blood flow velocities
  - Blood flow velocity at arterial anastomosis of synthetic graft
  - Blood flow velocity at venous anastomosis or synthetic graft
  - Blood flow velocity throughout the length of the graft
- If volume flow (blood flow velocity × cross sectional area) is reduced in the absence of stenosis, then arterial inflow must be assessed

**Table 1** Comparison between ultrasound and angiography as angiography is considered the gold standard

|  | Accuracy | Sensitivity | Specificity |
|---|---|---|---|
| Grafts | 86% | 92% | 84% |
| AV fistulas | 81% | 79% | 81% |
| Venous outflow stenosis | 96% | 95% | 97% |

- Regular surveillance is used to treat and prevent thrombosis
- Grafts with flow less than 800 mL/min have a 93% chance of thrombosis within 6 months
- Those with higher flow have a 25% chance of thrombosis within 6 months
- Elective revision of grafts with flow less than 800 mL/min reduced the 6-month thrombosis from 42% to 6%
- Ultrasound surveillance with elective revision for more than 50% stenosis increased patency rates at 6, 12, 24, and 36 months when compared with surveillance with physical examination alone
- Thus, ultrasound surveillance should be incorporated with access management programs.

## ■ HEMODIALYSIS CATHETERS AND PORTS

- Hemodialysis catheter is a device that allows blood withdrawal and infusion at high rates (Fig. 4).
- The permacath is used temporarily in patients with acute renal failure and permanently in patients who have exhausted all avenues (Fig. 5).

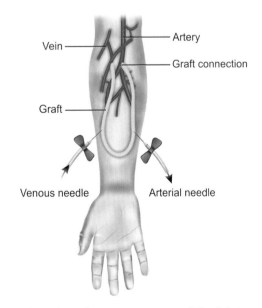

**Fig. 4** Sites where punctures are made for dialysis

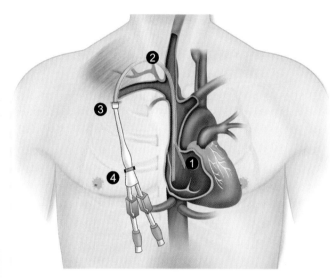

**Fig. 5** Permacath insertion

- The advantages are that there are no needle pricks and cannulation is easy.
- The disadvantages are a high degree of infection and thrombosis.
- The right internal jugular vein is the preferred site, as it offers a direct route into the right atrium. The complications are less compared with subclavian vein. There are less chances if stenosis—10% in jugular compared with 42% in subclavian vein. Rate of thrombosis is 3% in internal jugular vein compared with 14% in subclavian vein. The catheter tip must lie within the right atrium and must deliver more than 300 mL/min. Insertion by ultrasound guidance showed 100% success, while it was 88% by use of landmarks.

## Catheter Insertion Technique

- Cuffed and tunneled catheter is inserted under full aseptic precautions. Ultrasound is used to identify the vein prior to the preparation of the site. The vein is compressible and expands on Valsalva and shrinks on sniffing. Now, infiltrate the insertion site with a local anesthetic. IV sedation is given. A 21-gauge needle is inserted into the vein under ultrasound guidance. The syringe is removed and a guidewire inserted. After removing the needle, a 5F coaxial dilator is introduced over the guidewire. The inner 3F dilator is removed along with the guidewire and the 5F dilator is attached to a stopcock.
- Now, a subcutaneous pocket is created. A 1 cm incision is made extending laterally from the dilator. The subcutaneous tissue is bluntly dissected. Then, the exit site is identified on the patient's chest using a guidewire or catheter to know the distance to the right atrium. The exit site is infiltrated with local anesthetic. A tunnel is created using a tunneling device. The 5F dilator is removed over

a guidewire and multiple dilators are inserted in the vein over this guidewire. Lastly, a dilator with a peel sheath is inserted into the vein. The catheter is advanced through the peel away sheath. The sheath is then peeled away and removed. After ensuring that the tip of the catheter is within the right atrium, there are no kinks in the catheter and there is easy withdrawal of blood from the catheter when the venotomy is closed with sutures. The exit site is closed using a purse string suture over the catheter. Topical antibiotics may be used over the site. Finally, the lumen of the catheter is filled with heparin.

## Catheter Outcomes

- 100% technical success rate
- Infection is 0.08 per 100 catheter days
- Malfunction needing removal 0.22 per 100 catheter days
- Thrombosis needing removal 0.16 per 100 catheter days
- The alternative to the permacath is subcutaneous vascular port. The device is accessed through a subcutaneous pocket and accessed through the skin. A 14-gauge fistula needle activates a pinch valve that allows blood flow that stops once the needle is removed. With repeated punctures, a pain-free tissue tract develops. The mean duration of device survival was 6.8 months and the infection rate was 1.3 per 1000 patient-days compared with 3.3 per 1000 patient-days with permacath (cuffed tunneled catheter).

## ■ LIMITATIONS/COMPLICATIONS OF HEMODIALYSIS ACCESS

The failure of AV fistulas is due to:
- Infection—16–22% at 1 year
- Stenosis at the venous anastomosis or outflow vein due to neo-intimal hyperplasia
- Thrombosis—21–30% at 1 year
- These complications are more common in grafts than in AV fistulas.

## Dialysis Access-associated Steal Syndrome (DASS)

- This is a complication present in less than 4% but is a serious complication after creation of the AV fistula and is due to excess flow through the fistula. The arterial pressure distal to the access falls causing retrograde flow in the distal artery toward the access causing ischemia of the extremity. It may present as pain and clinical features of advanced tissue ischemia (Fig. 6).

It is corrected by:
- Closure of the fistula and repair of the artery
- Ligation of the artery distal to the access and a bridging bypass at some distance from the access

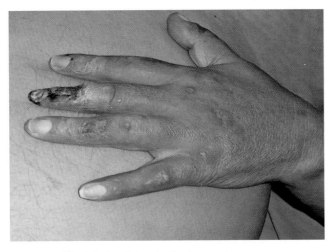

**Fig. 6** Ischemia hand with ulcers and gangrene

- Reduction of the shunt volume flow rate (banding)
- Thus, normal peripheral perfusion of the extremity takes place and avoids occurrence of the cardiac overload but is still sufficient to prevent thrombotic shunt occlusion.

## ■ SPECIAL ISSUES

### Endovascular Management of Hemodialysis Access Stenosis

- These are difficult to treat surgically because of their deep location and their tendency to recur and are best treated endovascularly. Percutaneous transluminal angioplasty (PTA) successfully treats 80% of the stenoses in both native fistulas and the synthetic grafts. It can be performed on the arterial and venous outflow tracts, on the anastomotic and proximal lesions. Angioplasty on the venous side improves fistula function and prolongs access survival.
- Angioplasty is done under fluoroscopic control and does not need heparinization. Needle is inserted antegrade into the fistula or the graft and a sheath inserted over a guidewire. A fistulogram is done to locate the site of stenosis where upon angioplasty is performed.
- The guidewire is passed beyond the lesion and a balloon catheter passed over the guidewire and is slightly larger than the affected vein. Usually, 6–8 × 4 balloons may be needed while a 12 mm balloon may be needed in a central vein. High pressure inflation is done at 10 atm and may go up to 20 atm. Each inflation is done for 1–2 minutes.
- Initial success rate for both grafts and fistulas is 80–95% and is 99% for forearm native fistulas. However, for native fistulas, it declines to 67–84% at 3 months and 8–40% at 1 year. Anastomotic lesions have patency of 8% at 1 year.

Stents are used:
- Venous rupture after angioplasty
- For elastic recoil after angioplasty

- If postangioplasty residual stenosis is more than 50%
- Only self-expanding stents are used. The diameter of the stent should be 1–2 mm larger than that of the largest balloon used for angioplasty. The stent should not protrude from the cephalic vein into the subclavian vein or from the subclavian into the superior vena cava (SVC).
- The primary patency rate at 1 year after stent implantation is 20%. After aggressive re-intervention, the secondary patency rate at 1 year is 70–80%.

Stents may be maintained by:
- Thrombolysis
- Repeated angioplasty
- Placement of a new stent
- Atherectomy
- The main reason for poor patency is neointimal formation. In future, drug-eluting stents may significantly reduce or eliminate the problem.

### Endovascular Management of Dialysis Fistula Thrombosis

- Dialysis fistula thrombosis is the most common complication of permanent vascular access accounting for 85–90% of the vascular accesses losses.

The reasons for this are:
- Venous stenosis (85%)
- Arterial stenosis
- Fistula compression
- Hypovolemia
- Hypercoagulable states.

Thrombosis can be treated by:
- Surgical thrombectomy
- Thrombolysis
- Mechanical modalities.

Endovascular therapy can be:
- Pharmacomechanical
- Purely mechanical.

In the pharmacomechanical technique, urokinase and heparin mixture is given through a catheter into the thrombus. This is delivered via a pulse-spray technique at every 30 s with 90% success.

Purely mechanical methods include clot extraction methods or balloon-based methods. The mechanical declotting devices available include—Angiojet, Amplatz thrombectomy device, Trerotola—percutaneous thrombectomy device and hydrolyzer. The main risk of purely mechanical devices is pulmonary embolism, and to reduce this risk, the hydrolyzer pulverizes the clot into tiny particles.

The initial success rate for both pharmacomechanical and purely mechanical devices are 90–95%, though the long-term patency rate is lower. The primary patency rates after declotting at 1, 3, 6, and 12 months is 74, 63, 52 and 27% in native fistulas, while in declotted PTFE grafts, it is only 8–10% at 1 year. Secondary patency rates are 75% with native AV fistulas and 50% with PTFE grafts. Mortality rates are less than 1% in AV fistulas while complication rates are 9% and include vessel rupture, injection, pseudoaneurysm, and bleeding in 1%.

## ■ CONCLUSION

- As the number of patients with ESRD grows, there will be an increased need for hemodialysis access.
- There are many types of hemodialysis access—each with advantages and disadvantages.

- AV fistulas have been used for several decades and are most trouble free once established.
- AV fistula must be created months before starting dialysis and needs surgical experts who are very familiar with the anatomy.
- AV grafts need less time to mature but are prone to infection and thrombosis.
- Catheters and ports are implanted with ease and can be used soon after placement but are mostly used on a temporary basis.

## PRACTICAL POINTS

- Autogenous AV fistula is best and most practical for dialysis.
- The normal maturation time for AV fistula is 2–4 months.
- History and examination provide crucial information in deciding location and type of hemodialysis access.
- Early detection and percutaneous treatment of stenosis of hemodialysis access can prolong the lifespan of shunts.
- The tip of the percutaneous placed dialysis catheter must be positioned in the mid-right atrium optimally.

# 26

# Perioperative Management of Patients with Peripheral Vascular Disease

*Jaisom Chopra*

Cardiovascular complications are the most common and a concern for any doctor and patient undergoing surgery. There are guidelines for evaluation and reduction of cardiac risk in noncardiac surgery.

## ■ PREOPERATIVE CARDIAC RISK ASSESSMENT

A cardiac clearance is generally asked preoperatively for patients undergoing surgery. An accurate assessment is a must so as to help in decision-making regarding surgery.
The perioperative cardiac risk is best assessed by:
- Clinical evaluation—history and physical examination
- Those patients whose risk is not clear (intermediate) on clinical evaluation alone should have a stress treadmill test and stress dobutamine test. Those who are at low or high risk do not need to undergo these tests.

The commonly used classification to assess the risk is—"The American Society of Anesthesiology Classification of Perioperative Risk."
- Normal healthy patient
- Mild systemic disease
- Severe systemic disease that limits activity
- Incapacitating systemic disease that is a constant threat to life
- Moribund patient not expected to survive more than 24 h, with or without surgery.

Patients with immediate life-threatening disease get 4–5 rating; those with active disease get 3 rating. The patients free of medical problems fall in category 1 while most patients generally fall in category 2.
However, this classification is being abandoned because:
- It poorly defines the perioperative risk.
- It provides little guidance as to the role of further testing.

- It does not point out to what is meant by systemic, severe, or incapacitating disease.

As this classification was very vague, further studies were conducted to identify the risk factors and scores were given to these risk factors. The high-risk clinical and cardiac factors identified were:
- Severe valvular heart disease
- Heart failure
- Recent myocardial infarction (MI)
- Older age
- Arrhythmias and
- Serious medical comorbidity.

A "revised cardiac risk index score" was given to each factor identified (Table 1). The factors identified were:

**Table 1** Revised cardiac risk index

| |
|---|
| High-risk surgery |
| Ischemic heart disease |
| History of congestive heart failure |
| History of cerebrovascular disease |
| Insulin therapy for diabetes |
| Preoperative serum creatinine >2 mg/dL |

Ischemic heart disease was defined as history of MI, positive stress test, angina, use of nitrates, or Q wave on electrocardiogram (ECG).

A lot of confusion prevailed while many attempts were being made to find the acceptable classification.

Eagle and associates limited their study to risk factors in peripheral vascular disease patients (Table 2).

**Table 2** Eagle clinical markers of perioperative cardiac risk

| |
|---|
| Age >70 years |
| Diabetes mellitus on medication |
| History of angina |
| History of MI or Q wave on ECG |
| Congestive heart failure (CHF)/Ventricular ectopic activity (VEA) requiring treatment |

In an attempt to find the suitable classification, "Five clinical variables" identified from various trials. They were:
- Advanced age
- Angina
- History of MI
- Diabetes mellitus
- History of congestive heart failure (CHF).

Thus, patients were put into low, moderate, and high-risk categories with observed cardiovascular events rate of 3, 8, and 18%.

On the basis of all these studies, the American Heart Association and American College of Cardiology formulated clinical markers for perioperative cardiac events:
- The clinical risk factors differ from the well-known markers for atherosclerosis. Factors such as high cholesterol, blood pressure, and tobacco abuse are well-known markers for atherosclerosis but do not figure as clinical risk factors for short-term cardiac events in the perioperative phase.

# ■ PREOPERATIVE TESTING

Thallium and dobutamine stress tests have consistently shown 100% negative predictive value, which means if the test is negative, there are no chances of a perioperative cardiac event. However, the positive predictive value is close to 12–15%, which shows that if the test is positive, 85% would not have a coronary event.

Therefore, how to pick up the cases at risk of a perioperative cardiac event?

Studies combined clinical evaluation and thallium stress test results:
- Those at clinically low risk did well irrespective of the thallium result.
- Those at clinically high risk all had high rates of perioperative cardiac events irrespective of the thallium results.
- Those at clinically moderate risk (having one or two of the five clinical markers) benefited from thallium testing—those in this category with a negative thallium had a 3% chance of perioperative event while those with positive thallium had a 15% chance.

The latest guidelines take into account:
- Patient's clinical risk
- Risk of surgery
- Patient's activity levels.

# ■ PERIOPERATIVE CARDIAC RISK REDUCTION (TABLE 3)

## Medical Treatment
- A study evaluating the effect of beta-blockers on perioperative cardiac events as well as long-term cardiac

**Table 3** Clinical markers of preoperative risk of cardiac complications

| |
|---|
| *Major* |
| • Unstable coronary syndromes |
| • Acute or recent MI with ischemic risk clinically or by tests |
| • Unstable or severe angina |
| • Decompensated heart failure |
| • Significant arrhythmias |
| • High grade AV block |
| • Symptomatic ventricular arrhythmia with heart disease |
| • Supraventricular arrhythmia with rapid ventricular rate |
| • Severe valvular disease |
| *Intermediate* |
| • Mild angina |
| • History of MI or pathologic Q waves |
| • Compensated or prior heart failure |
| • Diabetes mellitus (insulin dependent) |
| • Renal insufficiency |
| *Minor* |
| • Advanced age |
| • Abnormal ECG (left ventricular hypetrophy, left bundle branch block, ST-T abnormalities) |
| • Rhythm other than sinus (atrial fibrillation) |
| • Low functional capacity (inability to climb one flight of stairs with a bag or groceries) |
| • History of stroke |
| • Uncontrolled systemic hypertension |

events in patients undergoing noncardiac surgery was carried out. The results showed no difference in the perioperative cardiac events, but long-term follow-up over 2 years showed reduced rate of cardiac events with perioperative beta blockade.

- In another study, high-risk patients (with abnormal dobutamine stress echocardiogram facing major vascular surgery) were given perioperative beta-blockers and placebo. The results showed a dramatic reduction in MI and death if given beta-blockers. Thus, the study concluded that in high-risk patients undergoing high-risk surgery, the use of beta-blockers perioperatively reduces the incidence of serious cardiac events.
- The role of alpha-agonists given intravenously perioperatively was studied and showed a significant reduction in the perioperative MI and death in patients undergoing major vascular surgery.

## Recommendations for Perioperative Medical Therapy

*Class I*
- Beta-blockers needed in the recent past to control angina, symptomatic arrhythmias, or hypertension
- Beta-blockers: high cardiac risk patients with ischemia on preoperative testing who are to undergo vascular surgery

*Class IIa*
- Beta-blockers: preoperative checkup shows untreated hypertension, known coronary disease, or major risk factor for coronary disease

*Class IIb*
- Alpha 2 agonist: perioperative control of hypertension or known CAD or major risk factor for CAD

*Class III*
- Beta-blockers: contraindication to beta-blockade
- Alpha-2 agonists: contraindication to alpha-2 agonists

## ■ PERCUTANEOUS CORONARY INTERVENTIONS

- Perioperative heart failure and angina were more frequent among CAD patients who had not undergone percutaneous coronary intervention (PCI).
- There was no difference in the perioperative death and MI rates.

- For aortic surgery patients who underwent preoperative testing and PCI, the mortality was lower perioperatively.
- In peripheral bypass surgery, preoperative PCI showed higher mortality. This was due to the stent thrombosis because of the stoppage of vital drugs coupled with an increase in hypercoagulable state following noncardiac surgery.
- The freshly put stent takes time to endothelialize. Thus, noncardiac surgery should be performed 4–6 weeks after PCI to give adequate cover with antiplatelet drugs such as ecosprin and clopidogrel.

Current guidelines (Flow charts 1A to C) suggest that the indications for PCI are the same for operative and nonoperative settings, which are:
- Unstable angina
- High-risk stress test
- Large ischemic burden.

## Coronary Artery Bypass Surgery

- There are not many studies confirming the role of coronary artery bypass surgery (CABG) prior to major vascular surgery in high-risk CAD patients. However, according to Eagle and colleagues, patients with CAD and CABG had death and MI rates roughly half to one-third those of patients with CAD treated medically.
- After the introduction of the guidelines, 64% patients facing major aortic surgery underwent preoperative noninvasive testing and 58% received perioperative beta blockade. There was a dramatic reduction of perioperative MI.

## ■ CONCLUSION

- Preoperative evaluation and reduction of perioperative risk for PAD patients should be the same for any other patient undergoing nonvascular surgery.
- In the majority, history and examination can define risk in noncardiac surgery.
- Selective testing may identify increased risk or those who would benefit from coronary revascularization.
- Stress testing should be limited to moderate-risk patients.
- Beta-blockers reduce the perioperative risk of cardiac events in noncardiac patients with abnormalities on noninvasive testing.

**Flow chart 1A**

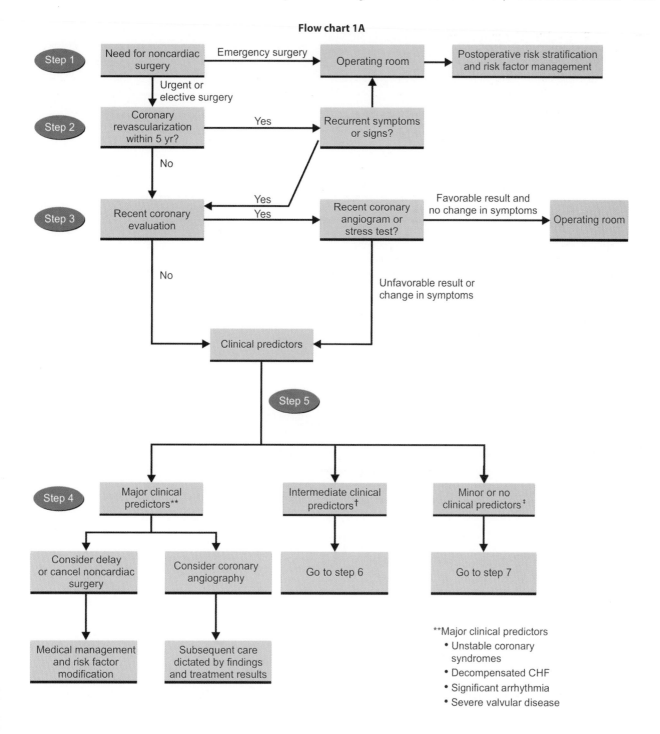

**Flow chart 1B**

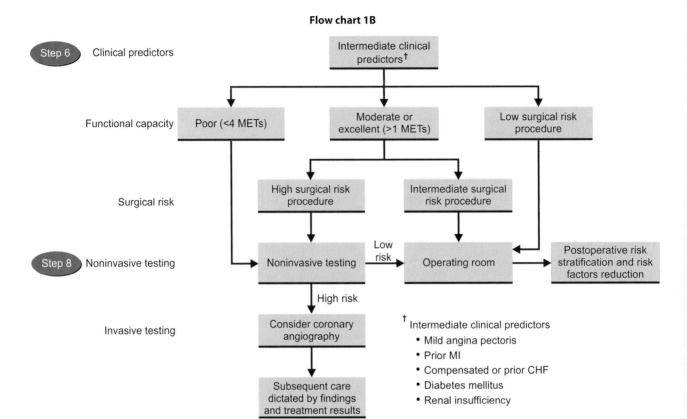

**Flow chart 1A to C** ACC/AHA guidelines for perioperative cardiovascular evaluation for noncardiac surgery

**Flow chart 1C**

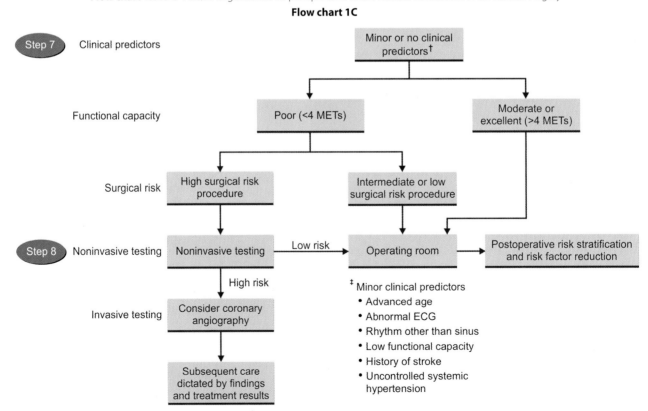

## PRACTICAL POINTS

- The goal of perioperative evaluation is not to clear patients for surgery but to accurately assess and minimize risk.
- Patients with favorable, noninvasive, and invasive testing in the last 2 years need no further cardiac workup if asymptomatic, since the test and functionally very active.
- Patients with changing clinical features of ischemia should have further evaluation.
- Poor functional capacity or combination of high-risk surgery and moderate functional capacity in patients with intermediate clinical predictors of cardiac risk (two or more) often need further noninvasive testing.

# 27
# Bypass Grafts: Surgical Aspects and Complications

*Jaisom Chopra*

## ■ VASCULAR CONDUITS (TABLE 1)

The success of vascular bypass graft depends upon:
- Quality of inflow
- Quality of outflow
- Characteristics of the bypass graft.

Grafts are placed in a thromboreactive state, which is defined in terms of intensity and duration. This state determines whether the graft will remain patent or occlude.

The characteristics of an ideal graft used are:
- Should be readily available
- Come in a variety of lengths and diameters
- Be antithrombogenic
- Provide long-term durability
- Easily sutured to the donor and recipient arteries
- Should be elastic to help pulsatility of the vascular system
- Should be impermeable to blood
- Luminal surface should be smooth and nonthrombogenic
- The graft should be biocompatible, as antigenicity can promote inflammatory response and thrombosis.

Such an ideal graft does not exist.

Types of vascular conduits are listed in Table 1.

**Table 1** Types of vascular conduit

| |
| --- |
| • Autogenous vein grafts |
| • Arterial autografts |
| • Biological grafts |
| • Umbilical vein grafts |
| • Cryopreserved grafts |
| • Prosthetic grafts |
| • Composite grafts |
| • Endovascular grafts |

## Vein Grafts (Fig. 1)

The sources of vein grafts are:
- Long saphenous vein
- Short saphenous vein
- Basilic vein
- Cephalic vein.

The most common used graft is the long saphenous vein (LSV) because of its:
- Length
- Easy access
- Suitable diameter.

The LSV is not suitable in 10–20% cases due to:
- Previous harvest for coronary bypass
- Superficial phlebitis
- Congenital absence.

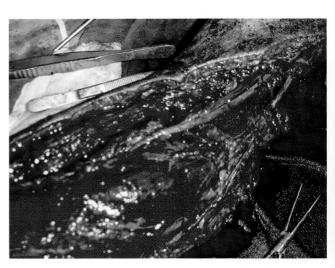

**Fig. 1** Vein bypass

- The contralateral LSV is a good alternative, if ipsilateral vein is not available. If this site not heal in peripheral vascular disease (PVD) that happens in 2%, then another bypass in indicated on that leg also.
- In case of short saphenous vein (SSV), avoid injury to sural nerve. This vein is harvested from the popliteal fossa to the lateral border of Achilles tendon.
- The arm veins—basilic and cephalic—are a good choice but may have had repeated venipuncture and so may be quite sclerotic.

Factors affecting the patency of the vein after harvesting:

- Pressure in which the vein is distended after the harvest. If over 200 mm Hg, endothelial cell dysfunction occurs.
- Use of vasoactive substances such as papaverine to distend the vein helps observe endothelial morphology.
- The temperature at which it is stored between the harvest and implantation—cold is harmful. Normal body temperature is ideal.
- Avoid undue tension or pressure on the vein during harvesting.
- Vein diameter less than 3 mm is not suitable due to lower patency rates. This is confirmed by duplex ultrasonography.
- If the length of the vein is not enough, then multiple small veins segments can be joined to make a longer vein, though the long-term durability is less than, if a single vein was used.
- Vein grafts are not inert, once they have been implanted.
- All autogenous vein grafts undergo morphological changes in response to the arterial circulation—venous arterialization.

    The vein graft may deteriorate in the first 30 days and is due to:
    - Poor selection
    - Technical errors
    - Initial quality of the vein.
- Between 30 days and 2 years, there could be neointimal hyperplasia at anastomotic site or site of valves incision. This is seen in 10%.
- After 2 years, changes occur due to progression of atherosclerosis. This can involve the venous conduit and occurs at a faster rate than arterial involvement.
- Aneurysmal dilation may occur in the vein over years.

## Arterial Autografts (Fig. 2)

These are the best bypass conduits currently available. Their advantages are:

- Maintain their viability
- Do not degenerate with time
- Are resistant to infection
- Have proportional growth when used in children.

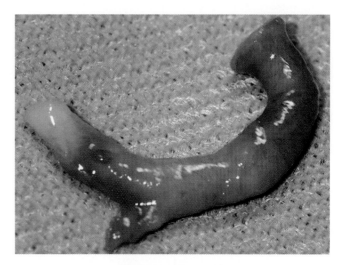

**Fig. 2**  Arterial autograft

Three common sites from where they are harvested:

- Internal iliac artery
- External iliac artery
- Superficial femoral artery.

    These sites can be reconstructed using a prosthetic conduit, as it is better tolerated at these sites.

    In children and young adults, the internal iliac artery has been harvested without mortality or long-term morbidity. Most of these grafts are used in the abdomen for visceral vessel reconstruction or in the groin region. These conduits are not used in the aortic region or lower limb bypasses.

## Biologic Grafts

These are generally used when vein or arterial grafts are not available.

### Umbilical Vein Grafts

The umbilical cord gives 50 cm of vein, which can be dilated up to 7 mm in diameter. These are unmodified heterogeneous grafts. There is immunological rejection of these grafts several weeks after their implantation. Rejection leads to thrombosis and graft degeneration. To avoid rejection, glutaraldehyde was used—tanned umbilical veins. The advantages are:

- These grafts maintain their basic architectural structure.
- The protein crosslinking increases the tensile strength of the graft.
- The tanning masks its antigenicity.
- There are some cases of umbilical vein aneurysms and so they are wrapped in polyester mesh.

## Cryopreserved Grafts

The harvested arterial and venous segments from cadavers can be stored by freezing for later use. The problems associated with these grafts are:

- Immunologically derived biological degradation
- Aneurysmal formation
- Calcification
- Rupture
- Occlusion.

Cryopreserved grafts can be kept for years and currently involves the use of dimethyl sulfoxide (DMSO), atraumatic harvest of the vessel, and storage at ultralow temperatures with liquid nitrogen. By this, the endothelium is preserved and there is reduced thrombogenicity. Intima is replaced by host endothelium, but until that happens, the graft is exposed to thrombosis.

## Prosthetic Grafts

These have been constructed keeping three things in mind:

- Graft porosity
- Graft thrombogenicity
- Graft compliance.

They are classified according to the method of construction and are either textile or non-textile grafts.

The textile grafts are from polymers, first spun into yarns, and then knitted or woven together to form the graft (Fig. 3).

Non-textile grafts are made of polytetrafluoroethylene (PTFE) or polyurethane, using precipitation or extrusion of polymer from sheets of the material.

The criteria the prosthetic graft must meet to be used as a conduit:

- Material must be biocompatible.
- Material must be free of toxicity, allergic reactions, and carcinogenic side effects.

- The graft must be durable and resist degradation and degeneration over time.
- Must be readily available in various sizes and diameters.
- Must be flexible and yet be resistant to kinking.
- It must have structural integrity so that it can be sutured in place.
- The graft must be impervious to blood but at the same time porous. It may be microporous as expanded PTFE (ePTFE) or macroporous such as loosely woven Dacron. These macroporous grafts need preclotting to prevent blood leakage. The greater the degree of porosity, the more the fibrous encapsulation of the graft. Autogenous tissue ingrowth through the pores would provide adherence for a stable intimal lining and improved patency.
- Graft thrombogenicity is a major concern. Upon exposure to blood, the graft becomes coated with serum proteins, mainly fibrinogen. This is followed by platelet adherence and activation that starts a local hemostatic reaction. The graft becomes lined by proteins and fibrinogen, which forms a pseudointima. If the process accelerates in an uncontrolled fashion, then the graft thrombosis occurs. However, in autogenous vein grafts, there is intimal lining along the length of the graft which prevents thrombogenicity and preserves patency. In prosthetic grafts, intimal lining covers only 2–3 cm at either end. This happens because of the finite ability of the endothelial cells to divide (Fig. 4).
- The faster the blood flow through the graft, the less chances of fibrin deposition and platelet adherence, reducing the chances of graft thrombosis. This is more important in long grafts as axillofemoral and leg bypasses.
- The narrower the size of the graft, the more the chances of thrombosis because the pseudointimal lining further will narrow the graft and make it more prone to thrombosis.

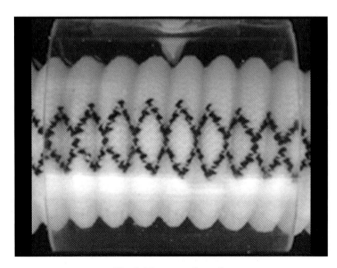

**Fig. 3** Woven textile grafts

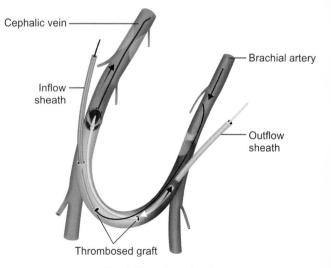

**Fig. 4** Thrombosed graft

- Graft compliance is important to prevent thrombogenicity. Compliance is the ability of the graft to expand in response to increased pressure. In vein grafts, it is dependent upon the elastin and collagen within the wall of the vein.
- The durability depends upon the material of the graft. PTFE and Dacron are the promising materials. Dacron grafts are knitted, woven, or braided to form the graft. Woven grafts have little or no stretch capacity and are tightly constructed, which reduces their porosity providing reduced blood leakage and decreased incidence of aneurysmal dilatation. These grafts flay at the cut edges and have reduced compliance. Knitted grafts have increased porosity that leads to better graft incorporation, better compliance, and better handling characteristics, though they have reduced strength compared with the woven type. Both these types can be velour surfaced to provide it improved elasticity and handling features. Velour surfacing increases the porosity with reduced hemorrhage and increases the grafts ability to incorporate into the surrounding tissue. It has not shown improved patency and durability.
- Crimping improves graft flexibility, elasticity, and shape retention. This however provides irregular luminal surface leading to increased fibrin deposit and thrombogenicity thus reducing the luminal diameter. To avoid this, no crimping is done, but external support is given via rings as in ePTFE grafts.
- PTFE is a non-textile synthetic graft, which is chemically inert, electronegative, and hydrophobic. There is a thin layer of outer reinforcement to prevent aneurysmal dilatation. It is more porous than the knitted or woven textile grafts with smaller pore size so that bleeding does not occur. However, there is little tissue ingrowth through the pores, though the graft becomes incorporated into the surrounding connective tissue. These grafts are more compliant being thinner and are supported by external rings or coils to prevent external compression and kinking (Fig. 5). The main disadvantage is that they have anastomotic healing abnormalities.

## Composite Grafts (Fig. 6)

These are considered in one-third of the cases where the vein is not suitable for bypass due to its caliber or its length or quality. Longer prosthetic grafts have a higher occlusion rate due to thrombosis than a same length vein graft due to:

- Exposure of blood to a longer prosthetic graft surface area
- Slower flow through these long grafts.

To overcome these problems, composite grafts were suggested. This consists of a proximal prosthetic graft anastomosed to a distal vein graft composing a single bypass graft. The prosthetic and vein parts are joined by end-to-end anastomosis.

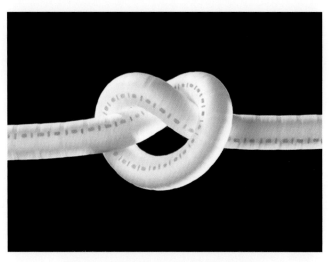

**Fig. 5** Inter-ring PTFE grafts showing flexibility

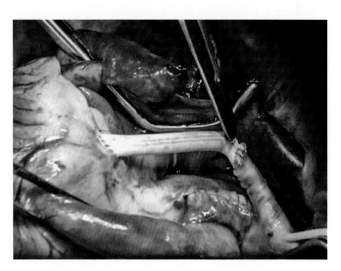

**Fig. 6** Composite graft showing PTFE graft attached to vein by end-to-end anastomosis

Then, there is a sequential—composite graft wherein the prosthetic graft is anastomosed distally and then a jump graft is taken from the prosthetic graft and anastomosed further distally to supply the blood (Fig. 7). The advantage is that in the distal portion thrombosis, the proximal portion may remain patent. The advantage of the composite and the sequential—composite grafts is that the compliant and flexible vein graft traverses the knee joint. The vein graft is anastomosed to the smaller diseased distal vessel, which reduces the incidence of anastomotic narrowing. Not enough data are available to compare composite and sequential—composite grafts with either prosthetic grafts alone, vein grafts alone, or synthetic grafts with miller cuff.

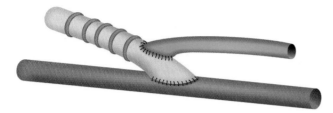

**Fig. 7** Polytetrafluoroethylene graft is attached to artery and a jump graft is from PTFE to artery distally

## Endovascular Grafts (Fig. 8)

These are mainly for the treatment of abdominal aortic aneurysm (AAA) and the various devices in the market differ in their delivery system and alterations in the different aspects of the graft.

## Delivery System

The device is placed through the common femoral arteries in the groin. The delivery system size, its flexibility, and deliverability are important factors in graft placement. The narrowing of the iliacs due to atheroma or calcification is important in preventing graft placement. The size of the delivery system depends on the internal diameter of the iliac arteries, which is 7–8 mm in diameter. The delivery system has got to be pliable to traverse a tortuous iliac artery.

## Endograft Features

There are two main types of endografts:
1. Unibody
2. Modular.

The former is a single graft including the limbs with reduced chances of endoleaks, as it is one piece, but it requires a larger delivery system and sizing may be more difficult (Fig. 9).

The modular device is composed of two to three pieces—the main body with one or two docking limbs. They are placed through a smaller docking system that provides more flexibility, but as there are multiple sites for docking, there are more chances of endoleaks (Fig. 10).

The graft material ranges from PTFE to polyester, which is supported by modified stainless steel framework—elgiloy or notional.

The graft is supported from inside the graft material (endoskeleton) or from outside (exoskeleton). They could be fully supported having stent material throughout or partially. The graft skeleton helps in:
• Graft fixation and obtaining a seal
• Hooks or barbs at the proximal end that anchor the graft into the aortic wall preventing migration (Fig. 11)
• Metallic skeleton provides columnar strength preventing migration
• Prevent kinking and occlusion of the limbs, as they traverse the aortoiliac anatomy.

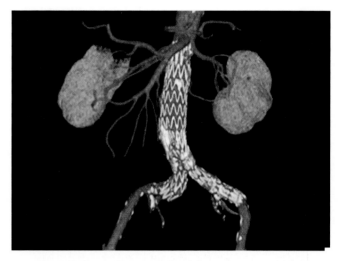

**Fig. 8** Endovascular stenting for abdominal aortic aneurysm

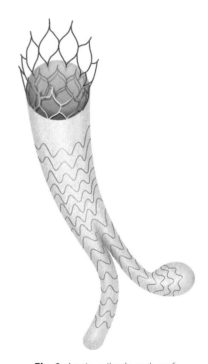

**Fig. 9** Aortic unibody endograft

## Graft Selection in Open Surgery

To select a graft, one must weigh the advantages and disadvantages and how it will behave in a particular situation.
• The factors the surgeon must look at before use are:
  – Graft patency
  – Convenience of use
  – Absence of complications
  – Cost
• In aortic surgery, we do not use venous or arterial autografts because of the length and size.

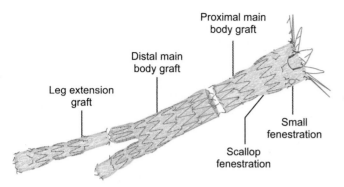

**Fig. 10** Modular endovascular graft

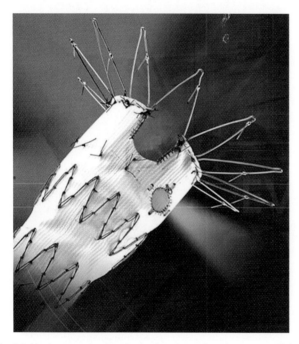

**Fig. 11** Hooks at proximal end to anchor the graft and prevent endoleaks

- In thoracic aorta, bleeding is of much concern and tightly woven Dacron grafts are preferred because of excellent dimensional integrity and prolonged patency rates (Figs 12A to C).
- In thoraco-abdominal reconstruction, multiple grafto-tomies are needed to implant the visceral vessels; the stiffness and poor conformability of the tightly woven Dacron graft hinders the operation. Here, ePTFE or coated knitted Dacron grafts are used.
- For AAA, Dacron grafts or ePTFE grafts have been recommended (Fig. 13).
- For lower extremity bypass, the long saphenous vein has always been preferred. This can be placed *in situ*, but valves have to be lysed. If placed reverse, then there can be a significant mismatch at the anastomotic site.
- In infra-inguinal bypasses, vein grafts are always preferred. Synthetic grafts are a poor alternative because of the low patency rates.
- In an infected field, vein grafts are always preferred over synthetic grafts due to increased resistance to infection compared with synthetic grafts.
- Most extra-anatomic bypasses—femorofemoral or axillo-femoral bypasses are performed using ePTFE grafts with external supporting rings.
  The advantage of using ePTFE is:
  - Less leaks from graft and so reduced hematoma formation under the skin
  - Resistant to kinking
  - Easy graft thrombectomy.

## ■ SURGICAL CONSIDERATIONS

To decide which conduit to use, the main consideration is appropriate size match. Where to look for the conduit?
- Autograft from within the same operative field
- Autograft from other location provided it does not add to the morbidity
- External synthetic conduit.

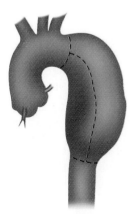
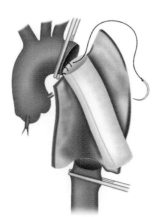
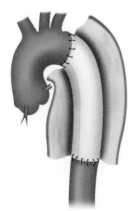

**Figs 12A to C** Thoracic aortic aneurysm with grafting

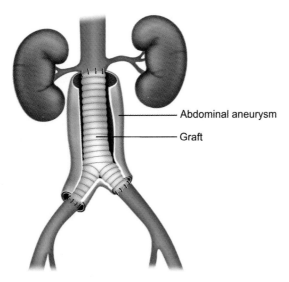

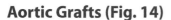

**Fig. 13** Open AAA surgery with grafting

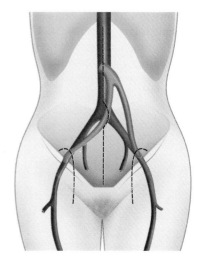

**Fig. 14** Aortobiiliac bypass

## Aortic Grafts (Fig. 14)

- These are required for the treatment of aortoiliac occlusive disease or aortoiliac aneurysmal disease.
- For occlusive disease, the aorta is approached through a midline incision transperitoneally or less frequently via the retroperitoneal approach, which is of big advantage in previous multiple abdominal surgeries.
- Bilateral groin incisions are made to approach the common femorals wherein the distal ends of the grafts are placed.
- The prosthetic graft is anastomosed to the aorta either end-to-end (Fig. 15) or end-to-side (Fig. 16). Both have advantages.

*End-to-end has the advantages:*
  - All blood flows through the graft with less competitive flow through the aorta and so less chances of graft thrombosis.
  - The high flow may reduce the risk of recurrent atheroma formation.
  - Reduces the risk of pseudoaneurysm formation at the site of the anastomosis.

*Advantages of end-to-side anastomosis:*
  - The aorta may not be totally occluded and a side biting clamp put. So, the flow is maintained even while anastomosing. This is a major advantage in patients with extensive atherosclerotic occlusive disease in external iliac arteries.
  - By this technique, flow is maintained through the internal iliac arteries to the pelvis.
  - If the proximal end of the graft is anastomosed to the thoracic aorta.
- The graft is tunneled retroperitoneally along the iliacs but behind the ureter.
- The lower ends of the graft are anastomosed to the common femoral or the profunda femoris artery.

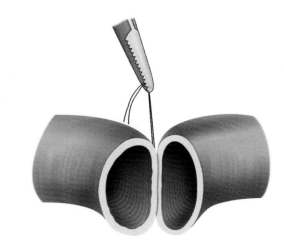

**Fig. 15** End-to-end anastomosis

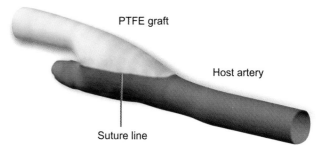

**Fig. 16** End-to-side anastomosis

- If there is a stenosis of the origin of the profunda, then the arteriotomy is extended from the common femoral into the profunda beyond the stenosis to perform a patch angioplasty.
- The anastomosis must be flawless at the femoral for good technical success.

- The outcome of this surgery is excellent with 5-year patency being 85–90% and 70–75% at 10 years.
- Thoracofemoral bypasses have similar patency rates.
- These procedures have few complications and 30-day mortality is 2–3%.
- Despite excellent long-term patency rates, the long-term survival in these patients is 60% at 5 years and 40% at 10 years due to comorbidities.

### *AAA Repair*

- In repair of AAA the approach is similarly midline or retro-peritoneal.
- The proximal anastomosis is performed end-to-end. The distal end of the graft is anastomosed end-to-end to the aorta or a bifurcated graft is put end-to-side onto the iliacs or the femorals as the situation demands.
- The long-term results are excellent and mortality is less than 5%.

## Endovascular Grafting in AAA

- An improved approach to the treatment of AAA is endo-vascular graft, which is inserted via a femoral cut-down.
- Endoleaks are high (15–20%) where blood partially continues to flow through the native aorta despite the endograft.
- The advantage of this procedure is that it is less stressful to the patient especially, those with coexisting cardiac or pulmonary problems.

## Extra-anatomic Grafts

These are the axillofemoral (Fig. 17) and the femorofemoral bypass grafts (Fig. 18).

They are performed in patients who are sick due to other problems and could not stand aortofemoral surgery (Fig. 19). The input is taken from the axillary artery by an infraclavicular incision. Preoperatively, brachiocephalic occlusive disease must be excluded. A ringed ePTFE graft is taken that is resistant to external compression and kinking. The graft is tunneled in the anterior axillary line and anastomosed to the common femoral artery. The 5-year patency is 30–70%. It is suggested that axillobifemoral bypass has a superior patency rate over axillounifemoral bypass.

Femorofemoral bypass is for patients with unilateral occlusive iliac artery disease.

The ringed graft runs from the donor femoral artery subcutaneously in the supra-pubic tunnel to the recipient femoral artery.

Mild iliac stenosis is treated with angioplasty and stenting (Figs 20A and B).

An 8-mm ringed PTFE graft is used. Vein grafts have not been shown to give better patency rates and are reserved for infected situations. Five-year patency rates range from

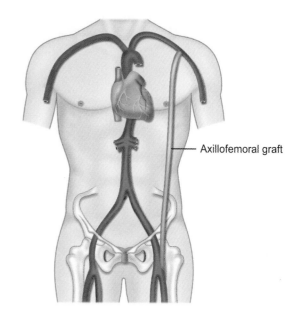

**Fig. 17** Left axillofemoral bypass

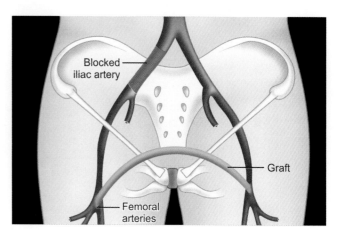

**Fig. 18** Femorofemoral graft

50% to 80%. If the profunda femoris is patent, then SFA occlusion does not adversely affect the long-term patency rates. In 10%, claudication in the donor limb may occur because of hemodynamic changes and infra-inguinal disease.

## Lower Extremity Grafts (Fig. 21)

In the lower extremity, mostly vein grafts are used that may be reversed or *in situ*. They are tunneled anatomically.

The advantages of the *in situ* or nonreverse vein graft are:

- It lies anatomically
- Does not need much dissection and so less chances of injury to the vein
- The anastomotic sites of the artery and the vein are well matched at the proximal and the distal end.

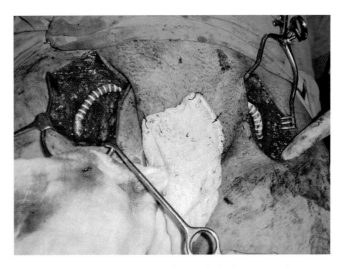

**Fig. 19**  Femorofemoral graft tunneled subcutaneously

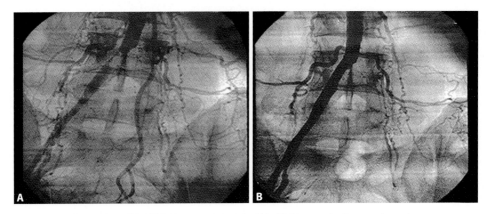

**Figs 20A and B**  (A) Tight stenosis in right CIA, (B) After angioplasty and stenting

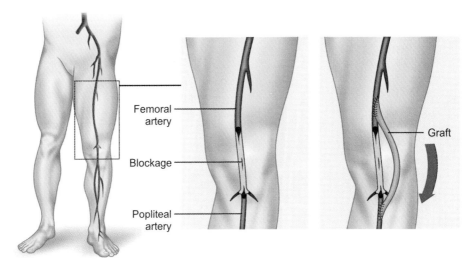

**Fig. 21**  Femoropopliteal bypass surgery

The main disadvantage is that during lysis of the valves, there could be injury to the intima leading to fibrosis, scarring, and subsequent narrowing. The cusp of the valve may be left intact despite lysis leading to partial narrowing.

The disadvantages of reverse vein grafts are:
- It needs more extensive dissection than *in situ* grafts
- There is a mismatch between the artery and the vein at the distal end, mainly below the knee.

The patency rates depend upon:
- Site of the distal anastomosis—the more distal the shorter the patency rate.
- Indications of surgery—worse for critical limb ischemia and then claudication.

Femoropopliteal above-knee bypasses have a 5-year patency rate of 80% while for below knee it is 60%. Limb salvage rates at 5 years are 80–90%.

Should autologous vein not be available, then one can consider glutaraldehyde-stabilized human umbilical vein graft. As it is very delicate, some technical points must be observed during the implantation:
- Poor handling may lead to intimal fracture and extensive mural dissection of blood.
- The vein wall may be very thick leading to difficulty during anastomosis.
- Care must be taken to include the intimal layer in the suture that can be easily missed in the thick wall.
- The toe and heel of the anastomotic site must be with interrupted sutures.
- These grafts must be tunneled through a rigid tunnel device to prevent venous injury to the polyester mesh.

The 5-year patency rates reported for femoropopliteal above knee are 61% while below the knee to the tibial fall to only 39%. Secondary patency rates however improve to 67% and 51% with limb salvage rates of 80% and 68% at 5 years. Thirty-six percent undergo aneurysmal formation at 5 years and 21% after 5 years.

Umbilical vein grafts have been used in aortorenal bypass and in extra-anatomic bypasses such as axillofemoral and femorofemoral bypasses but to no greater advantage over synthetic bypasses.

Cryopreservation vein grafts have shown no major advantage and 1-year patency is less than 50% due to rejection. Use of immunosuppressants has not been of much benefit.

Arterial autologous grafts—external iliac artery and superficial femoral artery are excellent conduits for bypassing the common femoral artery, profunda femoris artery, and popliteal artery. The length of occlusion is generally short and there are good diameter matches. The arterial homograft has advantages that it can grow and shows resistance to infection and is a good conduit in children and young adults for oncologic surgery.

Prosthetic grafts are used when no other conduit is available. The advantages are:
- Shorter operative time
- Operation performed through a small incision at two sites.

The 5-year patency rates for femoropopliteal above-knee bypass graft are 50% and secondary patency rates 60–70%. If the distal end is below the knee to the tibial artery, then a vein cuff or patch is required to improve the compliance. The patency rate at 4 years is 25–60%. If adequate vein is available and a composite or composite sequential graft is used, the patency at 4 years is 40–60%.

## ■ LIMITATIONS AND COMPLICATIONS

### Graft Thrombosis

This is seen not very infrequently depending on the anatomic location of the graft.
- In aorto-femoral bypass graft, early thrombosis is generally due to technical problems at the femoral anastomosis.
  - These patients present with acute limb ischemia.
  - Long-term graft thrombosis over 5 years occurs in 10% and they present with less severe symptoms.
  - Patients with acute limb ischemia are given anticoagulation with balloon catheter thrombectomy of the affected limb and subsequent revision of the distal anastomosis.
  - If the symptoms are not acute, then one could try thrombolysis that may also uncover the cause of graft thrombosis.

In the case of lower extremity and extra-anatomic graft thrombosis, the same principles hold true. In acute graft thrombosis, immediate anticoagulation is given. An on-table angiogram is done to see the inflow and outflow vessels. Balloon catheter thrombectomy is carried out. The graft must be checked for kinks. Thrombolysis is carried out, if the situation is not very acute.

In the STILE trial (Surgery versus Thrombolysis for Ischemia of the Lower Extremity), patency was restored in 81% of the occluded bypass grafts by thrombolysis without surgical intervention.

### Graft Infection

The diagnosis and the management of *aorta-iliac graft infection* can be very difficult. The presentation is very varied:
- Fever
- General malaise
- Anastomotic pseudoaneurysm
- Frank purulent discharge from the wound.

Investigations include:
- Angiogram
- Computed tomographic (CT) scan
- Magnetic resonance imaging (MRI).

Treatment is removal of the graft and reconstruction that can be a real challenge. It is generally performed in stages:

*Stage 1*—extra-anatomical bypass such as axillofemoral or axillobifemoral or axillopopliteal bypass.

*Stage 2*—complete graft removal.

Some recommend a single-stage procedure in which the superficial femoral and popliteal veins are harvested bilaterally and harvested to create a new aortic graft. Cryopreserved aortic allograft reconstruction after removal of the infected graft is being performed.

Treatment of the lower extremity graft (Fig. 21) infection involves:
- Antibiotics to control infection
- Excision of all infected tissue
- Removal of the infected graft
- Restoration of the blood supply.

The common organisms are—*Staphylococcus epidermidis, Staphylococcus aureus,* and *Escherichia coli.* The less virulent organisms such as *Staphylococcus epidermidis* can be treated by antibiotics and may eradicate infection and preserve the graft, whereas the more virulent organisms such as *Pseudomonas aeruginosa* are treated more aggressively with graft removal.

The usual presentation is draining sinus or mass.
The tests ordered are:
- Ultrasound
- CT scan
- MRI
- Radioisotope tagged white blood cell (WBC) scan.

The treatment includes:
- Antibiotics
- Removal of the infected graft and debridement
- Close anastomotic sites with vein patches
- Unless acutely threatened delay revascularization till the infection settles
- If the limb is threatened, venous bypass conduits are preferred and try to pass the new venous graft through healthy tissue
- Another option is use of arterial homograft used mainly in infected groin wounds and need a femorofemoral bypass
- If needed, the previously bypassed external iliac artery can be harvested and eversion endarterectomy performed to restore the patency. Recurrent infection rate is reported to be low
- Glutaraldehyde-treated human umbilical vein graft, though not immune to infection, is quite resistant due to the tanning process and is consistent with infection rates using saphenous vein (below 3%).

## Graft Aneurysm (Fig. 22)

Pseudoaneurysm occurs in less than 5% of the aortoiliac bypasses. The most common site is the femoral anastomosis. The common causes are:
- Suture failure
- Graft infection
- Graft dilatation
- End-to-side anastomosis
- Arterial degradation.

Most are asymptomatic and not picked up as an incidental ultrasound finding performed for another cause or when it is large enough to be palpated on physical examination.

Pseudoaneurysm can develop at any time following graft placement. Early development is mostly due to technical error or graft infection, whereas late development is due to arterial wall degeneration.

Repair is confined to the site of the aneurysm where the limb of the graft is anastomosed to the healthy arterial wall after treating it for infection.

Aortic pseudoaneurysm reconstruction is difficult and may need supraceliac clamping. Reimplantation of the visceral arteries may be needed which could be very difficult so endovascular techniques are being attempted with some promise.

True aneurysm degradation can occur in grafts. Dacron grafts dilate over time up to 10–20% from their original size immediately after implantation. Over time, this could increase from 23% to 94%. Although this dilatation of the graft does not affect adversely, but pseudoaneurysm at the anastomotic site could develop.

Aneurysmal degradation of the saphenous vein graft can occur in children, over time. This is because in children, the vein wall is nourished by network of vaso vasorum that are damaged during the vein harvest. In adults, these networks are not needed and so harvesting the vein has a little impact.

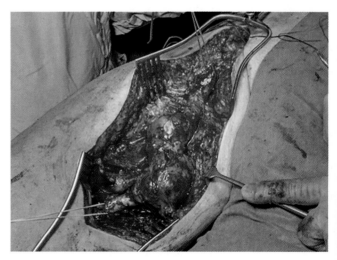

**Fig. 22** False aneurysm at the distal end of the graft

Umbilical vein grafts rarely dilate because of the superior tanning technology. If aneurysm forms and is more than 3 cm, it should be resected and replaced by an interposition graft or a new bypass graft.

## Lymph Leaks

This is estimated at 2–3%. This can be prevented with careful meticulous dissection and dividing and ligating all lymphatic channels helps prevent these leaks. Factors predisposing to formation of lymph fistula or lymphocele are:

- Advanced age
- Aortobifemoral bypass
- Repeated groin dissection
- Extensive profunda femoris exposure.

These patients present with a nontender and nonerythematous groin swelling.

Ultrasound shows a hyperechogenic mass.

Aspiration reveals yellow clear fluid with no blood cells or bacteria and a protein content of 0.5–2 g/L.

Treatment with aspiration has limited success and carries the risk of infection especially with underlying graft. Mostly, aspiration is done once or twice under complete aseptic precautions before surgical intervention wherein the groin is explored and all leaking lymphatics ligated. Vital blue dye is given in the webspace between the first and second toes to assist subcutaneous injection. This dye is carried by the lymphatics to the groin and seen pooling from the site of lymphatic leak.

Lymphatic leak occurs in the abdomen from aortic dissection resulting in chyloperitoneum. This is rare and patients present with abdominal distention, nausea, vomiting, and reduced appetite. Paracentesis is diagnostic. Initially, conservative management is done with patient on high protein, low fat diet supplemented with medium chain triglycerides. If this fails, then the patient is put on reduced oral intake with parenteral nutrition. Rarely do we need peritoneal venous shunt.

## ■ SPECIAL ISSUES

The most common cause of vein graft failure within 2 years of infra-inguinal revascularization is neointimal hyperplasia. It is seen in 10–30% of the grafts with majority in 12 months. These are detected on routine ultrasound used to monitor grafts in the postoperative period with the objective to correct these lesions before they compromise the blood supply. These lesions whether found on routine screening or after thrombolysis need correction, which is done by:

- Open surgical patch angioplasty
- Rebypass
- Percutaneous balloon angioplasty that has success rates of 90 and patency of 60% at 2 years. Short solitary lesions less than 15 mm have the best outcome. Secondary lesions respond less favorably to angioplasty than primary lesions.

Sanchez and colleagues studied vein graft stenosis treated by balloon angioplasty. The lesions were either simple or complex. Simple lesions were single, non-recurrent, and short (<15 mm long) within the vein graft that was more than 3 mm diameter. Complex lesions were recurrent, multiple, or long within a graft less than 3 mm diameter. Simple lesions treated with PTA had a 2-year patency of 66% compared with 17% in complex lesions. Surgical intervention of the failing graft had a patency of 84% at 2 years.

The results of in-graft stenosis of prosthetic grafts were similar to those of vein grafts.

## ■ CONCLUSION

- None of the bypass conduits are ideal.
- Large diameter prosthetic grafts are an excellent option for aortic reconstruction.
- Saphenous vein bypass is ideal for lower extremity bypass. Other conduits give significantly low patency rates.
- Both vein and synthetic grafts have complications that can be limited by meticulous surgical technique.

## PRACTICAL POINTS

- There is no ideal vascular conduit currently available.
- Saphenous vein is the bypass conduit of choice for lower limb.
- Prosthetic grafts and umbilical vein grafts can be used for lower limb but have significantly lower patency rates.
- Aortic reconstruction has high patency rates with large synthetic grafts.
- Extra-anatomic grafts are performed using synthetic grafts as they have low porosity and are resistant to kinking. Vein grafts have not shown improved patency and are reserved for an infected field.
- Multiple complications can occur with arterial reconstruction but these are limited by meticulous surgical technique.

# 28

# Computed Tomographic Angiography

*Jaisom Chopra*

It is a minimally invasive medical test that helps physicians to diagnose and treat medical conditions.

Computed tomographic angiography (CTA) uses the following:
- X-rays with catheters
- Computerized tomography (CT) (Fig. 1)
- Magnetic resonance imaging (MRI) (Fig. 2)
- Contrast material.

Iodine-rich contrast is injected into the vein, and as it flows throughout the blood vessels in various organs of the body, it is scanned. The images produced by the machine are processed through a special computer and software to view it in different planes and projections.

## ■ USES OF COMPUTED TOMOGRAPHIC ANGIOGRAPHY

Used to study the blood vessels and organs of the body such as:
- Brain
- Neck
- Lungs
- Heart
- Abdomen
- Legs.

It helps diagnose and evaluate blood vessel diseases such as:
- Injury
- Aneurysms
- Blockages (including those from clots or plaques)
- Blood supply to tumors and abnormal blood vessels
- Congenital anomalies of the heart and blood vessels.

CTA is ordered in the following conditions:
- Identify aneurysms in aorta and other arteries
- Detect atherosclerotic disease in carotid that can cause transient ischemic attacks (TIAs) and cerebrovascular accident (CVA)
- Identify aneurysms or arteriovenous (AV) malformations in the brain
- Detect stenoses or occlusions in leg arteries and plan endovascular or surgical intervention
- Detect renal artery disease and prepare for kidney transplant

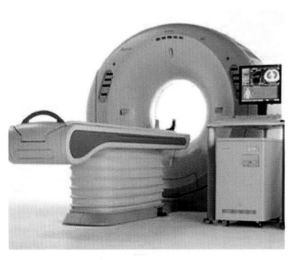

**Fig. 1** CT scan machine

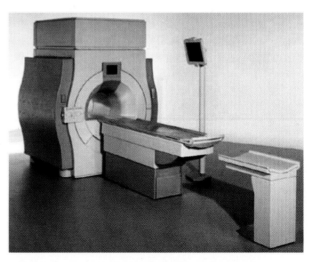

**Fig. 2** The magnetic field is created by passing electric current through wire coils

- Detect injury to arteries in trauma patients
- Evaluate arteries feeding tumors prior to surgery of chemo-embolization or selection internal radiation therapy
- Identify dissection in aorta or other vessels
- Show extent of atherosclerosis in coronary arteries and plan bypass or stenting
- Sample blood from specific veins to detect endocrine disease
- Detect clots in pulmonary artery in pulmonary embolism (PE)
- Look for congenital abnormalities in blood vessels.

In preparation for the test:

- The patient must be nil orally for 6 h prior to the test, if contrast is to be used
- The history of any allergies must be known
- If breastfeeding, pump out the milk prior to the test and keep it for use after the contrast is cleared from the body that takes 24 hour.

Breath-hold spiral CTA is being increasingly used to diagnose peripheral artery disease (PAD). This has a sensitivity of 93% and a specificity of 96% and an overall accuracy of 96% compared with digital subtraction angiography (DSA).

## Limitations of CTA

- Allergic to iodine
- Advanced kidney disease of severe diabetes—contrast may be harmful
- Very obese people.

## Risks

- A slight chance of cancer due to exposure to radiation. The benefit of accurate diagnosis outweighs the risk.
- If there is a history of allergic reaction, then steroids may be given few hours prior to test or a day before. Another option is doing MR angiogram instead of CTA.
- Leakage of contrast below the skin may lead to damage of the skin, blood vessel, and nerve.

## Benefits versus Risks

- CTA may eliminate the need for surgery or it may be performed more accurately.
- Stenosis or occlusion of blood vessels is visualized and corrective therapy performed.
- CTA may give accurate details about small vessels than MRA.
- CTA is less cumbersome, faster, and less invasive than conventional angiography.
- By CTA, arterial and venous phases can be seen, which is not possible on conventional angiography.
- CTA has a lower cost than conventional angiography.

## ■ MAGNETIC RESONANCE ANGIOGRAPHY

Magnetic resonance angiography (MRA) is a medical test helping physicians to diagnose and treat medical conditions related to blood vessels. In MRA, a powerful magnetic field, radiowaves, and a computer produce detailed images. MRA does not use ionizing radiations (X-rays).

## Common Uses

It examines blood vessels in various parts of the body such as:

- Brain
- Neck
- Heart
- Lungs
- Abdomen
- Pelvis
- Legs.

Physicians use the procedure to:

- Identify aneurysms in chest and abdomen
- Detect carotid artery disease which may cause TIA or stroke
- Identify small aneurysms and AV malformations in brain
- Detect peripheral disease causing narrowing or occlusion and help prepare for endovascular or surgical intervention
- Detect renal artery disease and visualize blood flow to prepare for kidney transplant
- Detect arterial injury in various parts of the body
- Evaluate arteries feeding tumor prior to surgery or embolization or selective internal radiation therapy
- Identify aortic dissection in chest or abdomen
- Show extent of coronary artery disease and plan stenting or coronary artery bypass grafting (CABG)
- Sample blood from specific veins to detect endocrine disease
- Examine pulmonary arteries for PE
- Look for congenital anomalies
- Screen for arterial disease in families.

## Before Scan

- Inform radiologist about allergic diseases such as asthma and allergies to drugs, iodine, food, and so on
- The contrast used in MRA is gadolinium that rarely causes allergic reaction
- Must inform about previous surgeries, as metal staples may have been used
- Radiologist must be informed about pregnancy, as the fetus will be in a powerful magnetic field
- Breastfeeding mothers must pump out the milk and keep it to be given to the baby. It takes 24 h for the dye to clear.

- It is safe to perform MRA in patients with metal implants except:
  - Internal implanted defibrillator or pacemaker
  - Cochlear (ear) implant
  - Clips on brain aneurysms
  - Metal coils placed in blood vessels

Although not a contraindication to MRA, the radiologist must be informed about:
- Artificial heart valves
- Implanted drug infusion ports
- Metallic joint prosthesis
- Implanted nerve stimulators
- Metal pins, screws, plates, stents, or surgical staples.

Metal objects implanted in orthopedic surgery pose no problems in MRA unless recently implanted. A plane X-ray is indicated prior to MRA if a metal object is implanted. Trauma with bullets or shrapnel injury must be informed. Tooth fillings and braces rarely are a problem, but the radiologist must be aware, as they could interfere with the images.

The differentiation between normal and diseased tissue is better with MRI than CT, X-ray, or ultrasound.

The blood vessels with contrast appear as white.

## Benefits versus Risks

- Catheter-based DSA is the gold standard for evaluating vascular disease. MRA is fast becoming the noninvasive investigation of choice to replace DSA. MRA is especially adapted to visualization of the lumen and the wall of the artery in question.
- Clinical use—it is used to study arteries in the head, neck, thorax, abdomen, and extremities. It has been less successful in studying coronary arteries than conventional angiography and CTA. Mostly, underlying disease is atherosclerosis, but aneurysms and AV malformations can also be diagnosed by MRA.
- The advantage over conventional angiography is that it is noninvasive.
  Compared with both CTA and conventional angiography:
  - Less ionization radiations are given to the patient.
  - The contrast used for MRA is less toxic because less quantity is used compared with the other two modalities.
- The disadvantages are:
  - The higher cost
  - Limited spatial resolution
  - Longer time taken
  - Patients with pacemaker, metal clips from previous surgery or metal in the eyes.

## ■ NONINVASIVE EVALUATION OF EXTRACRANIAL CAROTID ARTERY DISEASE

Significant internal carotid artery stenosis increases the risk of TIAs and strokes as well of myocardial infarction (MI) and cardiovascular death. Thus, it is important to diagnose this condition noninvasively.

## Duplex Ultrasonography

It provides excellent accuracy and reproducibility and is the investigation of choice. It identifies accurately plaques, stenosis, and occlusions of the internal, common, and external carotid arteries. It also identifies flow direction in the vertebral arteries. The indications for this test are:
- TIAs
- CVA
- Cervical bruit
- After surgical or endovascular revascularization
- Patients who are at high risk for carotid stenosis.

The carotid vessels are located in two planes—longitudinal and transverse noting plaques and alterations in flow. Doppler waveform and velocity are noted in common (CCA), internal (ICA), and external (ECA) carotid arteries. These velocities are noted using a constant Doppler angle of 60°. This helps to determine the degree of stenosis. The sensitivity is 85% and the specificity is 90%. It is 93% accurate in locating carotid occlusion. The limitations of this test are:
- Overestimation of ICA stenosis due to severe contralateral ICA disease
- Underestimation of ICA stenosis due to tight ipsilateral CCA stenosis
- Identifying ECA as the ICA
- Mistaking severe stenosis as occlusion

## Magnetic Resonance Angiography

MRA along with MRI of the brain provides excellent information on:
- Extracranial carotid circulation
- Symptomatic disease unexplained by duplex ultrasound
- Patients with suspected intracranial disease.

## ■ NONINVASIVE EVALUATION OF RENAL ARTERY STENOSIS (FLOW CHART 1)

Atherosclerotic renal artery stenosis (RAS) can be the cause of:
- Resistant hypertension
- Deterioration of renal function
- Recurrent "flash pulmonary edema"
- Long-term ill effects of poorly controlled hypertension
- If bilateral RAS or stenosis in a solitary kidney—develop end-stage renal disease
- Long-term survival in such patients is very poor.

The diagnosis of RAS is made on:
- Duplex ultrasound
- CT angiogram
- MRA
- Radionuclide scans

The investigation and treatment of RAS is given in Flow chart 1.

## Renal Artery Duplex Ultrasonography

This is an excellent test but only in experienced hands. The principle it is based on is comparing the peak systolic velocities within the renal arteries and the aorta called the renal: aortic ratio (RAR). The ultrasound findings are compared with angiography or MRA. The peak systolic velocity in the aorta is measured at the level of the superior mesenteric artery. The entire renal artery from the ostium to the hilum of the kidney is visualized. RAR over 3.5 means a RAS 60–99%. In a large comparative trial using angiography and duplex ultrasound, the sensitivity was 98%, the specificity 99%, and the positive predictive value 99% while negative predictive value 97%. It is useful for:

- Renal artery stenosis
- Renal artery occlusion
- Patency of renal artery stents

**Flow chart 1** Algorithm for the detection and treatment of renal artery stenosis

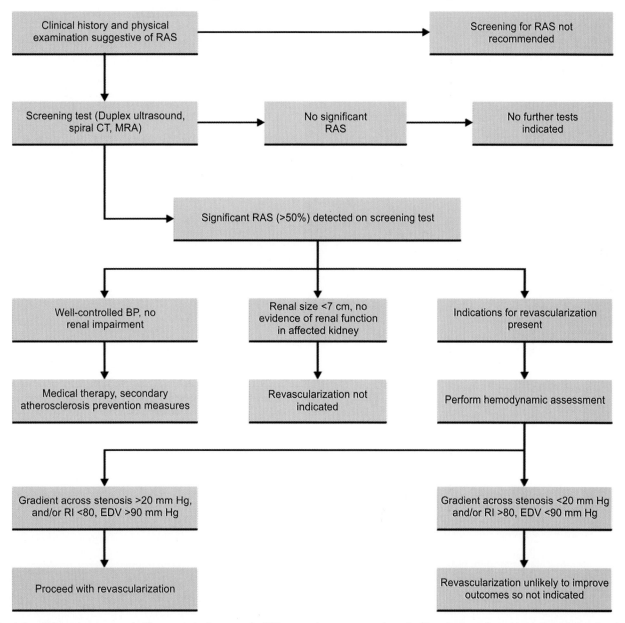

*Abbreviations:* RAS, renal artery stenosis; CT, computerized tomography; MRA, magnetic resonance angiography; RI, renal artery resistance index (1 − end-diastolic velocity divided by maximal systolic velocity) × 100; EDV, end-diastolic velocity. Adapted from Mukherjee D. Renal Artery Stenosis: Who to screen and how to treat? ACC Curr J Rev. 2003;12(3):70-75

- Early and late restenosis of renal artery stents
- Detect the degree of stenosis prior to stenting.

Patients have both renal artery and renal parenchymal disease; the addition of restrictive indices within the parenchyma may help us determine which patients will benefit from revascularization.

The limitation of this technique is:

- Bowel gas preventing proper identification of renal arteries.

## Magnetic Resonance Angiography

This is an extremely useful test in the work-up of secondary hypertension due to RAS. Gadolinium-enhanced MRA provides three-dimensional (3D) images with multiplane images of renal arteries.

## ■ EVALUATION OF AORTIC ANEURYSMAL DISEASE

The diagnosis of aneurysmal disease depends upon:

- Palpating a pulsatile abdominal mass
- Family history of aortic aneurysms in first-degree relatives
- Incidentally found on abdominal imaging performed for other unrelated causes.

Management is based on:

- The transverse diameter of the aneurysm
- Site of the aneurysm—suprarenal or infrarenal
- General health of the patient.

Investigative techniques are:

- Ultrasound study
- CT angiogram
- MRA.

CT angiogram and MRA are preferred because they provide anatomical and spatial details needed for endovascular management and the postoperative follow-up of these patients.

## Computed Tomographic Angiography

It is of value in determining:

- Growth rate of the aneurysm
- Timing of the surgery
- Precise extent of the aneurysm
- Aneurysmal wall integrity
- Location and amount of calcification within the wall
- Venous anomalies
- Retroperitoneal blood
- Aortic dissection
- Infection of inflammation of the wall
- Proximal and distal extent of the aneurysm
- Shows other intra-abdominal pathology
- Diagnosing and follow-up of endovascular leaks.

Limitations of CT angiography are:

- Need for nephrotoxic iodinated contrast
- Increased radiation exposure
- Increased cost.

It is performed by:

- Rapid intravenous bolus injection
- Timed breath-held spiral CT acquisition during peak arterial opacification
- 3D reformatting using maximal intensity projections (MIPs)
- Curved planar reformation
- Shaded surface displays.

## Magnetic Resonance Imaging

The advantages are:

- No iodinated contrast—risk of nephrotoxicity
- No catheter-based arteriography—risk of atheroembolism.

It provides information regarding the extent of the aneurysm and the involvement and relationship with the great vessels. It is quick taking less than 30 sec for 3D contrast. It is also of value in follow-up of endovascular stents provided the stents are made of nitinol that can be visualized.

## Duplex Ultrasonography

This is the most common test conducted primarily and provides reliable information regarding the size of the aortic abdominal aneurysm (AAA) and its periodic surveillance of expansion. A low-frequency (3.5 MHz) transducer is used. After an overnight fast, the test is done in supine reverse Trendelenburg position and aorta seen in the sagittal plane throughout its length and then in the coronal plane to record the transverse measurements in suprarenal, juxtarenal, and infrarenal positions. The normal infrarenal aortic diameter varies with age and sex being about 2 cm. The average growth rate is 0.21 cm per year. The chances of rupture are 0% per year if less than 4 cm diameter, 1% per year if 4–5 cm, and 11% per year if 5–6 cm. This screening has reduced the rupture rate by 49%. Recently, it is being used for detection of endoleaks.

Limitations are:

- Obesity
- Bowel gas.

## ■ CONCLUSION

- Vascular laboratory provides an accurate and noninvasive technique for arterial disorders.
- History and examination provide information to the type of test needed.
- Duplex ultrasound is the mainstay of noninvasive vascular imaging.
- MR and CT are very useful in evaluating AAA and cerebrovascular disease.

## PRACTICAL POINTS

- Ankle brachial index (ABI) is the first step to be performed in suspected PAD.
- Segmental limb pressures and pulse volume recording provide information about the location of the disease.
- Exercise tests help exclude disease in patients with lower limb discomfort and pseudoclaudication.
- RAS is detected by duplex ultrasound. An RAR more than 3.5 corresponds to 60–99% stenosis.
- Duplex ultrasound is useful to screen and follow-up of AAA.
- CT is superior to ultrasound in visualizing aortic wall integrity: dissection, calcification, venous abnormalities, retroperitoneal blood, anatomic extent of aneurysmal disease, and in the diagnosis and follow-up of endoleaks.

# Index

Page numbers followed by *f* refer to figure, *t* refer to table and *fc* refer to flow chart.

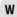